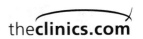

CLINICS IN PERINATOLOGY

Perinatal Causes of Cerebral Palsy

GUEST EDITOR
Marcus C. Hermansen, MD

June 2006 • Volume 33 • Number 2

SAUNDERS

An Imprint of Elsevier, Inc.
PHILADELPHIA   LONDON   TORONTO   MONTREAL   SYDNEY   TOKYO

W.B. SAUNDERS COMPANY
A Division of Elsevier Inc.

Elsevier, Inc., 1600 John F. Kennedy Blvd., Suite 1800, Philadelphia, PA 19103-2899

http://www.theclinics.com

CLINICS IN PERINATOLOGY   Volume 33, Number 2
June 2006   ISSN 0095-5108
Editor: Carla Holloway   ISBN 1-4160-3543-5

Clinics in Perinatology (ISSN 0095-5108) is published quarterly by W.B. Saunders, 360 Park Avenue South, New York, NY 10010-1710. Months of Publication are March, June, September, and December. Business and Editorial offices: 1600 John F. Kennedy Blvd., Suite 1800, Philadelphia, PA 19103-2899. Accounting and circulation offices: 6277 Sea Harbor Drive, Orlando, FL 32887-4800. Periodicals postage paid at New York, NY and additional mailing offices. Subscription prices are $165.00 per year (US individuals), $250.00 per year (US institutions), $195.00 per year (Canadian individuals), $310.00 per year (Canadian institutions), $225.00 per year (foreign individuals), $310.00 per year (foreign institutions), $80.00 per year (US students), and $110.00 per year (foreign students). Foreign air speed delivery is included in all Clinics subscription prices. All prices are subject to change without notice. **POSTMASTER:** Send address changes to *Clinics in Perinatology*, Elsevier Periodicals Customer Service, 6277 Sea Harbor Drive, Orlando, FL 32887-4800. **Customer Service: 1-800-654-2452 (US). From outside of the US, call 1-407-345-4000.** E-mail: hhspcs@harcourt.com.

Clinics in Perinatology is also published in Spanish by McGraw-Hill Interamericana Editores S.A., P.O. Box 5-237, 06500 Mexico D.F., Mexico.

Clinics in Perinatology is covered in *Index Medicus, Current Contents, Excerpta Medica, BIOSIS,* and *ISI/BIOMED.*

Printed in the United States of America.

GUEST EDITOR

MARCUS C. HERMANSEN, MD, Associate Professor of Pediatrics, Adjunct Associate Professor of Obstetrics and Gynecology, Department of Pediatrics, Dartmouth Medical School, Lebanon, New Hampshire; Southern New Hampshire Medical Center, Nashua, New Hampshire

CONTRIBUTORS

VINOD K. BHUTANI, MD, Professor, Departments of Neonatal-Developmental Medicine and Pediatrics, Lucile Packard Children's Hospital, Stanford University, Stanford, California

LARISSA T. BILANIUK, MD, Professor of Radiology, University of Pennsylvania School of Medicine; Staff Neuroradiologist, The Children's Hospital of Philadelphia, Philadelphia, Pennsylvania

EVE BLAIR, PhD, Adjunct Associate Professor, Centre for Child Health Research, University of Western Australia, Perth, Western Australia

GABRIELLE DE**VEBER, MD, MHSc, FRCPC,** Associate Professor, Pediatrics and Neurology, Faculty of Medicine, University of Toronto; Scientist, Population Health Sciences Program, The Hospital for Sick Children Research Institute; Director, Children's Stroke Program, Division of Neurology, The Hospital for Sick Children, Toronto, Ontario, Canada

JAMES J. FILIANO, MD, Associate Professor, Department of Pediatrics, Section of Critical Care and Neurology; Section Chief, Pediatric Critical Care, Dartmouth Medical School Children's Hospital at Dartmouth Hitchcock Medical Center, Lebanon, New Hampshire

LAURA FLORES-SARNAT, MD, Division of Pediatric Neurology, Alberta Children's Hospital, Calgary, Alberta, Canada

SVETLANA V. GLINIANAIA, MD, Senior Research Associate, School of Population and Health Sciences, University of Newcastle, Newcastle upon Tyne, United Kingdom

MARCUS C. HERMANSEN, MD, Associate Professor of Pediatrics, Adjunct Associate Professor of Obstetrics and Gynecology, Department of Pediatrics, Dartmouth Medical School, Lebanon; Southern New Hampshire Medical Center, Nashua, New Hampshire

MARY GOETZ HERMANSEN, CRNP, Southern New Hampshire Medical Center, Nashua, New Hampshire

TING HONG, MD, MSc, Departments of Epidemiology and Pediatrics and Human Development, College of Human Medicine, Michigan State University, East Lansing, Michigan

J.L. HUTTON, PhD, CStat, Professor, Department of Statistics, The University of Warwick, Coventry, United Kingdom

STEPHEN JARVIS, MD, Professor Emeritus, Institute of Child Health, University of Newcastle, Newcastle upon Tyne, United Kingdom

LOIS JOHNSON, MD, Clinical Professor, Department of Pediatrics, Pennsylvania Hospital, University of Pennsylvania School of Medicine, Philadelphia, Pennsylvania

ADAM KIRTON, MD, MSc, FRCPC, Clinical Research Fellow, Children's Stroke Program, Division of Neurology, The Hospital for Sick Children, Toronto, Ontario, Canada

STEVEN KORZENIEWSKI, MSc, Departments of Epidemiology and Pediatrics and Human Development, College of Human Medicine, Michigan State University, East Lansing, Michigan

JOHN H. MENKES, MD, Professor Emeritus, Department of Neurology and Pediatrics, David Geffen School of Medicine at UCLA, Los Angeles, California; Director Emeritus, Department of Pediatric Neurology, Cedars-Sinai Medical Center, Los Angeles, California

MICHAEL E. MSALL, MD, Professor of Pediatrics, University of Chicago Pritzker School of Medicine; Chief of Development and Behavioral Pediatrics, Kennedy Mental Retardation Center, Comer Children's and LaRabida Children's Hospitals, Chicago, Illinois

MICHAEL J. NOETZEL, MD, Professor, Department of Neurology and Pediatrics, Director, Clinical Services, Division of Pediatric Neurology, Washington University School of Medicine, St. Louis, Missouri; Medical Director, Clinical and Diagnostic Neuroscience Services, St. Louis Children's Hospital, St. Louis, Missouri

NIGEL PANETH, MD, MPH, Departments of Epidemiology and Pediatrics and Human Development, College of Human Medicine, Michigan State University, East Lansing, Michigan

JEFFREY M. PERLMAN, MB ChB, Department of Pediatrics, Weill Cornell Medical Center, New York, New York

PETER O.D. PHAROAH, MD, MSc, FRCP, FRCPCH, FFPHM, Department of Public Health, FSID Unit of Perinatal and Paediatric Epidemiology, University of Liverpool, Liverpool, United Kingdom

TONSE N.K. RAJU, MD, DCH, Medical Officer/Program Scientist, Pregnancy and Perinatology Branch, CDBPM, National Institute of Child Health and Human Development, National Institutes of Health, Bethesda, Maryland

RAYMOND W. REDLINE, MD, Professor of Pathology and Reproductive Biology, Case School of Medicine; Co-Director, Pediatric and Perinatal Pathology, University Hospitals of Cleveland, Cleveland, Ohio

STEVEN M. SHAPIRO, MD, Professor of Neurology, Pediatrics, Physiology, Otolaryngology-Head and Neck Surgery, and Physical Medicine and Rehabilitation, Division of Child Neurology, Department of Neurology, Virginia Commonwealth University Medical Center, Virginia Commonwealth University, Richmond, Virginia

ROBERT A. ZIMMERMAN, MD, Professor of Radiology, University of Pennsylvania School of Medicine; Chief, Division of Neuroradiology, The Children's Hospital of Philadelphia, Philadelphia, Pennsylvania

CONTENTS

very preterm (< 32 weeks) and extremely preterm (< 28 weeks) babies. Despite these advances in prenatal care, neurodevelopmental motor impairment remains a substantial sequela. This article describes the major progress and challenges in understanding pathways of preterm children who go on to have one of the cerebral palsy syndromes. The contributions of chronic lung disease, intraventricular hemorrhage, retinopathy of prematurity, and postnatal steroids are analyzed. Management can then be directed to limiting the comorbidities that are associated with threats to survival and to improving protection of central nervous system functions that are involved in moving, manipulative skills, feeding, communication, and learning.

285

When birth weight for gestation is used as a surrogate for intrauterine growth, the prevalence of cerebral palsy varies continuously in a reversed J shape, with steep increases in the risk for infants lighter and heavier than the optimum size. Patterns of size-at-birth specific risk for cerebral palsy differ between male and female infants, as do the patterns for more severe versus milder cases. Although these excess risks with abnormal size at birth imply antenatal precursors, it is not clear whether or how intrauterine growth is involved in any of the suspected causal pathways resulting in cerebral palsy. The implication for clinicians is that serial measures of in utero growth may provide an important indicator of fetal health.

301

Multiple compared with singleton gestations have a five- to tenfold increased risk of CP. The increased risk associated with MC placentation has been variously ascribed to transfer of thromboplastin or thromboemboli from the dead to the surviving fetus, exsanguination of the surviving fetus into the low pressure reservoir of the dead fetus, or hemodynamic instability with bidirectional shunting of blood between the two fetuses. An increased risk of CP in assisted reproductive technology gestations is to be expected because of the higher proportion of preterm births. The increase in risk of CP associated with monochorionic placentation will not be observed except for the minority of assisted reproductive technology gestations that undergo monozygotic splitting.

315

Infections of the mother, the intrauterine environment, the fetus, and the neonate can cause cerebral palsy through a variety of mechanisms. Each of these processes is reviewed. The recently proposed theory of cytokine-induced white matter brain injury and the systemic inflammatory response syndrome with multiple organ dysfunction syndrome is critically evaluated.

Perinatal hypoxic-ischemic cerebral injury, secondary to interruption of placental blood flow that results in cerebral palsy (CP), is a rare event. The ability to link an intrapartum event to subsequent CP should include a history of a sentinel event during labor, followed by the delivery of a depressed acidemic infant, and the subsequent evolution of neonatal encephalopathy, systemic organ injury, and acute neuroimaging abnormalities.

In this article "perinatal trauma" is restricted to injuries that are sustained by the infant during the labor and delivery primarily as a result of mechanical factors, with the understanding that even under optimal circumstances, the process of birth is traumatic. Mechanical insults to the perinatal brain may result in primarily a hypoxic or ischemic injury to the cerebral tissues; those conditions are not discussed in this article. Although there are multiple types of perinatal trauma, this article is restricted mainly to those types that impact upon the subsequent development of cerebral palsy, although when applicable, other adverse developmental outcomes are mentioned.

Congenital hemiplegia is the most common form of cerebral palsy in children born at term, and stroke is the number one cause. Neonatal ischemic stroke includes perinatal arterial ischemic stroke, presumed pre- or perinatal stroke, and cerebral sinovenous thrombosis, all of which have emerged as important contributors to cerebral palsy. Of increasing interest is how the overlapping list of associations and risks for stroke and cerebral palsy relate to each other. Stroke-induced injury is focal, and the preservation of normal areas of brain may afford unique opportunities for plastic adaptation. The implications of this essential difference are stressed in a discussion of how the epidemiology, pathophysiology, diagnosis, and therapeutic advancements in perinatal stroke relate to the outcome of cerebral palsy.

pathology are the "sentinel lesion," the high prevalence of thromboinflammatory lesions affecting large fetal placental vessels, the significance of underlying placental reserve, and the realization that placental findings can serve as markers for processes occurring in the mother or fetus.

MRI can demonstrate and differentiate the various insults and anomalies that can be responsible for cerebral palsy. Recent advances have resulted in techniques and sequences that allow prompt detection of cytotoxic edema and evaluation of brain perfusion. MRI precisely demonstrates the various patterns of injury, distinguishing insults owing to profound asphyxia, partial prolonged asphyxia, and mixed partial prolonged and profound asphyxia. Infants and children can be studied with MRI, and ultrafast MRI permits evaluation of the fetal central nervous system. In the fetus, the cause of ventriculomegaly can be determined, such as cerebrospinal fluid flow obstruction, brain malformation, or brain destruction with or without hemorrhage. Results from fetal MRI have led to better understanding of many brain abnormalities.

The life expectancy of people who have perinatally acquired cerebral palsy can be similar to that of the general population, or it can be reduced substantially. The most important factors that are associated with reduced survival are disabilities of motor, cognitive, or visual functions. Prematurity and low birth weight are associated with lower rates of disability, and better survival. A 2-year-old who has severe cerebral palsy has about a 40% chance of living to age 20, in contrast to a child who has mild cerebral palsy, for whom the chance is 99%. Cerebral palsy, respiratory diseases, epilepsy, and congenital malformation are the most commonly recorded causes of early death.

GOAL STATEMENT

The goal of *Clinics in Perinatology* is to keep practicing neonatologists and maternal-fetal medicine specialists up to date with current clinical practice in perinatology by providing timely articles reviewing the state of the art in patient care.

ACCREDITATION

The *Clinics in Perinatology* is planned and implemented in accordance with the Essential Areas and Policies of the Accreditation Council for Continuing Medical Education (ACCME) through the joint sponsorship of the University of Virginia School of Medicine and Elsevier. The University of Virginia School of Medicine is accredited by the ACCME to provide continuing medical education for physicians.

The University of Virginia School of Medicine designates this educational activity for a maximum of 60 category 1 credits per year, 15 category 1 credits per issue, toward the AMA Physician's Recognition Award. Each physician should claim only those credits that he/she actually spent in the activity.

The American Medical Association has determined that physicians not licensed in the US who participate in this CME activity are eligible for AMA PRA category 1 credit.

Category 1 credit can be earned by reading the text material, taking the CME examination online at http://www.theclinics.com/home/cme, and completing the evaluation. After taking the test, you will be required to review any and all incorrect answers. Following completion of the test and evaluation, your credit will be awarded and you may print your certificate.

FACULTY DISCLOSURE/CONFLICT OF INTEREST

The University of Virginia School of Medicine, as an ACCME accredited provider, endorses and strives to comply with the Accreditation Council for Continuing Medical Education (ACCME) Standards of Commercial Support, Commonwealth of Virginia statutes, University of Virginia policies and procedures, and associated federal and private regulations and guidelines on the need for disclosure and monitoring of proprietary and financial interests that may affect the scientific integrity and balance of content delivered in continuing medical education activities under our auspices.

The University of Virginia School of Medicine requires that all CME activities accredited through this institution be developed independently and be scientifically rigorous, balanced and objective in the presentation/discussion of its content, theories and practices.

All authors/editors participating in an accredited CME activity are expected to disclose to the readers relevant financial relationships with commercial entities occurring within the past 12 months (such as grants or research support, employee, consultant, stock holder, member of speakers bureau, etc.). The University of Virginia School of Medicine will employ appropriate mechanisms to resolve potential conflicts of interest to maintain the standards of fair and balanced education to the reader. Questions about specific strategies can be directed to the Office of Continuing Medical Education, University of Virginia School of Medicine, Charlottesville, Virginia.

The authors/editors listed below have identified no professional or financial affiliations for themselves or their spouse/partner:

Vinod K. Bhutani, MD; Larissa T. Bilaniuk, MD; Eve Blair, PhD; Gabrielle deVeber, MD, MHSc, FRCPC; James J. Filiano, MD; Laura Flores-Sarnat, MD; Svetlana V. Glinianaia, MD; Marcus C. Hermansen, MD, Guest Editor; Mary Goetz Hermansen, CRNP; Carla Holloway, Acquisitions Editor; Ting Hong, MD, MSc; Steve N. Jarvis, MD; Lois Johnson, MD; Adam Kirton, MD, MSc, FRCPC; Steven Korzeniewski, MSc; Michael E. Msall, MD; Michael J. Noetzel, MD; Nigel Paneth, MD, MPH; Jeffrey M. Perlman, MB ChB; Peter O. D. Pharoah, MD, MSc, FRCP, FRCPCH, FFPHM; Tonse N. K. Raju, MD, DCH; Raymond W. Redline, MD; Steven M. Shapiro, MD; and Robert A. Zimmerman, MD.

The author listed below identified the following professional or financial affiliations for himself/herself, his/her spouse/partner:

Jane L. Hutton, PhD, CStat is a consultant for McMahon O'Brien Downes, Conway Kelleher Tobin & Comyn, Beauchamps, A&L Goodbody, Capsticks, Welsh Legal Health Services, Mintons, Greenwoods, Healds, Forbes, Kennedys.

John H. Menkes, MD holds stock in Elan.

Disclosure of Discussion of non-FDA approved uses for pharmaceutical products and/or medical devices: The University of Virginia School of Medicine, as an ACCME provider, requires that all faculty presenters identify and disclose any "off label" uses for pharmaceutical and medical device products. The University of Virginia School of Medicine recommends that each physician fully review all the available data on new products or procedures prior to instituting them with patients.

TO ENROLL

To enroll in the *Clinics in Perinatology* Continuing Medical Education program, call customer service at 1-800-654-2452 or visit us online at www.theclinics.com/home/cme. The CME program is available to subscribers for an additional fee of $195.00

FORTHCOMING ISSUES

RECENT ISSUES

ELSEVIER
SAUNDERS

CLINICS IN
PERINATOLOGY

Clin Perinatol 33 (2006) xv–xvi

Preface

Perinatal Causes of Cerebral Palsy

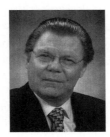

Marcus C. Hermansen, MD
Guest Editor

Although cerebral palsy is rarely diagnosed in the fetus or newborn infant, the etiology is nearly always from a perinatal or neonatal cause. This issue of the *Clinics in Perinatology* brings together an impressive multinational group of authorities to review the etiologies of cerebral palsy. After analyzing each for this publication, this Guest Editor estimated the contribution of each process toward the total population of patients with cerebral palsy as follows:

Prematurity and intrauterine growth rate restriction: 40% to 50%
Birth asphyxia or birth trauma: 25% to 30%
Neonatal stroke: 5% to 10%
Toxoplasmosis, rubella, cytomegalovirus, herpes simplex, other infections: 5% to 10%
Chromosomal abnormalities: 5% to 10%
Inborn errors of metabolism: 5% to 10%
Other known causes: 5% to 10% (neonatal sepsis/meningitis, kernicterus, hypoglycemia, environmental toxins, drug and alcohol exposure, maternal thyroid disease, postnatal infections and trauma, and others)
Idiopathic: 5% to 10%

There are some obvious difficulties in producing such estimates. Many cases of cerebral palsy may be considered to have more than one cause. For example,

doi:10.1016/j.clp.2006.03.015
perinatology.theclinics.com

if a premature infant suffers severe birth asphyxia, followed by a large intra-parenchymal hemorrhage, and ultimately cerebral palsy, the case can be attributed to both prematurity and birth asphyxia. If another infant with sepsis suffers protracted hypoglycemia with seizures, that case might be attributed to both sepsis and hypoglycemia. For this reason the estimates may produce a total greater than 100%.

Recently the association between chorioamnionitis and cerebral palsy has drawn much attention, but chorioamnionitis does not appear on the list of etiologies. The cases in which chorioamnionitis caused cytokine-induced periventricular leukomalacia in the preterm infant are classified as cases of prematurity in the estimates. In term babies the most likely mechanism of damage from chorioamnionitis is placenta dysfunction with subsequent birth asphyxia. These cases are classified as birth asphyxia in the estimates.

One of the more controversial estimates is birth asphyxia. The contribution attributed to asphyxia depends on the criteria used to define the condition. For example, the presence of marginally low Apgar scores alone would be considered an unacceptably liberal definition of "birth asphyxia as a cause of cerebral palsy" and would produce an excessively high estimate attributed to asphyxia. As one imposes increasingly stringent criteria for defining birth asphyxia as a cause of cerebral palsy, the contribution of asphyxia to cerebral palsy decreases accordingly. Perhaps the most stringent criteria are those proposed by the American College of Obstetricians and Gynecologists' Task Force on Neonatal Encephalopathy and Cerebral Palsy. The use of such stringent criteria will produce an inaccurately low estimate of the risks of cerebral palsy following birth asphyxia.

It is noteworthy that the contribution attributable to an idiopathic process continues to decrease with advances in diagnostic testing. This issue of the *Clinics in Perinatology* presents the recent advances in neuroimaging, placenta pathology, chromosomal analysis, and metabolic testing that now explain cases of cerebral palsy previously classified as idiopathic.

I have been honored to work with this outstanding group of contributors. I believe you, the readers, will appreciate and benefit from every article in this collaboration.

Finally, I would like to acknowledge the support I have received from my friends, family, and colleagues in producing this work. I offer special thanks to my children and grandchildren—Sloan, Ian, Vanessa, Lauren, Caitlin, Dawson, Luke, and Quincy—for their love and support.

Marcus C. Hermansen, MD
Southern New Hampshire Medical Center
8 Prospect Street
Nashua, NH 03061-2014, USA
E-mail address: Marcus.Hermansen@SNHMC.org

CLINICS IN
PERINATOLOGY

Clin Perinatol 33 (2006) 233–250

Historical Perspectives on the Etiology of Cerebral Palsy

Tonse N.K. Raju, MD, DCH

*Pregnancy and Perinatology Branch, CDBPM, National Institute of Child Health and
Human Development, National Institutes of Health, 6100 Executive Boulevard, Room 4B03,
Bethesda, MD 20892-MS7510, USA*

But I, that am not shaped for sportive tricks . . .I, that am curtailed of this fair
proportion, cheated of feature by dissembling nature, deformed, unfinished, sent
before my time into this breathing world scarce half made up, and that so lamely
and unfashionable that dogs bark at me as I halt by them.

—Shakespeare, Act I, The Tragedy of Richard III

We cannot be sure whether the Duke of Gloucester, the man who would be the
King, was really "sent before his time" and so "deformed and unfinished" that
he could not play sports or dogs barked at him. Nevertheless, we can be certain
that the Bard's brilliant description relating prematurity to later deformities of the
body and the deficiencies of intellect remains one the oldest of such associations
in history [1,2].

About 250 years later, another Londoner made a more compelling argument
for such an association. In 1861, William John Little (Fig. 1A), an orthopedic
surgeon, lectured at the Obstetric Society of London and asserted that prematurity and adverse events leading to perinatal asphyxia could cause poor outcomes
later in life [3]. Without mincing words, Little described case after case from his
practice that supported his thesis. The stunned audience, some of the most
eminent obstetricians of the day, politely applauded but sternly disagreed with

Some sections of this article were previously published in 2002 in the chapter, "Cerebral palsy
and its causes: historical perspectives" in the monograph *Birth Asphyxia and the Brain* edited
by S. Donn, S.K. Sinha, and M.L. Chiswick and published by Futura Publishing, New York
(ISBN 0-87993-499-9). I am indebted to Blackwell Scientific International, the current holders of
the copyrights, for permission to reproduce those sections.

E-mail address: rajut@mail.nih.gov

him. Thus began more than a century of controversy about the association between prematurity, birth injury, perinatal asphyxia, and cerebral palsy [4–13].

In this essay, I present the early history on the evolution of concepts about the etiology of cerebral palsy, especially the contributions of the early pioneers. This attempt to describe how they derived their hypotheses, including the errors they made, will help one understand the complex processes of deciphering etiologic associations.

William Little: his early life and training

William Little was born in London where his father owned the famous Red Lion Inn, the supposed hangout for the notorious highwayman Dick Turpin. William was a sickly child. He suffered from measles, pertussis, and other childhood ailments. At the age of 4 years, he developed poliomyelitis which left him with a clubfoot deformity. He recuperated in a village near Dover where he continued schooling [14–16].

His schooling was not pleasant. Little's classmates called him "Canard Boitu," "lame duck," and other epithets [11]. Such humiliations must have led him to

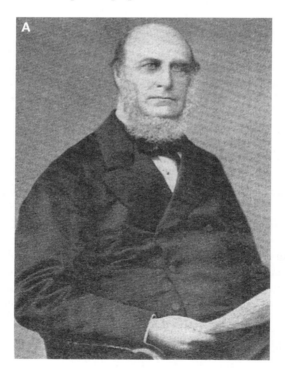

Fig. 1. (*A*) William John Little (1810–1894). (*B*) The first page of Little's famous article published at the Transactions of the Obstetric Society of London in 1861 [3].

B   INFLUENCE OF ABNORMAL PARTURITION, ETC.   293

Dr. TYLER SMITH observed that the object of the author seemed to be to show that his (Dr. Smith's) view of the cause of retroversion of the gravid uterus had been anticipated by Morgagni and others. His own paper, which had been referred to, was exclusively directed to the subject of retroversion; but it was remarkable that in the quotations given by Dr. Aveling there was not a single practical observation upon retroversion of the gravid uterus. The displacements referred to were the different forms of lateral obliquity of the pregnant organ. Only one of the authors cited spoke at all of retroflexion, and then in a purely speculative manner. His own view, as opposed to that of William Hunter, that retroversion of the gravid uterus was caused by the impregnation and development of the previously retroverted uterus, was published in 1856, and it had not yet been shown that this fact had been understood by previous writers.

ON THE INFLUENCE OF ABNORMAL PARTURITION, DIFFICULT LABOURS, PREMATURE BIRTH, AND ASPHYXIA NEONATORUM, ON THE MENTAL AND PHYSICAL CONDITION OF THE CHILD, ESPECIALLY IN RELATION TO DEFORMITIES.

By W. J. LITTLE, M.D.

SENIOR-PHYSICIAN TO THE LONDON HOSPITAL; FOUNDER OF THE ROYAL ORTHOPÆDIC HOSPITAL; VISITING-PHYSICIAN TO ASYLUM FOR IDIOTS, EARLSWOOD; ETC.

(Communicated by Dr. TYLER SMITH.)

PATHOLOGY has gradually taught that the fœtus in utero is subject to similar diseases to those which afflict the economy at later periods of existence. This is especially true if we turn to the study of the special class of abnormal conditions, which are termed deformities. We are acquainted, for example, with abundant instances of deformities arising *after* birth from disorders of the nervous system—disorders of nutrition, affecting the muscular and osseous structures, —disorders from malposition and violence. Each of these classes of deformity has its representative amongst the de-

Fig. 1 (*continued*).

resolve to help himself and others with disabilities. After studying French at the celebrated Jesuit College in St. Omer, he decided to become a doctor. Two years of apprentice work under James Sequeira, a local surgeon, and 3 more years of study at the London Hospital qualified him to become a surgeon. He obtained a licentiate from the Society of Apothecaries of London in 1831, and the next year was admitted to the Royal College of London.

Little continued surgical training in London, Berlin, Leipzig, and Dresden. While in Berlin, he persuaded Dr. Louis Stromeyer to perform "subcutaneous tenotomy," a new surgical procedure of incising the Achilles tendons to release contractures. Reportedly, the procedure completely cured Little's foot deformity.

Delighted by the results, Little learned the surgical procedure and perfected it. By the age of 27 years, he was performing tenotomy on his patients and soon became an authority on clubfoot. He built a thriving practice in London and was instrumental in founding the Royal Orthopedic Hospital, which received the Royal Charter in 1845. Here Little saw many children with a variety of physical deformities and intellectual impairments.

Little on cerebral palsy

At the Orthopedic Hospital, Little taught medical students. Between 1843 and 1844, he delivered several lectures on neurologic deformities in children and published them in the journal *Lancet* [17]. In 1853, he collected and published the lectures in a monograph entitled, *"On the Nature and Treatment of the Deformities of the Human Frame"* [18].

This text was perhaps the first book dedicated entirely to the subject of deformities in children, which later came to be known as cerebral palsy [18]. Although Little did not use the term *cerebral palsy* (which came 34 years later), he gave a wealth of clinical details and suggested an etiologic association between birth injury, perinatal asphyxia, and cerebral palsy as follows:

- **On the nature of illness in the newborn:** "A peculiar distortion which affects the new-born children which has never been elsewhere described...the spasmodic tetanus-like rigidity and distortion of the limbs of new-born infants..."
- **On the causes of cerebral palsy:** "...I have seen so many cases of [mental and physical] deformity traceable to causes operative at birth ... [some of which are] traced to asphyxia neonatorum and mechanical injury to the foetus immediately before or during parturition..."
- **On the observation that all infants with perinatal asphyxia do not get cerebral palsy:** "It is obvious that the great majority of apparently stillborn infants, whose lives are saved by the attendant accoucheur, recover unharmed from that condition."
- **On prematurity as a risk factor:** "...the subjects were born at the seventh month, or before the end of the eighth month of utero-gestation."
- **On the risk for term infants:** "...[two infants were term, who...] owing to the difficulty and slowness of parturition, were born in a state of asphyxia, resuscitation having been obtained at the expiration of two and four hours....."
- **On previous literature on birth injury and hemiplegia:** "...[while others are silent about the later effects of asphyxia neonatorum] Duges...is the only one who distinctly enunciates that hemiplegia and idiocy may follow injury received at birth."
- **On treatment:**"...tenotomy has now been added to every part of the frame..."

As one can see, Little had already described cerebral diplegia as a consequence of premature birth and "congenital hemiplegia" and its association with birth injury in this monograph [18]. The latter was probably the first reported case of perinatal arterial stroke. He proposed that prolonged labor, birth injuries, and severe asphyxia could lead to later neurologic disabilities. Unfortunately, this monograph was ignored by historians. Even obstetricians did not read it, perhaps because they regarded it as a book written by an orthopedic surgeon for orthopedic surgeons.

Little continued to accumulate similar cases with chronic orthopedic problems and, over the next decade, studied and treated them. With superb history taking and observational skills and an impeccable physical examination technique, he was able to make brilliant, well-reasoned deductions, albeit, with caution. He analyzed birth histories and clinical courses and pieced together a plausible hypothesis to account for the neurologic deficits seen in all of his patients with deformities and intellectual impairments. By the early 1860s, Little was ready to share his thoughts with obstetricians—a group that needed to know.

Little managed to get himself invited to deliver a talk at the Obstetrical Society of London on October 2, 1861 [3]. The title of the talk was long (Fig. 1B). He began by saying that just as "strange evil forces" may harm the fetus before and after birth, they can also harm the fetus during birth. The nature and the severity of such "evils" would determine the outcome. He noted that many infants died of asphyxia but normal survival was possible. He observed that there could be a third type of outcome, one in which the infants suffered from "apoplexy" or "congenital paralysis," and that, if they survived, they might manifest mental deficiencies and physical deformities.

Little was one of the first physicians to introduce the taking of birth histories in pediatrics. He stressed the importance of obtaining the history of pregnancy duration and labor, including whether the latter was normal or prolonged, and determining whether any instruments were used. He attempted to ascertain the infant's status at birth and whether any resuscitation was performed. He argued that such histories were important because they could be associated with injury to the brain and spinal cord.

He began to hypothesize that, even without obvious external trauma, an inadequate supply of "oxygen and materials for nutrition" from the placenta to the fetus or an "insufficient removal of carbon and other residues" from the fetus through the placenta could lead to brain injury. If there was a delay in initiating "pulmonary respiration" after birth, he maintained that the same set of adverse processes could lead to brain injury.

Like the title of his talk, the lecture too was long. It was 33 pages in print with an additional 20 pages of appendix describing the birth histories and clinical features of 63 cases. He provided two illustrations. Little's presentation and the discussion that followed were published in the *Transactions of the Obstetric Society of London* in 1861 [3]. These materials can now be accessed on the Internet through the *Neonatology on the Web* site [19].

How many of Little's 63 patients suffered from cerebral palsy? In 1989, Accardo addressed this question [7] and concluded that 57 of the 63 patients

(90%) did indeed sustain cerebral palsy, a record that most of us would be happy with in our own practice. Thirty-four of the 57 patients had cerebral diplegia; 13 had hemiplegia (right, 9; left, 4); 8 had quadriplegia; and 1 each had double hemiplegia and choreoathetosis. Twenty-six of the 57 patients (46%) were preterm, and 33 of 57 (54%) had a positive history for prolonged labor or difficulties during birth.

Little's presentation was so powerful and the evidence so compelling that his audience was dumbfounded. They agreed that a "novel concept worthy of serious consideration" had been proposed. Nevertheless, some obstetricians recounted having seen infants with asphyxia who had recovered completely. Even apparently stillborn or nearly dead infants had survived and had been doing well. One obstetrician asserted that it was teething that caused convulsions and hemiplegia during infancy. Another cited the paradox of the celebrated scholar Samuel Johnson, who was "born almost dead and did not cry" yet became "synonymous with intellectual grandeur." The obstetrician challenged Little to suggest an alternative diagnosis for Samuel Johnson's "nervous disorder," implying that it was not cerebral palsy.

Box 1. Little's minor errors

Cerebral palsy and mental development

Indicated that most patients with spastic paralysis were intellectually impaired.

Spinal versus cerebral pathology

Because of a lack of personal experience in neuropathology, he was unable to correlate clinical findings in his patients with neuropathology. He relied upon the autopsy findings reported by others. He concluded that, in cerebral palsy cases, the most common pathology would be in the medulla oblongata.

Prenatal and postnatal causes

Although he stated that other disorders might lead to paralytic conditions in children, he could not specify which prenatal or postnatal causes might lead to cerebral palsy. Nevertheless, during his time, most of the other causes of cerebral palsy, such as kernicterus in the neonatal period and encephalitis, poliomyelitis, and meningitis during infancy, had not been identified as specific clinical entities.

Little agreed that other "cerebrospinal" causes might lead to "infantile spastic and paralytic contractions." He was even conciliatory, suggesting that "for each congenital case of spasticity, there may be twenty or more from other causes incidental to later life" [3,19]. It is remarkable that in this anecdotal statement Little implies that approximately 5% of cerebral palsy can be due to perinatal asphyxia, a figure lower than contemporary estimates [20]. Little's lecture was an historic milestone and a "learned bombshell" [5]. His hosts thanked him for drawing their attention to this important theory but were not eager to accept the seemingly farfetched conjectures (Box 1). They were naturally reluctant to accept that, somehow, the failures of the members of their craft could lead to such horrible long-term disabilities.

Little continued to practice and write into his 70s. Increasing deafness forced him to retire at Kent, where he died at the age of 84 years just as he had lived—quietly and with dignity.

William Osler and Sigmund Freud

No history on cerebral palsy would be complete without recognizing the contributions of two of Little's contemporaries, namely, William Osler and Sigmund Freud. William Osler (1849–1919) (Fig. 2A) pursued his interest in neurology upon becoming a Professor of Clinical Medicine at the University of Penn-

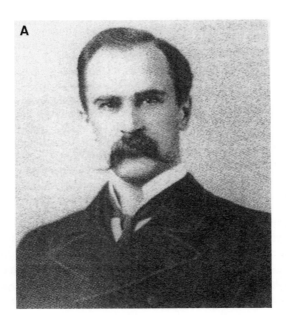

Fig. 2. (*A*) Sir William Osler (1849–1919). (*B*) Osler's monograph on cerebral palsy in children [23].

B

THE

CEREBRAL PALSIES

OF

CHILDREN

A CLINICAL STUDY FROM THE INFIRMARY FOR NERVOUS DISEASES, PHILADELPHIA.

BY

SIR WILLIAM OSLER

FELLOW OF THE ROYAL COLLEGE OF PHYSICIANS, LONDON;
PROFESSOR OF CLINICAL MEDICINE IN THE UNIVERSITY OF PENNSYLVANIA; PHYSICIAN
TO THE UNIVERSITY HOSPITAL, TO THE PHILADELPHIA HOSPITAL, AND
TO THE INFIRMARY FOR NERVOUS DISEASES

FIRST PUBLISHED 1889

Fig. 2 (*continued*).

sylvania in Philadelphia in 1884 [21,22]. Based on the experience of seeing 151 children with neurologic deformities at the Philadelphia Infirmary for Nervous Diseases, Osler published a monograph entitled "*The Cerebral Palsies of Children*" (Fig. 2B) [23]. A visionary wordsmith, Osler introduced the phrase *cerebral palsy* to describe this nonprogressive neuromuscular disease in children. In his monograph, Osler reported 120 children who had hemiplegia and 20 others who had bilateral hemiplegias. Besides the usual oslerian wit and clarity, this work also provides an excellent classification of cerebral palsy.

To some extent, Osler agreed with Little on the etiology of cerebral palsy. He observed that cerebral palsy "usually dates from birth." Nevertheless, he favored the hypothesis that trauma leading to "meningial hemorrhage and compression of brain and spinal cord" was a major cause of cerebral palsy. Osler's opinion was influenced by the reports from other well-known scientists of the day, including Sarah McNutt, Warton Sinkler, and William Gowers [24–29]. Ever cautious, Osler stressed that it was nearly impossible to be sure about the causes of cerebral palsy.

The third major contribution to the cerebral palsy literature in the nineteenth century was that of Sigmund Freud (1856–1939) (Fig. 3A) [21,30]. Before his famous career in psychiatry, Freud was deeply interested in neurology. In 1885 he went to Salpêtriére in France on a traveling fellowship and trained under the legendary neurologist Jean-Martin Charcot (1825–1893). Over the next decade, Freud became a superb clinician and practiced in Vienna. He studied and wrote on many neurologic problems in children and adults. Between 1891 and 1897, Freud published three monographs and many articles on spastic diplegia in children (Fig. 3B) [21]. Contemporary reviewers soon noted that those works were "masterly and comprehensive." Before long, Freud was considered an authority on children's paralytic conditions.

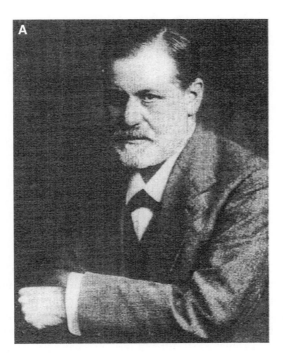

Fig. 3. (*A*) Sigmund Freud (1856–1939). (*B*) The monograph in which Freud's article on spastic diplegia in children appeared (from Accardo [30]).

B

REVUE

NEUROLOGIQUE

ORGANE SPÉCIAL D'ANALYSES

DES TRAVAUX CONCERNANT LE SYSTÈME NERVEUX
ET SES MALADIES

 onmé par

E. BRISSAUD et P. MARIE

PROFESSEURS AGRÉGÉS A LA FACULTÉ DE MÉDECINE DE PARIS
MÉDECINS DES HOPITAUX

Secrétaire de la Rédaction : Dr H. LAMY

PARIS

G. MASSON, ÉDITEUR

120, BOULEVARD SAINT-GERMAIN, 120

—

1893

Fig. 3 (*continued*).

Agreeing with Little and distancing himself from Osler, Freud asserted that asphyxia and birth trauma could lead to brain damage; however, Freud went a step further. Extending Little's explanations, he noted that "...since the same abnormal processes of birth frequently produce no effects...diplegia still may be of congenital... [In some cases] difficult birth ... may be merely a symptom of deeper effects influencing the development of the fetus." He proposed that "difficulties during labor and delivery, including asphyxia" might be the result of

Table 1
Milestones in the early history of cerebral palsy

Year	Names	Comments
1812–1820	Reil, and later Cazauvielh	Reported "cerebral atrophy" in an adult who had "congenital paralysis".
1830–1831	Billard, Cruveilhier, Breschet, Lallemand, and Rokitansky	Presented isolated cases of "cerebral atrophy" in children.
1820–1830	Andrey, Heine, and Depeck	Some clinical features of cerebral diplegia described under the title "cerebral spastic paralysis."
1828	Joerg	Said that "...too early and unripe born children may present a state of weakness and stiffness in the muscles persisting until puberty or later."
1843–1844	Little	Presented 11 lectures at the Royal Orthopedic Hospital published in the Lancet (1843–1844) [17]. In the eighth and ninth lectures, described the clinical features of spastic diplegia in children and implied, but did not elaborate, on its etiology.
1853	Little	Published a monograph based on the previous lectures entitled "On the Nature and Treatment of Deformities of Human Frame." Noted an association between prematurity, prolonged labor, asphyxia, neonatal convulsions, and the use of obstetric forceps with later spastic diplegia in children.
1861	Little	After years of study and contemplation, spoke at the Obstetric Society of London, during which he boldly proposed an association between difficult delivery, prematurity, and asphyxia with cerebral palsy. The lecture was later called a "learned bombshell."
1889	Osler	Published "The Cerebral Palsies of Children" in which he used for the first time the term cerebral palsy for a specific group of nonprogressive neuromuscular disabilities in children. Also gave an excellent classification.
1891–1897	Freud	Published three monographs and many papers on cerebral palsy. Agreed with Little about abnormal parturition and spastic diplegia but extended the concept to include prenatal factors dating back to early pregnancy and to the period of fetal brain development. Argued that spastic diplegia was "cerebral" not "spinal." Also gave one of the most comprehensive classifications on spastic diplegia.

Data from Refs. [11–13,21].

Table 2
Other milestones related to cerebral palsy and its etiology

Year	Name	Comments
1885	McNutt	In two influential articles, McNutt presented autopsy findings of infants manifesting cerebral hemorrhages. Concluded that all developmental delays and mental retardation occurred from birth trauma with brain hemorrhage.
1885–1888	Gower	Described "birth palsies" and attributed "first-born" children being at risk; noted that other physicians attributed it to teething.
1860–1880	Various authors	Expressed much uncertainty about the clinical aspects and varieties of cerebral palsy; the importance of pre- and perinatal factors was debated.
1875–1885	Mitchell, Wharton, and Sinkler	Suggested that injury to the brain may occur from forces used with forceps during labor, possibly leading to trauma of the brain.
1900–1924	Collier, Phelps, and others	Suggested "arrested brain development" as additional causes for cerebral palsy. Clarified that most cerebral palsy infants were intellectually normal. Improved upon the classification.
1953	Apgar	First to standardize the "language of asphyxia." With a set of scores, Apgar gave a means for communicating an infant's condition at birth. This system led to the ritual of giving an "Apgar" and erroneously designating the score as suggestive of asphyxia, and considering any brain damage later in life to be due to a low Apgar score at birth.
1981	Nelson and Eleenberg	Using Collaborative Perinatal Project cohort and follow-up data, these investigators showed that, in this half of the twentieth century, Apgar scores did not have a predictive value for cerebral palsy. Showed that although severely asphyxiated infants were at a higher risk for poor outcomes, in the United States, birth-related events accounted for only a small fraction of all cerebral palsy cases, and an overwhelming majority of infants with cerebral palsy had normal birth histories.
1990s	Modern MRI scans	Revealed that over one-half of cerebral palsy may be due to developmental defects of the brain, implying that "fetal distress" and poor Apgar scores may be symptoms, not causes, of early brain damage.
1992	ACOG and AAP	Proposed the contemporary definition of perinatal asphyxia.

Data from Refs. [11–13,21].

early developmental defects of the brain rather than the causes of cerebral palsy [21,30].

This assertion was brilliant. With a stroke of genius, Freud had dismissed the hypothesis of the "spinal pathology" of cerebral palsy and made it truly a disease of cerebral origin. With regard to the etiology of cerebral palsy, Freud was in the same camp as Little, stating that some cases of cerebral palsy might arise from brain damage owing to asphyxia, difficult labor, and abnormal parturition. Freud

---

Box 2. Contributions of Little to the subject of cerebral palsy

Clinical description

- Provided an accurate description of the various types of cerebral palsy, particularly spastic diplegia.
- Recognized the early symptoms of cerebral palsy, such as eating and swallowing difficulties and excessive drooling.
- Reiterated that most infants with asphyxia recovered completely—an assertion that was not widely noted by others.
- Described the association between microcephaly in infancy and cerebral palsy later in infancy.
- Was the first to suggest that neonatal convulsions increased the risk of a poor outcome.

Causes

- Showed beyond a doubt that prolonged and complicated labor or a delay in establishing "pulmonary respiration" led to asphyxia, and that these events were risk factors for neuromotor disability.
- Noted that most infants with cerebral diplegia were born prematurely.
- Noted that brain damage could occur even in the absence of obvious overt external injury to the head, neck, or body. Argued that just as "abnormal factors" could damage the fetus, brain damage could occur in the absence of overt damage to the skull or the external surface of the body.

Pathogenesis, pathology, and susceptibility

- Theorized that "fine lesions" occur in the brain substance, with one region being affected more than the other.
- Recognized that, in comparison with adults and children, newborn infants have greater resistance to asphyxia.

added two caveats. First, because one does not always find a history of asphyxia at birth, one must look for causes beyond the intrapartum period. The second and most important caveat was that even obvious intrapartum asphyxia could be due to developmental abnormalities of the brain. About 100 years later, Freud's latter assertion that, in some cases, abnormal brain development may be the proximate cause of cerebral palsy has become accepted [20,21,30]. Freud was also one of the earliest scientists to provide a comprehensive classification of cerebral palsy [21].

Why was Little mistaken?

At the dawn of the twentieth century, 2 decades since Little's famous lecture at London's Obstetric Society [3], confusion about the terminology persisted, with a plethora of phrases greeting the student of cerebral palsy. Terms such as *Little's disease, birth palsy, spinal sclerosis,* and *spastic tabes in childhood* continued to be used for over a century [11–13,24–29].

Yet, by then, the battle lines had been drawn concerning the etiology and classification of cerebral palsy. There were two sets of theories to explain cerebral palsy. One theory agreed with Little's suggestion that adverse perinatal events and asphyxia can lead to brain damage. The other maintained that asphyxia was not a cause for cerebral palsy in any patient; instead, the theory held that "congenital" cases were due to "inheritance" and "acquired" cases to infections or teething. Tables 1 and 2 outline some of the major milestones in the early history of cerebral palsy and the evolution of the concepts of its etiology.

Clearly, Little was not wrong concerning the etiology of cerebral palsy, especially in the context of the status of knowledge at his time and when one looks at the cases he reported. Although he erred in some minor details, he was accurate about the main features of cerebral palsy (Box 2). A retrospective kaleidoscope helps us to see why so many brilliant scientists were led astray when attempting to elucidate the cause of cerebral palsy well through the twentieth century.

- The neuronal doctrine of cerebral function was not known in Little's time; therefore, it was difficult to explain the complex clinical features of cerebral palsy, particularly its changing signs and symptoms as the child got older.
- Being an orthopedic surgeon, Little had no access to autopsies. He relied upon the neuropathology reports of others to correlate pathologic findings with clinical features in his cases.
- In the mid-nineteenth century, hospitals rarely maintained written medical records; therefore, objective prenatal and perinatal histories were not available. Little obtained such histories from parents or caregivers of institutionalized children, which might have been incomplete, inadequate, or biased.
- Rather than asphyxia, other postnatal disorders common in those days, such as poliomyelitis, encephalitis, and meningitis, might have caused neurologic disabilities in some of his patients.

- Little's research was essentially "retrospective." It traced the birth histories of children who were already manifesting disabilities; therefore, the research suffered from the limitations of retrospective research, namely, recollection bias and ascertainment bias, the lack of normal healthy controls, and the limitations of making causal associations from observational studies.
- Statistical concepts such as multivariate analyses, odds ratio, and relative risks had not evolved during Little's time; therefore, he could only give descriptive explanations for his observations.
- The state of obstetric practice left much to be desired during the mid-nineteenth century. Even x-rays had not been discovered. Assessing the size of the pelvic outlet, the fetal weight, and head circumference was an educated guess. Rickets and a contracted pelvis were common in women of reproductive age; therefore, prolonged and obstructed labors were frequent. These complications often led to fetal and maternal death. Obstetricians regularly dealt with newborn infants sustaining severe asphyxia and birth trauma.
- Although cesarean sections were being performed, obstetricians tended to avoid them for fear of maternal death from peritonitis. Obstetric forceps of all sorts (high, mid, and outlet) were commonly used to assist in obstructed labors. This practice naturally increased the risk for trauma to the mother and the fetus. Furthermore, in the absence of antiseptics, antibiotics, or safe anesthetic agents, any instrument-assisted delivery carried an increased risk of infection and trauma to the mother and the newborn infant, and severe perinatal complications were the order the day.
- During Little's time, the diagnosis of "perinatal asphyxia" was made using empiric clinical criteria and not uniformly applied. There was no consensus about the definition of asphyxia, nor was there a process to obtain such consensus. There were no laboratory tests that could even provide a hint of the possibility of asphyxia neonatorum.
- Most importantly, Little was attempting to convince a group of obstetricians that severe asphyxia and iatrogenic trauma during labor and delivery could (and might) lead to fetal injury and subsequent neurologic deficits. Such an argument was difficult to make, especially since he was a guest speaker at the Obstetric Society. He must have felt compelled to muster as much evidence as he could, yet be diplomatic, mixing delicacy with firmness. He knew that his conjecture would be unpopular because it implicated an entire profession.

Summary

In the annals of the history of cerebral palsy, Little remains a quintessential pioneer. He described the condition with impeccable accuracy and drew attention to a set of factors others had not even considered. In the process, he opened the eyes of an entire generation of scientists. Besides Little, the seminal contributions of Osler and Freud cannot be ignored. A study of the reasons why these scientists erred also will help us understand the complex process of discovery.

After nearly150 years, it is clear that cerebral palsy results from the "final common pathway" due to numerous etiologies, not the least of which remain "abnormal parturition," major fetal trauma, and severe perinatal asphyxia. We also know that prematurity increases the risk for cerebral palsy and cerebral diplegia.

In 1992, the American College of Obstetricians and Gynecologists and the American Academy of Pediatrics recommended that the term *perinatal asphyxia* be reserved for newborn infants who manifest a set of severe clinical and biochemical markers of asphyxia [31]. It is also noteworthy that it took 150 years after Little's suggestion that perinatal events were causally associated with cerebral palsy for a comprehensive definition of cerebral palsy to evolve [32]. Recently, MRI studies have vindicated Little by showing that adverse events during or immediately preceding the infant's birth (acute or subacute in nature) remain the most frequent causes of severe encephalopathy in the neonatal period and neurologic morbidity during infancy [33].

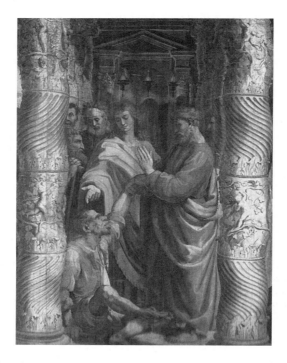

Fig. 4. A detail from the cartoon *The Healing of the Lame* (c 1515–16) by Raphael (Raffaello Sanzio, 1483–1520). The scene is based on a Biblical account of St. Paul and St. Peter healing the lame. Raphael was commissioned in 1515 by Pope Leo X to draw cartoons for the production of tapestries for the newly built Sistine Chapel in the Vatican. This figure and six others from the original are now part of the Royal Collection and are on loan since 1865 at the Victoria and Albert Museum in London [34]. The original tapestries are in the Vatican Museum in Rome.

Cerebral palsy in literature and the arts

I believe Raphael's *The Healing of the Lame* (Fig. 4) [34] is probably one of the oldest paintings of a "cripple." Raphael used models as well as subjects from real life for his drawings before painting. The "lame" in this picture, who seems to exhibit rigidity in contracture deformity in his lower limbs, was probably suffering from cerebral palsy.

After his talk and during discussion, Little quoted from Shakespeare's famous soliloquy of King Richard in the play *Richard III*. As if to add levity to an otherwise heavy discourse, Little noted that even Sir Thomas Moore had stated that Richard was born prematurely with "feet forward" and had neonatal teeth. Both of these conditions were supposedly "bad omens," forecasting Richard's deformity of the frame and famously cruel character. Little concluded that King Richard III was an historical example of a man with cerebral palsy who was born "before his time" [3].

This quote by Little has been noted by others when referring to prematurity as a risk factor for cerebral palsy. Nevertheless, some historians have raised doubts about King Richard's physical deformity. It has even been claimed that Richard was a noble man [35]. Accardo has argued that King Richard had hemiplegia, not diplegia [36].

References

[1] Kail AC. The medical mind of Shakespeare. Balgowlha (Australia): Williams and Wilkins, ADIS Pty Limited; 1986. p. 101.

[2] Byrne R. 1911 best things anybody ever said. New York: Fawcett, Columbine; 1988. p. 128.

[3] Little WJ. On the influence of abnormal parturition, difficult labours, premature births and asphyxia neonatorum on the mental and physical condition of the child, especially in relation to deformities. Trans Obstet Soc London 1861–62;3:293.

[4] Cameron HC. Spasticity and the intellect: Dr. Little versus the obstetricians. Cerebral Palsy Bulletin 1958;1(2):1–5.

[5] Neale AV. Was Little right? Cerebral Palsy Bulletin 1958;1(2):23–5.

[6] Beller FK. The cerebral palsy story: a catastrophic misunderstanding in obstetrics. Obstet Gynecol Surv 1995;50:83.

[7] Accardo P. William John Little and cerebral palsy in the nineteenth century. Journal of the History of Medicine 1989;44:56–71.

[8] MacKeith RC, Mackenzie ICK, Polani PE. The Little Club memorandum on the terminology and classification of "cerebral palsy." Cerebral Palsy Bulletin 1959;2(5):27–35.

[9] Polani PE. 1. Classification of cerebral palsy: yesterday and today. Cerebral Palsy Bulletin 1959; 2(5):36–9.

[10] Grisoni-Coli A. Our point of view on the standardisation of terminology. Cerebral Palsy Bulletin 1959;2(5):40–58.

[11] Collier JS. The pathogenesis of cerebral diplegia. Brain 1928;47:1–21.

[12] Cameron HC. Intracranial birth injuries. Lancet 1922;2:1292–5.

[13] Phelps WM. The etiology and diagnostic classification of cerebral palsy. Nerv Child 1950; 7:10.

[14] Bishop WJ. William John Little, 1810–1894: a brief biography. Cerebral Palsy Bulletin 1958; 1:34.

[15] Schoenberg DG, Schoenberg BS. Eponym: William John Little and his large contribution to medicine. South Med J 1978;71:1296–7.

[16] Dunn PM. Dr. William Little (1810–1894) of London and cerebral palsy. Arch Dis Child 1995; 72:F209–10.

[17] Little WJ. Courses of lectures on the "Deformities of the Human Frame." Lancet 1843–44;1: 5–7;38–44;70–74;209–12;230–33;257–60;290–93;318–20;346–9;350–54.

[18] Little WJ. On the nature and course treatment of deformities of human frame. Being a course of lectures delivered at the Royal Orthopedic Hospital in 1843 and 1844. London: Longman, Brown, Green, and Longmans; 1853.

[19] Little WJ. On the influence of abnormal parturition, difficult labours, premature birth, and asphyxia neonatorum, on the mental and physical condition of the child, especially in relation to deformities. Neonatology on the Web. Available at: http://neonatology.org/classics/little.html. Accessed April 17, 2006.

[20] Nelson KE, Gretehr JK. Causes of cerebral palsy. Curr Opin Pediatr 1999;11:487–91.

[21] Longo LD, Ashwal S. William Osler, Sigmund Freud and the evolution of ideas concerning cerebral palsy. J Hist Neurosci 1993;2:255–82.

[22] McHenry LC. William Osler: a Philadelphia neurologist. J Child Neurol 1993;8:416–21.

[23] Osler W. The cerebral palsies of children: a clinical study from the infirmary for nervous diseases. Philadelphia: P. Blakiston; 1889. [Facsimile reprinted: Classics in developmental medicine, No. 1. Oxford (England): Blackwell Scientific; 1987].

[24] McNutt SJ. Apoplexia neonatorum. Am J Obstet 1885;1:73–81.

[25] McNutt SJ. Double infantile spastic hemiplegia, with the report of a case. Am J Med Sci 1885;89:58–79.

[26] Sinkler W. On the palsies of children. Am J Med Sci 1875;69:348–65.

[27] Sinkler W. The different forms of paralysis met with in young children. Med News (Philadelphia) 1885;51:521–3.

[28] Sinkler W. Discussion. In: Parvin T, editor. Injuries of the foetus during labor. Med News (Philadelphia) 1885;51:561–80.

[29] Gower WR. Birth palsies. Lancet 1888;1:709–11.

[30] Accardo P. Freud on diplegia. Am J Dis Child 1982;136:452–5.

[31] American Academy of Pediatrics and American College of Obstetricians and Gynecologists. Guidelines for perinatal care. 3rd edition. Elk Grove Village (IL): American Academy of Pediatrics; 1992. p. 221–4.

[32] Bax M, Goldstein M, Rosenbaum P, et al, and the Executive Committee for the Definition of Cerebral Palsy. Proposed definition and classification of cerebral palsy, April 2005. Dev Med Child Neurol 2005;47:571–6.

[33] Miller SP, Ferriero DM, Leonard C, et al. Early brain injury in premature newborns detected with magnetic resonance imaging is associated with adverse early neurodevelopmental outcome. J Pediatr 2005;147:609–16.

[34] Fermor S. The Raphael tapestry cartoons: narrative decoration and design. London: Scala Books and Victoria and Albert Museum; 1996. p. 67.

[35] Norwich JJ. King Richard III [1471–1485]. In: Shakespeare's kings: the great plays and the history of England in the Middle Ages. 1337–1485. New York: Scribner; 1999. p. 355–88.

[36] Accardo PJ. Deformity and character: Dr. Little's diagnosis of Richard III. JAMA 1980;244: 2746–7.

ELSEVIER
SAUNDERS

CLINICS IN
PERINATOLOGY

Clin Perinatol 33 (2006) 251–267

The Descriptive Epidemiology of Cerebral Palsy

Nigel Paneth, MD, MPH[a,b,*], Ting Hong, MD, MSc[a],
Steven Korzeniewski, MSc[a]

[a]*Department of Epidemiology, College of Human Medicine, B 636 West Fee Hall,
Michigan State University, East Lansing, MI 48823, USA*
[b]*Department of Pediatrics and Human Development, College of Human Medicine,
B 636 West Fee Hall, Michigan State University, East Lansing, MI 48823, USA*

Methodologic issues in ascertaining the frequency of cerebral palsy

The first question that epidemiologists ask about a disease is "How much?". Before resources can be allocated toward the prevention or control of any disease or health condition, it is essential to weigh the importance of a disease in the context of competing public health priorities. The importance that is assigned to CP is a function of its severity; the consequent burden that it places on affected children, their families, and societies; and of its high frequency as a cause of activity limitation in childhood. This article reviews the evidence about the frequency of CP, how this frequency varies in different places, and whether CP is becoming more or less prevalent.

Measuring the frequency of a disease in a population is not an easy task. We have no good ongoing count of the frequency of cardiovascular disease (CVD), even though it is the major cause of death and disability in the western world. The difficulty of accurately counting the variety of manifestations of incident CVD (eg, sudden death, onset of angina, heart attack, abnormal angiogram)

This work was supported by the Training Program in Perinatal Epidemiology at Michigan State University, Grant No.1 T32 HD046477-01A1 from the National Institutes of Health, and United Cerebral Palsy Grant No. R-735-02.

* Corresponding author. Department of Epidemiology, College of Human Medicine, B 636 West Fee Hall, Michigan State University, East Lansing, MI 48823.

E-mail address: paneth@msu.edu (N. Paneth).

perinatology.theclinics.com

requires epidemiologists to default to mortality data to monitor CVD time trends in most populations.

Counting cases of disease in a population requires having a good operational case definition, sound sources of information about cases, and a system for collecting and systematizing that information. At the same time, the population at risk for the disease in question must be enumerated accurately. Fortunately, because CP is such an important cause of childhood disability, and because its close links to pregnancy and the perinatal period have suggested to many investigators that its frequency may reflect perinatal care, efforts to measure its frequency in populations are ongoing in several parts of the world.

Case definitions in cerebral palsy

CP is a clinical diagnosis; no laboratory test or tissue histology defines its presence or absence. In addition, despite the usefulness of CT and MRI scanning, no single neuroimaging pattern or group of patterns fully encompass the diagnostic findings that are possible in CP. In fact, some children who have CP have normal brain imaging findings. Diagnostic language to describe CP has been developed by many authorities, most recently by the International Committee on Cerebral Palsy Classification [1]; however, all clinical diagnoses are subject to some degree of observer variability, no matter how carefully a clinical entity is defined. Unless a single highly skilled observer diagnoses all cases of CP in a population—clearly an impossible task—population counts of CP must rely on existing clinical records. It has been shown that with enough information, especially if that information includes aspects of motor functioning and not just motor examination findings, experienced clinicians can classify children reliably based on medical records [2].

Some degree of motor dysfunction is essential to the concept of CP. The skilled child neurologist may detect Achilles tendon hyperreflexia and slight hypertonia in some young children who have clumsiness but no real impairment of motor functioning. But should such children be referred to as having CP? This argument is not easy to settle, but from a public health perspective, the decision is clear. Such cases do not carry the personal, familial, and social burden that we associate with CP, and, moreover, are unlikely to be recorded as having CP using the usual methods that are available for population enumeration. Therefore, although it can be accepted that CP can exist in a nearly subclinical state, subject to diagnosis by skilled and experienced clinicians, it is not useful for public health action to include such cases in the CP rubric. The CP that is described in this article, and which is recorded in CP registries, is disabling CP (ie, CP with enough motor disability to interfere clearly with ordinary tasks, such as walking, running, jumping or climbing stairs). The useful Gross Motor Function Classification Scale [3,4] would classify all children who have disabling CP at level 2 or above.

At some point in the future, perhaps through further advances in neuroimaging, we may learn that such mild cases share features in common with CP as conventionally understood, and that expanding the definition of CP to include such children will lead to advances in understanding etiology, analogously to the way in which the concept of asymptomatic infection has clarified much about infectious disease epidemiology. But we are not there yet.

Age at diagnosis is also important to case definition. A well-known phenomenon in child neurology is that some signs that appear to be surprisingly severe, including hypotonia and hypertonia, can be seen in infants, but disappear with age. Such findings are especially common in very premature infants. For this reason, the diagnosis of CP should not be made before the age of 24 months, unless the child has an unusually severe case or other supporting information (eg, severe neuroimaging abnormalities) is available.

Typology

An issue that is subsidiary to the subject of case definition is whether the different subtypes of CP also can be enumerated well. It is likely that some subtypes of CP come to clinical attention more readily than do others. A mild hemiplegia in which age of walking is not delayed may be missed in population counts, as will some cases of spastic diplegia. At the same time, severe spastic quadriplegia or dramatic choreoathetosis is unlikely to be missed. Thus, the distribution of subtypes of CP in any population study may provide clues to the thoroughness with which CP is being ascertained in a population. A higher than average proportion of quadriplegia may signal a passive reporting system.

What is the appropriate denominator population for reporting the frequency of cerebral palsy?

A fundamental concept in epidemiology is that all measures of disease frequency in a population should, to the extent possible[1], be denominatored to the population that is actually at risk for acquiring the disease. For example, prostate and uterine disorders are denominatored to men and women, respectively, and not to the entire population. CP is a disease that can be acquired only once in a lifetime, and then only during a specific period of risk (ie, from early in pregnancy until about age 1 or 2 years). Because newborns and infants constitutes the only population at risk, it makes sense to use the birth cohort from whence the case arose as the denominator, and this is the common, although not universal, practice in CP registries.

If a prevalence survey of all 5- to 10-year-old children who have CP is performed in a community, using the total number of 5- to 10-year-old children in the community as the denominator population seems to be a reasonable choice. It

---

[1] In disease rates that are denominatored to populations enumerated in censuses, it surely happens that some cases of disease did not arise from the enumerated population because of inmigration of people with disease, and vice versa; however, the error that is introduced is generally small.

must be remembered that 5- to 10-year-old children are, by definition, at zero risk for developing CP (brain damage to head injury in a child of that age will not be termed CP). Moreover, using school-age children as the denominator risks causing confusion, because family patterns of movement across geographic boundaries may be related to having a child with a disability. If a region is rich in health care facilities and schools that are known to accommodate children with disabilities, families with CP may migrate to it preferentially. Conversely, having a child who has CP may preclude some movement by families from one region to another.

An illustration of this point can be seen in two CP surveys that were made during roughly the same period of time by the Metropolitan Atlanta CP Surveillance Program. Each reported a different prevalence of CP. When live births were used as the denominator, the prevalence of CP ranged from 1.7 to 2.0 per 1000 live births between 1975 and 1991 [5]. But when 5-year-old children in Atlanta were used as the denominator, CP prevalence was reported as 3.1 to 3.6 per 1000 between 1996 and 2000 [6]. It is unlikely that the higher figure represents an increase in CP over time. Comparison with population-based data from other Western countries (Table 1) indicates that the second figure is the outlier. Therefore, it seems likely that families with children who have CP move to Atlanta for services, which inflates the numerator when place of birth is ignored. Such children have emerged from birth cohorts outside of Atlanta, and should be denominatored to the populations in which they were born.

Should the denominator be live births or survivors?

Consistent with the view that the population at risk should be the denominator, it might be argued that survivors of the neonatal period are a better denominator than are live births, because deaths are not at risk for CP. When neonatal mortality is low (currently <5/1000 in the United States [7]), the difference to too small to matter; however, for VLBW infants ($\leq$1500 g at birth), the difference between CP rates per live births and per neonatal survivors is substantial. When survival rates are improving rapidly, as they have been in the United States for the past 30 years, the public health is better served by examining CP rates per live births in VLBW infants. This is the only way to obtain a sense of the net contribution of improving survival to the prevalence of CP in the population. Rarely, CP in VLBW infants has been reported per 1000 total live births of all weights [8]. This figure gives a sense of the net contribution of VLBW births to total CP prevalence, but does not represent the risk accurately.

Incidence or prevalence?

When a cohort of births is under effective surveillance, and the appropriate diagnostic information is sought at regular intervals, one is in a position to describe the cumulative incidence of a disease within the cohort. A registry system, by contrast, inevitably produces cross-sectional information—the num-

Table 1
Cerebral palsy prevalence per thousand live births (unless otherwise specified) in population-based registry studies

Location	Reference	Period covered	No. of cases of CP	Population denominator (live births unless indicated)	CP prevalence per 1000
UK: Birmingham	Griffiths & Barrett, 1967, [16]	1950–1959	302	186,125	1.62
Iceland: Eastern Health Board area	Gudmundsson, 1967 [17]	1953–1962	102	46,036	2.28
Australia: Western Australia	Stanley, 1982 [11]	1956–1975	903	377,824	2.39
Sweden: Gothenberg region	Hagberg et al, [8,14,18–24] & Himmelmann et al, 2005 [25]	1954–1998	1824	935,367	1.95
Ireland: counties of Cork & Kerry	Cussen et al, 1978 [26]	1966–1975	254	98,648	2.57
UK: Mersey	Pharoah et al, 1987 [27]	1966–1977	685	453,146	1.51
Italy: northeast region	Bottos et al, 1999 [28]	1965–1989	610	334,598	1.82
UK: northeast England	Colver et al, 2000 [29]	1964–1993	584	308,488 neonatal survivors	1.89
US: metropolitan Atlanta	Yeargin-Allsopp et al, 1992 [30]	1975–1977; 1981–1991;	815	431,760	1.89
UK: Avon	MacGillivray & Campbell, 1995 [31]	1969–1988	489	236,920	2.06
Norway: Vestvold	Meberg & Broch, 1995 [32]	1970–1989	110	45,976	2.4
Netherlands: Gelderland	Wichers et al, 2001 [33]	1977–1988	127	172,376 survivors to age six	0.74
Japan: Shiga	Suzuki & Ito, 2002 [34]	1977–1991	325	242,293 survivors to age six	1.34
UK: northeast Thames region	Williams & Alberman, 1998 [35]	1980–1986	584	486,666 neonatal survivors	1.2
Denmark: eastern region	Topp et al, 1997 [36] Topp et al, 2001 [37]	1979–1990	908	342,198	2.66
UK: Scotland & 5 English counties	Pharoah et al, 1998 [38]	1984–1989	1649	782,600 neonatal survivors	2.10
US: metropolitan Atlanta	Winter et al, 2002 [6]	1985–1987	206	102,000	2.0
Slovenia	Kavic & Perat, 1998 [39]	1981–1990	768	258,585	3.0
Northern Ireland	Parks et al, 2001 [40]	1981–1993	982	445,464	2.20
Sweden: southern region	Nordmark et al, 2001 [41]	1990–1993	167	65,514	2.2
US: metropolitan Atlanta	Bhasin et al, 2006 [5]	1996–2000	268	80,815 5-year-olds	3.32

ber of cases in existence at the time of ascertainment—a figure that is referred to as "prevalence." Some epidemiologists would argue that even a figure that is based on follow-up of a birth cohort is best viewed as a prevalence rate, because all disease estimates that are denominatored to live births are prevalence figures. The logic is that incidence requires a specific time period in which cases emerge, and cases/live births do not carry the concept of time as does true incidence, or cases/unit time. Conversely, birth rates vary over time, and the number of cases of CP in the community must vary as birth rates go up and down, even if the prevalence of CP per live births is unchanging. The number of new cases of CP in the population is thus a function of the birth rate. However, the proportion of births that develop CP — a prevalence rate — is the figure of greatest importance both for public health and clinical medicine.

Longitudinal assessment versus a registry approach

Assessing the frequency of CP in the general population through periodic longitudinal assessment of all births is unrealistic, and has been reserved historically for special populations, such as low birth weight infants. In such infants, the high prevalence of CP justifies the resources that are needed to use the specialized trained personnel that are required to make the diagnosis of CP in timely fashion. The National Collaborative Perinatal Project (NCPP) was the only effort in which longitudinal assessment of a mostly unselected (although not population-based) and large (>40,000 children) cohort of births was followed and assessed through early childhood [9].

The practical approach to estimating the frequency of CP, and the only one in current use, is to ascertain all cases of CP that are known to service providers in an enumerated population. When population surveillance of CP is ongoing, it is common practice to assemble a registry that continuously records all cases of CP known in a region. The ongoing surveillance of CP that is performed in metropolitan Atlanta (see Table 3) is the closest approximation to a CP registry in the United States but is actually an intermittent population survey program. The registry approach requires intensive surveillance of all locations in which children who have CP might be seen, such as in the clinics of primary care practitioners, neurologists, and physiotherapists, and increasingly, in the school system. A particular difficulty that is faced by such efforts is that sufficient identifying information must be collected about each case so that the inevitable duplicate reports can be consolidated to avoid overcounting. A second difficulty is that reliance on service providers means that the registry data are only as good as the diagnostic acumen of the overall pool of providers in the region. Although case notes can be perused by experts, who can (if the records are complete enough) confirm or deny caseness, the system will miss cases that are not ascertained yet by service providers.

Two kinds of cases of CP are likely to be missed by registries. Some milder cases of CP (even those with real disability) may not be included in registries because they may not be diagnosed in the community. At the other end of the severity spectrum, infants who have severe CP may die before their CP is diagnosed formally, and may be missed by registry data collection. In the NCPP, children who were described as "neurologically abnormal" at age 12 months had a 50% risk for having CP at age seven, if they survived to that age. But 15% of these children died before their seventh birthday and probably would not have been enumerated in a population registry [10].

For all of the above reasons, the cumulative incidence of CP based on serial examinations of a cohort will always be higher than the prevalence of CP ascertained through registry work. The prevalence of CP in most registry studies (see Table 1)—about 2 per 1000 live births—is about 25% lower than the NCPP prevalence of 2.6 cases per 1000 live births that was found from longitudinal assessment of that large cohort [9].

It is important to keep in mind that registry data may be delayed. In the community, even moderately severe cases may be included years after their diagnosis could have been made by expert observers. For this reason, the prevalence of CP from registries should be viewed with caution in children who are under the age of five [11].

The registry work that is needed to count CP only can be performed in societies in which concerns about privacy generally are outweighed, in the public mood, by the potential value of such enumeration. Registries also are facilitated greatly by having a common identifying number that is used in all health care settings. Not surprisingly, the European, and especially the Scandinavian countries, have been leaders in counting CP, whereas the United States has lagged behind.

Registries of cerebral palsy around the world

Last's [12] dictionary of epidemiology defines a registry as a file of information concerning all cases of a particular disease in a defined population such that the cases can be related to a population base. Registries of CP are important because they facilitate population-based studies, whose epidemiologic findings are more secure than those that are based on convenience samples [13].

Table 2 provides a list of all CP registries that the authors could find that have published data in the peer-reviewed literature, with contact information where possible. Many CP registries emerged in Europe during the 1970s; this development was prompted, in part, by advances in neonatal care that led to increased attention to population trends in developmental disabilities, and especially CP, whose prevalence might be expected to change in light of improvements in perinatal care. The pioneer CP registry, in Gothenburg, Sweden, was developed by Bengt and Gudrun Hagberg and has reported continuously on CP since the 1950s [14].

Recently, 14 registries from eight European countries formed a network, Surveillance of Cerebral Palsy in Europe (SCPE). This pooling of data from several registries has facilitated interesting and useful epidemiologic investiga-

Table 2
Registries of cerebral palsy around the world

Country and region	Registry name	Contact information
United Kingdom		
Mersey region (Merseyside and Cheshire)[a]	Mersey Region CP Register	Mary Jane Platt, Dept of Public Health, University of Liverpool, Whelan Building, Quadrangle, Liverpool L69 3BX
Northern region[a]		Allan Colver, University of Newcastle upon Tyne, Sir James Spence Institute, Royal Victoria Infirmary, Queen Victoria Road, Newcastle NE1 4LP
		Tel: ++44 (0) 191 219 6672 (Secretary)
		allan.colver@ncl.ac.uk
York	York Register of children claiming Family Disability Allowance	P.O.D. Pharoah, FSID Unit of Paediatric and Perinatal Epidemiology, Dept. of Public Health, University of Liverpool, Liverpool L69 3GB
		p.o.d.pharoah@liverpool.ac.uk
Oxford[a]	Oxford region Register of Early Childhood Impairments	Jenny Kurinczuk, 4Child, National Perinatal Epidemiology Unit, Old Road Campus, Old Road, Headington, Oxford OX3 7LF
Scotland[a]	Cerebral Palsy Register for Scotland	James Chalmers, Information & Statistics Division, Trinity Park House, South Trinity, Edinburgh EH5 3SQ; Cerebral Palsy Register for Scotland, Napier University, 10 Colinton Road, Edinburgh EH10 5DT
		cprs@napier.ac.uk
Avon	Avon Handicap Register	Ian MacGillivray, Dept. of Obstetrics and Child Health, University of Bristol, Bristol. Contact Mrs Rita Ritchie; Tel: Ext 59376 or (01224) 559376 (direct line);
		Fax: (01224) 684880;
		r.m.ritchie@abdn.ac.uk
London	North East Thames Regional Health Authority (NETRHA)	Katrina Williams, Dept. of Paediatrics and Child Heath, the Royal Alexandra Hospital for Children, P.O. Box 3515, Parramatta, NSW 2124, Australia.[b]
Birmingham	Midland Spastic Association	N.M. Barrett, Midland Spastic Association, Victoria Road, Harborne, Birmingham 17.[b]
Denmark		
East Denmark[a]	Danish CP register	Monica Topp, P Udall, Piletoften 27, DK-2630 Taastrup, Denmark
		Monica.topp@dadlnet.dk
Sweden		

Gothenberg[a]	Swedish CP registry	B. Hagberg, Goteborg University, the Queen Silvia Children's Hospital, SE-416 85 Goteborg, Sweden Tel: +46 31 3435168; Fax: +46 31 257960 hagberg@pediat.qu.sc
Ireland Northern Ireland[a]	Northern Ireland CP Register (NICPR)[b]	Jackie Parkes, Room 1.36, Mulhouse Building, the Queens University of Belfast, Institute of Clinical Science, Grosvenor Road, Belfast BT12 6JB. Tel: 028 9063 5045 j.parkes@qub.ac.uk
Cork and Kerry[a]	Centers for Mentally Handicapped Children	V. McManus, G. Cussen; 32F Rosemount Park Drive, Rosemount Business Park, Ballycoolin Road, Dublin 11; Tel: 353 (0)1 872 7155; Fax: 353 (0)1 866 5222; communications@enableireland.ie
France Isere[a]		Christine Cans, RHEOP, 23, Av Albert 1er de Belgique 38000 Grenoble, France. E-mail: christine.cans@imag.fr
Haute Garonne[a]	Registre des Handicaps de l'Enfant	C Arnaud, F Baille[b]
Germany Tübingen district[a]		I. Krägeloh-Mann, University Hospital of Tubingen, igkraege@med.uni-tuebingen.de
Italy Viterbo[a]	The Register of Infantile Cerebral Palsy	[b]
Netherlands Gelderlands[a]		[b]
Australia Australia	Australian Cerebral Palsy Register	Telethon Institute for child Health Research, 100 Roberts Rd, Subiaco, WA 6008. Tell: (08) 9489 7766; Fa: (08) 9489 7700 linda@ichr.uwa.edu.au
Western Australia	The Western Australian Cerebral Palsy Register	Telethon Institute for Child Health Research, 100 Roberts Rd, Subiaco, WA 6008; Tel: (08) 9489 7766; Fax: (08) 9489 7700 linda@ichr.uwa.edu.au

(continued on next page)

Table 2 (*continued*)

Country and region	Registry name	Contact information
Australia		
New South Wales/Australian Capital Territory	New South Wales / Australian Capital Territory Cerebral Palsy Register	The Spastic Centre, 189 Allambie Rd, Allambie Heights, NSW 2100 Tel: (02) 9451 9022; Fax: (02) 9451 4877 cpregister@tscnsw.org.au
Queensland	Queensland Cerebral Palsy Register	55 Oxlade Drive, New Farm, QLD 4005 Tel: (07) 3358 8122; cpregister@cplqld.org.au
Victoria	Victorian Cerebral Palsy Register	C/O Department of Child Development & Rehabilitation, Royal Children's Hospital, Flemington Rd, Parkville, VIC 3052 Tel: (03) 9345 4808; Fax: (03) 9345 5871; vic.cpregister@rch.org.au
South Australia	South Australian Cerebral Palsy Register	Catherine Gibson, Women's and Children's Hospital, Level 8 Rieger Building, 72 King William Road, North Adelaide SA 5006 Tel: (08) 8161 7242; Fax: (08) 8161 6088; cpregister@mail.wch.sa.gov.au
Canada		
British Columbia	Alberta Congenital Anomaly Surveillance System	Barbara Sibbald, Manager, Alberta Congenital Anomalies Surveillance System, Department of Medical Genetics, Alberta Children's Hospital 1820 Richmond Road S.W., Calgary Alberta T2T 5C7, Tel: (403) 943-7367; barbara.sibbald@calgaryhealthregion.ca
Slovenia	National Cerebral Palsy Register	Milivoj velickovie Perat, Dept. of Developmental Neurology, Paediatric Hospital, University Medical Centre, SI-1525 Ljubljana.

[a] Part of the Surveillance of Cerebral Palsy in Europe.

[b] Surveillance of Cerebral Palsy in Europe contact provided in lieu of specific registry contact information. (SCPE contact) Christine Cans, RHEOP, 23, Av Albert 1er de Belgique 38000 Grenoble, France. E-mail: christine.cans@imag.fr.

tions of CP [15]. Funded by the European Commission, the network monitors trends in the CP prevalence rate, and provides a basis for collaborative research and service planning. The SCPE has provided new information concerning the impact of interregistry methodological variance on prevalence reports. Results of a workgroup that was intended to harmonize data collection methods revealed differences in overall CP rates, and particularly large differences among birth weight–specific rates, across the registries. These differences were related to variation in the definition of CP that was used, case ascertainment strategies, age of inclusion, and the classification of subtypes. Consensus on these issues now allows for valid interregistry comparisons among SCPE participants, and highlights the need for an internationally accepted classification schema for CP [1].

The Metropolitan Atlanta Surveillance Program for Developmental Disabilities is the only study in the United States that is registry-like, but there have been gaps in its coverage since it began in 1975. Two large cross-sectional population-based surveys have been performed in the United States: in northern California and by extracting data from the National Health Examination Survey (Table 3).

Geographic variation in cerebral palsy prevalence

The authors reviewed 50 reports of CP prevalence rates from many regions in the world published in the past 20 years and covering cohorts that were born since the 1950s. Reports that are based on registries are summarized in Table 1, whereas reports from intermittent surveillance efforts or cross-sectional surveys are listed in Table 3. The tables consolidate reports from the same registry published as separate installments over time. All reports are from developed countries in Europe, North America, or Asia, and it is not possible to draw conclusions about the prevalence of CP in less developed nations. Registries tend to use live births as the denominator, or, less commonly, neonatal or infant survivors. Cross-sectional surveys often use childhood populations as the denominator.

CP prevalence is remarkably similar in developed countries. Nineteen of the 27 reports show prevalences between 1.5 and 2.5 per 1000 live births or child survivors, and all studies show prevalences between 1.2 and 3.0 per 1000 live births. There is no suggestion of a systematic difference in prevalence in any geographic location. The cross-sectional surveys (see Table 3) produce virtually identical figures. The generalization that each 1000 births generally produces two children with CP, or that about 1 in every 500 children has CP, is a good approximation of the truth.

Time trends in cerebral palsy prevalence

The change in perinatal care over the past 30 years or so has been expected to have an impact on the prevalence of CP. One perspective posits that better

Table 3
Cerebral palsy prevalence per 1000 children or live births in cross-sectional population-based surveys

Location	Reference	Period covered	No. of cases of CP	Population denominator (children unless indicated)	CP prevalence per 1000
Eastern Health Board region of Iceland	Gudmundsson, 1967 [17]	1953–1962	102	46,036 live births	2.28
Malta and Gozo	Sciberras et al, 1999 [42]	1981–1990	134	55,200 live births	2.4
Three northern California counties	Cummins et al, 1993 [43]	1983–1985	192	155,636 3-year olds	1.23
Kashmir, India	Razdan et al, 1994 [44]	Cases found on November 1, 1986	79	63,645 total population	1.24
Metropolitan Atlanta	Yeargin-Allsop et al, 1992 [30]	1985–1987	206	103,000 10-year-old children	2.0
United States	Boyle et al, 1994 (National Health Interview Survey) [45]	1988	43	17,110 children ≤17 years	2.3
Alberta, Canada	Robertson et al, 1998 [46]	1985–1998	248	96,359 3-year-olds	2.57
China	Liu et al, 1999 [47]	May–July 1997	622	388,192 children younger than age 7	1.6

management of maternal complications, more intensive surveillance of fetuses in labor, and improved ventilatory management of premature newborns should be reflected in fewer cases of CP. An alternative perspective suggests that these improvements have been translated into much better neonatal survival, especially in very premature infants, and the price of increased survival is a larger number of children who have CP [48].

In an attempt to answer these questions, the authors have plotted CP prevalence per 1000 live births (or in a few cases, per 1000 survivors or children) using bubble charts that plot each study according to its size, and weight the study accordingly. The center of each bubble corresponds to the prevalence point-estimate, and bubble size is proportional to the size of the denominator population. A spline smoothing line was fitted to each figure to more easily visualize the secular trend.

For CP at all birth weights (Fig. 1), the overall impression is stability over time, but with a slight increase in prevalence in the 1980s. There is a suggestion that this increase may be on the decline. CP prevalence per 1000 liveborn infants who weigh less than 1500 g exhibited a sharp increase in the 1980s which seems to be on the decline (Fig. 2). A similar, but slightly less pronounced, trend was found for infants who weigh between 1500 g and 2499 g (data not shown). Finally, the time trend for infants who weigh more than 2500 g (Fig. 3) shows an up-and-down pattern with no obvious trend. It is

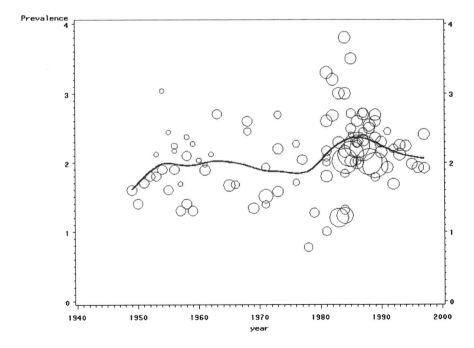

Fig. 1. Trend of cerebral palsy at all birth weights.

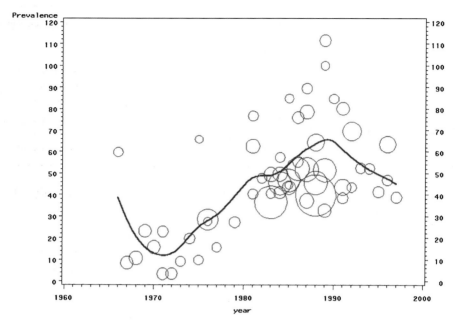

Fig. 2. Birth weight–specific cerebral palsy prevalence (birth weight <1500 g).

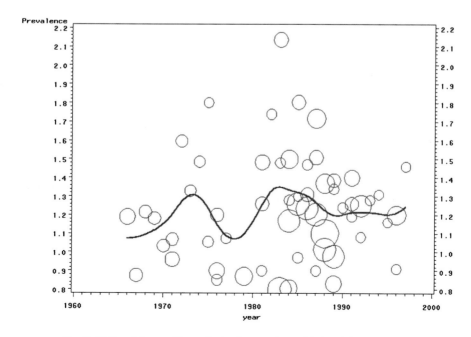

Fig. 3. Birth weight–specific cerebral palsy prevalence (birth weight ≥2500 g).

likely that the variations in the low rates of CP that are seen in normal weight infants—about 1 per 1000 live births—are simply sample variance, and that there is no real change in their CP prevalence. It also is apparent that the slight increase in CP prevalence that is seen in all infants reflects the increase in CP in VLBW infants, which is entirely a consequence of their increasing survival. The decline in CP in such infants recently may reflect improvements in care of VLBW infants that are beginning to affect rates of CP or it simply may be sample variance. Only time will tell.

Summary

CP is enumerated regularly in several parts of the world, and its prevalence ranges from 1.5 to 2.5 per 1000 live births. There is no suggestion of any major difference in prevalence among western nations, although data from the Americas are sparse. Time trends in overall CP prevalence for the past 40 years are most notable for their stability, but a modest increase in prevalence probably occurred in the last decades of the twentieth century. This increase in prevalence can be attributed to the substantial increase in the prevalence of CP per 1000 VLBW infants, which, in turn, is attributable to their increased survival that results from newborn intensive care. There are signs that this recent increase in prevalence of CP in VLBW infants may have leveled off and may be on the decline.

References

[1] Bax M, Goldstein M, Rosenbaum P, et al. Proposed definition and classification of cerebral palsy, April 2005. Dev Med Child Neurol 2005;47(8):571–6.

[2] Paneth N, Qiu H, Rosenbaum P, et al. Reliability of classification of cerebral palsy in low-birthweight children in four countries. Dev Med Child Neurol 2003;45(9):628–33.

[3] Palisano R, Rosenbaum P, Walter S, et al. Development and reliability of a system to classify gross motor function in children with cerebral palsy. Dev Med Child Neurol 1997;39(4):214–23.

[4] Russell D, Rosenbaum P, Avery L, et al. The Gross Motor Function Measure (GMFM-66, GMFM-88). User's manual, vol. 159. Cambridge (UK): Mac Keith Press; 2002.

[5] Bhasin TK, Brocksen S, Avchen RN, et al. Prevalence of four developmental disabilities among children aged 8 years—Metropolitan Atlanta Developmental Disabilities Surveillance Program, 1996 and 2000. MMWR Surveill Summ 2006;55(1):1–9.

[6] Winter S, Autry A, Boyle C, et al. Trends in the prevalence of cerebral palsy in a population-based study. Pediatrics 2002;110(6):1220–5.

[7] National Center for Health Statistics: Health, United States, 2005. With chartbook on trends in the health of Americans. Hyattsville (MD): National Center for Health Statistics; 2005.

[8] Hagberg B, Hagberg G, Beckung E, et al. Changing panorama of cerebral palsy in Sweden. VIII. Prevalence and origin in the birth year period 1991–94. Acta Paediatr 2001;90(3):271–7.

[9] Nelson KB, Ellenberg JH. Antecedents of cerebral palsy. I. Univariate analysis of risks. Am J Dis Child 1985;139(10):1031–8.

[10] Nelson KB, Ellenberg JH. Children who "outgrew" cerebral palsy. Pediatrics 1982;69:529–36.

[11] Stanley FJ. Using cerebral palsy data in the evaluation of neonatal intensive care: a warning. Dev Med Child Neurol 1982;24(1):93–4.

[12] Last J. A dictionary of epidemiology. 3rd edition. Oxford (UK): Oxford University Press; 2002.

[13] Cans C, Surman G, McManus V, et al. Cerebral palsy registries. Semin Pediatr Neurol 2004; 11(1):18–23.

[14] Hagberg B, Hagberg G, Olow I. The changing panorama of cerebral palsy in Sweden 1954–1970. I. Analysis of the general changes. Acta Paediatr Scand 1975;64(2):187–92.

[15] Jarvis S, Glinianaia SV, Torrioli MG, et al. Cerebral palsy and intrauterine growth in single births: European collaborative study. Lancet 2003;362(9390):1106–11.

[16] Griffiths MI, Barrett NM. Cerebral palsy in Birmingham. Dev Med Child Neurol 1967;9(1): 33–46.

[17] Gudmundsson KR. Cerebral palsy in Iceland. Acta Neurol Scand 1967;43(Suppl 34):31–2.

[18] Hagberg B, Hagberg G. The changing panorama of infantile hydrocephalus and cerebral palsy over forty years—a Swedish survey. Brain Dev 1989;11(6):368–73.

[19] Hagberg B, Hagberg G, Olow I. The changing panorama of cerebral palsy in Sweden. IV. Epidemiological trends 1959–78. Acta Paediatr Scand 1984;73(4):433–40.

[20] Hagberg B, Hagberg G, Olow I. The changing panorama of cerebral palsy in Sweden. VI. Prevalence and origin during the birth year period 1983–1986. Acta Paediatr 1993;82(4): 387–93.

[21] Hagberg B, Hagberg G, Olow I, et al. The changing panorama of cerebral palsy in Sweden. VII. Prevalence and origin in the birth year period 1987–90. Acta Paediatr 1996;85(8):954–60.

[22] Hagberg B, Hagberg G, Olow I, et al. The changing panorama of cerebral palsy in Sweden. V. The birth year period 1979–82. Acta Paediatr Scand 1989;78(2):283–90.

[23] Hagberg B, Hagberg G, Zetterstrom R. Decreasing perinatal mortality—increase in cerebral palsy morbidity. Acta Paediatr Scand 1989;78(5):664–70.

[24] Hagberg G, Olow I. The changing panorama of cerebral palsy in Sweden 1954–1970. II. Analysis of the various syndromes. Acta Paediatr Scand 1975;64(2):193–200.

[25] Himmelmann K, Hagberg G, Beckung E, et al. The changing panorama of cerebral palsy in Sweden. IX. Prevalence and origin in the birth-year period 1995–1998. Acta Paediatr 2005; 94(3):287–94.

[26] Cussen GH, Barry JE, Moloney AM, et al. Cerebral palsy: a regional study. Ir Med J 1978; 71(17):568–72.

[27] Pharoah P, Cooke R, Rosenbloom L, et al. Trends in birth prevalence of cerebral palsy. Arch Dis Child 1987;62:379–84.

[28] Bottos M, Granato T, Allibrio G, et al. Prevalence of cerebral palsy in north-east Italy from 1965 to 1989. Dev Med Child Neurol 1999;41(1):26–39.

[29] Colver AF, Gibson M, Hey EN, et al. Increasing rates of cerebral palsy across the severity spectrum in north-east England 1964–1993. The North of England Collaborative Cerebral Palsy Survey. Arch Dis Child Fetal Neonatal Ed 2000;83(1):F7–12.

[30] Yeargin-Allsopp M, Murphy CC, Oakley GP, et al. A multiple-source method for studying the prevalence of developmental disabilities in children: the Metropolitan Atlanta Developmental Disabilities Study. Pediatrics 1992;89(4 Pt 1):624–30.

[31] MacGillivray I, Campbell DM. The changing pattern of cerebral palsy in Avon. Paediatr Perinat Epidemiol 1995;9(2):146–55.

[32] Meberg A, Broch H. A changing pattern of cerebral palsy. Declining trend for incidence of cerebral palsy in the 20-year period 1970–89. J Perinat Med 1995;23(5):395–402.

[33] Wichers MJ, van der Schouw YT, Moons KG, et al. Prevalence of cerebral palsy in The Netherlands (1977–1988). Eur J Epidemiol 2001;17(6):527–32.

[34] Suzuki J, Ito M. Incidence patterns of cerebral palsy in Shiga Prefecture, Japan, 1977–1991. Brain Dev 2002;24(1):39–48.

[35] Williams K, Alberman E. The impact of diagnostic labelling in population-based research into cerebral palsy. Dev Med Child Neurol 1998;40(3):182–5.

[36] Topp M, Uldall P, Langhoff-Roos J. Trend in cerebral palsy birth prevalence in eastern Denmark: birth year period 1979–86. Paediatr Perinat Epidemiol 1997;11:451–60.

[37] Topp M, Uldall P, Greisen G. Cerebral palsy births in eastern Denmark, 1987–90: implications for neonatal care. Paediatr Perinat Epidemiol 2001;15(3):271–7.

[38] Pharoah PO, Cooke T, Johnson MA, et al. Epidemiology of cerebral palsy in England and Scotland, 1984–9. Arch Dis Child Fetal Neonatal Ed 1998;79(1):F21–5.

[39] Kavic A, Perat MV. Prevalence of cerebral palsy in Slovenia: birth years 1981–1990. Dev Med Child Neurol 1998;40:459–63.

[40] Parkes J, Dolk H, Hill N, et al. Cerebral palsy in Northern Ireland; 1981–1993. Paediatr Perinat Epidemiol 2001;15:278–86.

[41] Nordmark E, Hagglund G, Lagergren J. Cerebral palsy in southern Sweden. I. Prevalence and clinical features. Acta Paediatr 2001;90(11):1271–6.

[42] Sciberras C, Spencer N. Cerebral palsy in Malta 1981 to 1990. Dev Med Child Neurol 1999; 41(8):508–11.

[43] Cummins SK, Nelson KB, Grether JK, et al. Cerebral palsy in 4 northern California counties, births 1983 through 1985. J Pediatr 1993;123(2):230–7.

[44] Razdan S, Kaul RL, Motta A, et al. Prevalence and pattern of major neurological disorders in rural Kashmir (India) in 1986. Neuroepidemiology 1994;13:113–9.

[45] Boyle CA, Decoufle P, Yeargin-Allsopp M. Prevalence and health impact of developmental disabilities in US children. Pediatrics 1994;93(3):399–403.

[46] Robertson CM, Svenson LW, Joffres MR. Prevalence of cerebral palsy in Alberta. Can J Neurol Sci 1998;25(2):117–22.

[47] Liu JM, Li S, Lin Q, et al. Prevalence of cerebral palsy in China. Int J Epidemiol 1999;28(5): 949–54.

[48] Bhushan V, Paneth N, Kiely JL. Recent secular trends in the prevalence of cerebral palsy. Pediatrics 1993;91:1094–100.

CLINICS IN
PERINATOLOGY

Clin Perinatol 33 (2006) 269–284

The Panorama of Cerebral Palsy After Very and Extremely Preterm Birth: Evidence and Challenges

Michael E. Msall, MD

University of Chicago, Pritzker School of Medicine, Kennedy Mental Retardation Center,
Comer Children's and LaRabida Children's Hospitals, 5841 South Maryland Avenue,
MC0900, Chicago IL 60637, USA

During the past 25 years, major advances in maternal-fetal medicine, neonatology, and translational developmental biology have resulted in unprecedented survival rates for extremely preterm (≤28 weeks of gestation) or extremely low birth weight (ELBW) infants (≤1000 g) who received neonatal intensive care [1–3]. Although there has been success in improving survival, preventing adverse neurodevelopmental outcomes in early childhood for these high-risk survivors remains a major challenge [3–5]. This article reviews model multicenter or national follow-up studies of extremely preterm/ELBW infants who survived neonatal intensive care. Whenever possible, studies that follow children beyond early childhood and through their preschool years are reviewed to understand neurodevelopmental and functional pathways of risk and resiliency.

Frameworks for understanding cerebral palsy in the context of early childhood disability

Two frameworks have been developed to describe the complex web of children's health and well-being and include dynamic perspectives on early childhood neuromotor disability. The first framework, the "International Classification of Functioning" (ICF) model, describes a child's health and well-being in terms of four components: body structures, body functions, activities, and

---

E-mail address: mmsall@peds.bsd.uchicago.edu

participation [6]. Body structures are anatomic parts of the body, such as organs and limbs, as well as structures of the nervous, visual, auditory, and musculo-skeletal systems. Body functions are the physiologic functions of body systems, including psychologic functions, such as being attentive, remembering, and thinking. Activities are tasks that are done by children and include learning, communicating, walking, climbing, feeding, dressing, toileting, bathing, drawing, and grooming. Participation means involvement in community life, such as playing with peers, preschool education experiences, and attending family activities (eg, visiting relatives, attending religious services, going shopping). The ICF model also accounts for contextual factors in a child's life, including environmental facilitators and environmental barriers as well as personal factors. Environmental facilitators include family leave policies, day care and early education accessibility, and comprehensive health insurance. Environmental barriers include negative attitudes of others, lack of legal protections, and discriminatory practices. Personal factors include age, gender, interests, and sense of self-efficacy; these can be facilitators or barriers . Fig. 1 illustrates application of the ICF model to a 2-year-old girl who has diplegic cerebral palsy (CP).

The second framework is the "Developmental Kaleidoscope Model," which views children's health as a multifactorial interactive system that includes biology and behavior, physical and social environment, and policy and services [7]. This model allows for descriptions of the child's developmental strengths, challenges with functioning during daily activities, and potential. It also includes the use of medical services (glasses, hearing aides, inhalation medications for asthma, medications for gastroesophageal reflux, anticonvulsants, medications for spasticity, orthopedic and neurologic consultation, nutrition supports, public health nurse home visitation), rehabilitative and compensatory services (physical therapy, occupational therapy, speech-language therapy, alternative mobility supports, augmentative communication, robotic assistants), educational supports (early intervention and special education services), behavior supports (counsel-

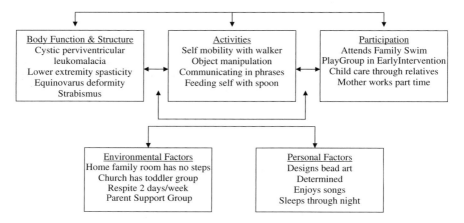

Fig. 1. International classification of functioning model; a 2-year-old girl who has cerebral palsy.

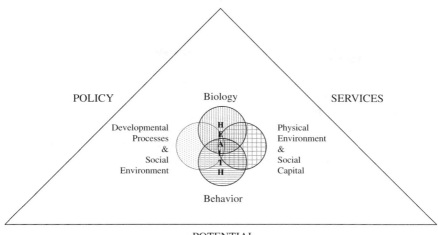

Fig. 2. Developmental kaleidoscope model for a 2-year-old boy who has triplegic cerebral palsy and visual disability. A 2-year-old boy is unable to use his right arm. He was born at 25 weeks' gestation and weighed 750 g. *Biology:* Vulnerability of extremely preterm infants to hemorrhagic perinatal infarction (intraventricular hemorrhage 4) and severe retinopathy of prematurity. He requires medications for reflux and asthma. *Physical environment and social capital:* Home visitation reveals that he lives in substandard housing. There are no toddler toys or children's books. His mother did not finish high school and has limited family support and financial resources. *Behavior:* Child is a fussy eater and has intense tantrums to gain attention. *Developmental processes and social environment:* Points with left hand, knows three body parts, jargon, but no words. Cannot attend day care because he vomits easily when caregivers try to feed him too quickly. Bilateral spasticity with inability to long sit or crawl; restricted visual fields with legal blindness. *Child health:* Child requires a medical home with access to quality pediatric subspecialists who can help with family support and care coordination. *Policy:* Gaps in skills of early childhood professionals and their ability to engage the family, prioritize interventions, and collaborate with medicine, especially with family supports. *Services:* Quality early childhood language and motor development programs are scarce resources for children with multiple challenges. *Potential:* With combination interventions for asthma control, medications for reflux, family support, and quality preschool services, he will learn more functional skills despite having developmental challenges.

ing, stimulant medication), and community context (parent training, family networks, neighborhood resources, adult employment). The Developmental Kaleidoscope Model is illustrated in Fig. 2 for a boy who was born weighing 750 g who is multiply neurologically impaired with triplegic CP, legal blindness, developmental delays, and is struggling in language development.

Measuring neuromotor impairments and describing cerebral palsy syndromes in the first 2 years of life

To understand the dynamic nature of the CP syndromes, one should examine risk factors, timing, and type of CP closely [8]. In this respect, very low birth weight and ELBW survivors have a high prevalence of all types of CP; it is important to report their gestational age and the timing of the first abnormality of the appearance of their central nervous system using cranial sonography or MRI [9–12]. Many centers perform sequential sonograms during the first few week of life, and subsequently, during the times of critical illness; however, cystic periventricular leukomalacia—the lesion that is most responsible for diplegia—often does not become visualized until 32 to 34 weeks postmenstrual age (PMA) [13]. Another option is to obtain a cranial MRI at 36 weeks PMA. De Vries and colleagues [14] demonstrated the value of sequential ultrasounds for all infants up to 32 weeks PMA, and showed a sensitivity of 95%, a specificity of 99%, and a positive predictive value of 48% for CP at age 2 years. Laptook and colleagues [15] examined the outcomes of children at age 18 to 24 months who were born weighing less than 1000 g and had normal cranial ultrasound. They discovered that ultrasound missed 9% of those who had CP and 25% of children with cognitive impairment defined as a Bayley mental development index (MDI) of less than 70. Mirmiran and colleagues [16] at Stanford compared cranial MRI at near term (36–40 weeks PMA) with cranial ultrasound in infants who weighed less than 1250 g and were less than 30 weeks' gestation. MRI was 86% sensitive and 89% specific for predicting CP at 31 months using the Amiel-Tison standardized neurodevelopmental examination. In comparison, ultrasound was 43% sensitive and 82% specific for detecting CP at 31 months. Thus, despite advances in imaging, no technology can detect 95% or more children who go on to have CP. Also, no imaging technology limits false reassurance of freedom from CP to less than 5%.

Much dynamic change in posture and voluntary motor control occurs in the first year of life [17]. These changes include rostral to caudal pattern of myelination; establishment of visual tracking, reaching, and eye–hand manipulation; and dynamic mobility underlying rolling, maintaining sitting position, crawling, pulling to stand, cruising, and walking. Allen and Alexander [18] compared milestones of preterm infants with full-term peers and demonstrated that correcting for prematurity in the first year of life resulted in similar developmental patterns of postural skills. Historically, CP was defined as a disorder of movement and posture due to a lesion or dysfunction in the developing brain, and included a topography based on the number of affected limbs. This topography includes monoplegia (one lower extremity), hemiplegia (one side of body, arm more than leg), diplegia (bilateral lower extremity involvement), triplegia (combination of diplegia and hemiplegia), and quadriplegia or tetraplegia (four-limb involvement). Fig. 3 indicates a topography with functional descriptors that can be combined with the gross motor function measure [19], oral motor, and communicative skills in the first 3 years of life. More recently, an expert panel defined CP as a group of (developmental) disorders of movement and posture, which cause activity limitations that are attributed to nonprogressive disturbances that occurred in the developing fetal or infant brain. The motor disorders of CP are accompanied often by disturbances of sensation, cognition, communication, perception, or behavior, or by a seizure disorder [20]. This expert

Type of Cerebral Palsy	Classification / Description
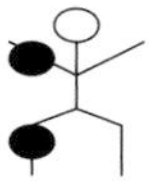 One Sided-Hemiplegia	Mild: difficulty with performing pincer task on an involved side. Moderate: Intermittently fisted, unable to manipulate objects in hand. Severe: Fisted, unable to use hand to assist.
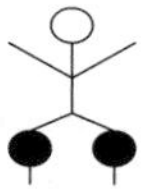 Leg dominated-Diplegia	Mild: Tall kneeling, spasticity at ankle. Moderate: walks with crouched gait difficulty climbing stairs. Severe: scissoring, hip tightness, unable to stand.
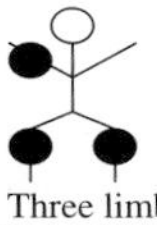 Three limb dominated-Triplegia	Mild: One upper extremity with pincer. Moderate: Upper extremity with ability to use first and third digits Severe: Raking with best upper extremity
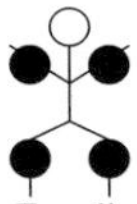 Four limb dominated-Quadriplegia	Mild: Pulls off socks, self-mobility in prone, sits with hands free. Moderate: Assisted sitting, some rolling. Severe: Unable to sit, or roll.

Fig. 3. Topography of cerebral palsy at 18 to 30 months.

panel also included anatomic and radiologic findings as well as considerations of causation and timing as key components of the classification system.

Early neuromotor assessment has been described in detail from several perspectives [17,21,22]. The robust observational traditions of Gesell and colleagues [23], Bayley [24], Illingworth [25], Griffiths [26], Neligan and Prudham [27], and Capute and Biehl [28] allow for descriptions of a child's movements and hand skills, as well as elicitation of problem-solving skills with blocks, toys, puzzles, crayons, and dolls—all of which are helpful in the assessment of young children [54].

It should be emphasized that experience with sequential assessment of ELBW survivors is preliminary. The key is not to burden families unnecessarily when their child's development is going smoothly, and to comprehensively support a family of a child who has diplegic CP and faces challenges in communicative skills. Specifically, outcomes at 2 years must allow for classification that includes functional skills, such as crawling, walking, running, climbing, sitting with hands free, reaching, transferring, manipulating, communicating in words and gestures, understanding verbal requests, and taking turns with peers. Some of these indicators are shown in Box 1 [55].

Box 1. Key mobility, manipulative, and cognitive functioning indicators in early childhood

Moving about and manipulating objects

Does the child sit with hands free, crawl or scoot, cruise or walk with one hand held, walk without help, stack two blocks, mark on paper with crayon, crawl up stairs, walk up stairs holding rail, walk down stairs putting both feet on each step, ascend and descend to pick up object on floor, kick a ball, run, open a door, and open a jar by unscrewing the lid?

Caring for Self

Does the child hold bottle or sippy cup, drink from an open cup, use a straw, feed self cookie or cracker, use a spoon to feed him/herself, take off socks, remove all clothes, urinate in toilet or potty chair, have bowel movements in toilet or potty chair, and wash hands?

Acquiring and using information

Does the child use gestures, such as waving ''hi'' and ''bye''; shake head for ''no''; respond to the request to ''give me'' an object; follow simple directions (''come here,'' ''sit down''); say 1 to 3 words; say 4 to 10 words; say more than 10 words; put 2 words together; point to or name a few body parts; point to a few pictures; name a few pictures; or talk in short sentences?

Attending to and completing tasks

Does the child look at someone who speaks to him/her, listen and pay attention to a simple story being read, play with toys for a few minutes, change activities without getting upset, or sing parts of a song?

Interacting and relating to others

Does the child give objects or point to objects to show them to others, use names for at least two people, smile or laugh when others say something funny or nice (''good work,'' ''that's a pretty hat''), try to please other people, play a simple game with another person (hiding, chasing), play ''make believe'' (feed dolls, put dolls to bed, pretend to go shopping), or enjoy having stories read to him/her?

Model multicenter outcomes

During the 1990s, infants with birth weights of 501 to 1000 g continued to have major neurodevelopmental impairments in the first 2 years of life. This section reviews several studies that suggested how outcomes might be framed to address the impact of biomedical interventions on early childhood neuromotor disability.

Schmidt and colleagues [29] examined three neonatal complications—bronchopulmonary dysplasia, parenchymal brain injury on serial cranial sonograms, and severe retinopathy of prematurity (ROP)—in 910 children who were less than 1000 g birth weight and enrolled in the international study of prophylactic indomethacin to prevent intraventricular hemorrhage (IVH). Among survivors at 18 months of age, 13% had CP and 26% had development disability; however, rates of CP increased to 36% for those who had parenchymal brain injury that was defined as IVH grade 3 or 4, ventriculomegaly, or cystic periventricular leukomalacia. Also, 24% of those who had severe ROP (stage 4 or 5) and 17% of those who had bronchopulmonary dysplasia (supplemental oxygen at 36 wks PMA) had CP. Among the neonates who were free of these three morbidities, the rate of death or neurodevelopmental impairment at 18 months was 18%. This occurred in a setting of mortality between 1.2% and 3%. In contrast, the rates of death or neurodevelopmental disability were 88% if all three of these impairments were present. This occurred in a setting of mortality between 9% and 10%. More than half of the children who had parenchymal brain injury or severe ROP had neurodevelopmental disability. Although the numbers were small, 78% of those who had severe brain injury and ROP had neurodevelopmental disability.

Several regional multicenter studies have examined 18- to 24-month outcomes in extremely preterm infants (Table 1). In the six largest multicenter studies by Schmidt and colleagues [36], Vohr and colleagues [30,31], Stoll and colleagues [32], Hintz and colleagues [33], and Wood and colleagues [34], rates of CP exceeded 12% for infants less than 28 weeks gestational age, the prevalence of developmental disability (Bayley Scores more than two standard deviations below the mean for corrected age) was more than 20%, sensorineural hearing impairment that required amplification was 1% to 4%, and visual impairment worse than 20/200 was 1% to 4%. For perspective, the rates of these impairments in term children are 0.2% for CP, 2% to 3% for developmental cognitive disability, 0.1% to 0.3% for hearing loss, and 0.1% for severe visual impairment [35].

A different strategy was undertaken by Doyle [3] who examined 2-year outcomes for ELBW infants who were born in 1997 in the Victorian Infant Collaborative Group. In comparing neurodevelopmental status in survivors of the 1997 group with those in the 1979–1980, 1985–1987, 1991–1992, and 1997 groups, rates of child survival increased from 25% to 38% to 56% and to 73% with advances in neonatology. Although early child disability initially decreased from 61% to 45%, it subsequently plateaued at 45% and 49% [3]. Concurrent

Table 1
Extremely low birth weight survivors: neurodevelopmental outcomes in the 1990s

Study	Sample	CP	DD	HI	VI
Schmidt et al 1996–1998 [41]	N = 467 INDO 500 – 999 g	12%	27%	2%	2%
	N = 477 PBO 500 – 999 g	12%	26%	2%	1%
Schmidt et al 1996–1998 [29]	BPD = 193	17%	38%	3.5%	1.9%
	No BPD = 130	9.3%	19%	1.4%	1.8%
	IVH 3 – 4 = 116	36%	42%	2.9%	2.9%
	No IVH 3 – 4 = 207	6.7%	23%	2.2%	1.6%
	Severe ROP = 58	24%	49%	3.8%	15%
	No severe ROP = 265	12%	25%	2.2%	0.5%
Mikkola et al 1996–1998 [49]	206 <1000 g	14%	9%	4%	2.6%
Vohr et al 1995–1998 [30]	N = 1860	15.2%	31%	2%	10%
Vohr et al 2 1995–1998 [30]	N = 1434	No CP	2.4%	0.6%	0.2%
	N = 120	Quad CP	89%	6.7%	5.8%
	N = 160	DHM CP	61%	4.3%	0.6%
Aziz et al 1987–1990 [50]	N = 567 (nl SONO) 500 – 1249 g	5.6%	2.6%	1.1%	0.9%
	N = 79 (abnl SONO) 500 – 1249 g	30.4%	20.2%	3.8%	15.2%
Jacobs et al 1990–1994 [37]	N = 274 23 – 26 wk	15%	26%	4%	4%
Vohr et al 1993–1998 [31]	N = 2291 22 – 26 wk	19%	37%	2.4%	1%
	N = 1494 27 – 32 wk GA	11.6%	26%	1%	0.7%
Wood et al 1995 [34]	N = 283 22 – 25 wk	16%	30%	2%	2%
Doyle et al 1997 [3,36]	N = 170 500 – 999 g	11%	22%	1.8%	2.4%
Finnstrom 1990–1992 [51]	N = 362 500 – 999 g	7%	15%	1%	4%
	N = 157 23 – 26 wk	12	23	1	2
	N = 185; ≥27 wk	3	8	0.3	1
Stoll et al 1993–2001 [32]	No infection N = 2161 400 – 999 g	8	22	1	5
	Sepsis N = 3460 400 – 999 g	16	35	2.5	15
	NEC/Men N = 392 400 – 999 g	20	40	3.2	16
Hintz et al 1995–1998 [33]	No NEC N = 2699 400 – 1000 g	15	31	1.5	1.0
	Med NEC N = 121 400 – 1000 g	12	37	0.8	0.8

(continued on next page)

Table 1 (*continued*)

Study	Sample	CP	DD	HI	VI
	Surg NEC N = 124 400 – 1000 g	24%	44%	4.1	4.1
Mestan et al 1998–2001 [38]	INO, N = 70 27.5 wk GA	8.6%	18.8	0	0
	N = 68 27.2 wk GA	10.3%	35.8	1.5	2.9
Shankaran et al 1993–1999 [43]	N = 246 ; ≤750 g ≤24wk;Ap1 ≤3	30%	46%	5%	2%
Wilson-Costello et al 1990–1998 [42]	N = 417 500 – 999 g	14%	26%	7%	1%
Wilson-Costello et al 1982–1989 [42]	N = 214 500 – 999 g	8	20	3	3
Fily et al 1997 [52]	N = 545 < 33wk	9	4.7	0.8	0.2
Shinwell et al 1993–1996 [53]	PBO, N = 79	15	29	1 SI	1 SI?
	DEC, N = 80	48	55	5 SI	5 SI?

Abbreviations: abnl, abnormal; Ap1, 1-minute Apgar score; BPD, bronchopulmonary dysplasia; DD, developmental diasability: MDI/PDI < 70; DEC, decadron; DHM, diplegic/hemiplegic/monoplegic CP; GA, gestational age; HI, hearing impairment requiring aides; INDO, indomethacin; INO, inhaled nitric oxide; Med NEC, medically managed NEC; Men, meningitis; nl, normal; PBO, placebo; Quad, quadriplegic, triplegic or extrapyramidal CP; SONO, sonogram; Surg NEC, surgically managed NEC; VI, visual impairment worse than 20/200 corrected.

rates of CP were 13.5%, 6.6%, 9.3%, and 10.7%, whereas rates of moderate to severe disability were 28%, 18%, 19%, and 26%.

Several strategies have been used to examine functional disability. In the 14-center 1995–1998 neonatal network study by Vohr and colleagues [30], 11% of hemiplegics, 8% of diplegics, 31% of triplegics, and 76% of quadriplegics could not sit as indicated by a gross motor functional classification system (GMFCS) level of 3 to 5. With respect to taking 10 steps at 18 months, 60% of hemiplegics, 38% of diplegics, 19% of triplegics, and 1.5% of quadriplegics could not perform this activity. In the EPICure Study, functional observations at 30 months revealed that 10% were unable to walk, 3% were unable to sit, 4% were unable to feed self a cracker, and 6% could not communicate in speech. Overall, 50% were free of disability, 26% had mild to moderate disability, and 24% had severe disability [34]. Subsequently, Marlowe [4] demonstrated that these key functional activity descriptors were highly predictive of educational and community disability in middle childhood.

In the Toronto surfactant cohort, 274 survivors of 23- to 26-week gestational age who had received surfactant in 1990–1994 were followed. Overall, 23% of the survivors had mild neuromotor impairments defined as (ie, GMFCS level 1) moderate (ie, GMFCS level 2) disability with concurrent cognitive impairments that were reflected in MDI scores of 70 to 84. Twelve percent were severely disabled, which was characterized by an inability to sit (ie, GMFCS level 4 or 5), blindness, sensorineural hearing loss that required amplification, cognitive disability (MDI scores <70), or shunted hydrocephalus [37]. Almost two thirds were free of neurodevelopmental disability at age 18 to 24 months.

Box 1 provides additional indictors that would help to define dimensions of functional skills in children who are receiving new technologies. The value of this approach is that it allows feedback to parents and professionals about precursors to communication, social, and adaptive tasks of the preschool years. Specifically, one can describe the individual child as becoming more independent or continuing to be dependent on his/her caregivers in daily tasks and more complex learning.

Cohort studies: pathways in neuromotor disorders with multiple disabilities

Several recent studies have examined postneonatal processes that might be amenable to intervention, such as infection control, necrotizing enterocolitis (NEC), use of inhaled nitric oxide (INO), and postnatal steroids (see Table 1) [32,33,38]. Stoll and colleagues [32] examined the role of postnatal infection on neurodevelopmental impairments among 6093 survivors who weighed between 401 and 1000 g and were born between 1993 and 2001 in the U.S. Neonatal Network. In this study, three major types of infants were identified: infants who did not have infection during their hospital stay [n = 2161]; infants who had clinical infection and received parental antibiotics for at least 5 days [n = 1538] or infants who had sepsis [n = 1922]; and infants who had NEC [n = 279] or meningitis [n = 193].

Almost two thirds of survivors had postnatal infections, the overwhelming majority of which were late onset. Among those who did not have infection, 8% had CP. Approximately one in five infants who had sepsis, NEC, or meningitis had CP. One of the disquieting outcomes of Stoll and colleagues' [32] study was the high rate of cognitive developmental disability (defined as a Bayley MDI <70 at 18 months). Cognitive disability occurred in 22% of infants who did not have infection and in 33% to 42% of those who had infection. The relationship between infection status and neurodevelopmental disability held when adjusting for bronchopulmonary dysplasia, postnatal steroids, and sonographic parenchymal brain injury—three major determinants of adverse outcomes in ELBW survivors [29,39].

Hintz and colleagues [33] examined the impact of NEC on ELBW survivors who required medical or surgical management and compared them with ELBW survivors who did not have NEC. Almost one in four patients who had surgically managed NEC had CP and more than two in five children had developmental disability. Rates of CP were 12% in children who did not have NEC. Thus, the combined impact of NEC is more than gastroenterological and has substantial contributions to neuromotor and cognitive disability in early childhood.

A different approach was undertaken by Mestan and colleagues [38] who examined 2-year neurodevelopmental outcome in very preterm children who had been part of a randomized clinical trial of INO for respiratory failure. Among infants who received INO, CP occurred with a frequency of 8.6%, whereas the rate was 10.3% among infants who had not received INO; however, the risk of neurodevelopmental disability in the survivors who received INO was 53% less than controls because of the favorable impact on cognitive and developmental outcome. Thus, the studies by Stoll and colleagues [32], Hintz and colleagues [33], and Mestan and colleagues [38] suggest the importance of examining CP outcomes when evaluating strategies to decrease sepsis, NEC, and chronic lung disease. Multicenter interventional studies that are aimed at decreasing chronic lung disease in ELBW have not occurred. Furthermore, the international Trial of Indomethacin Prophylaxis in Preterms and the New England IVH prevention study demonstrated that when more severe grades of IVH are decreased, rates of CP and cognitive disability do not decrease [29,39]. This suggests that IVH is not the predominant pathway to CP, and that other mechanisms are involved in the pathways of cognitive disability.

Doyle [40] undertook a meta-analysis of very low birth weight and ELBW infants who had received postnatal steroids to hasten extubation and who had neurodevelopmental follow-up. Rates of CP were 23% for infants who had received steroids and 15% for controls. It must be pointed out that only five studies had more than 100 infants enrolled. An interesting observation occurred in an Israeli study of very preterm infants; 79 children who had received placebo were compared with 80 children who had received Decadron to facilitate ventilator weaning [41]. For children in the group who received Decadron the rates of CP increased from 15% to 48%, and rates of developmental disability increased from 29% to 55% compared to children in the placebo group. Thus, the neonatal management strategies that might enhance short-term pulmonary outcome need to have neurodevelopmental end points so that the proper assessment of risks and benefits is understood.

Vohr and colleagues [31] compared children who were born at 22 to 26 weeks' gestation and weighed less than 1000 g with children who were born at 27 to 32 weeks' gestation and weighed less than 1000 g in the National Institute of Child Health and Human Developement Neonatal Network between 1993 and 1998. Rates of CP were 19% and 12%, respectively. Wilson-Costello and colleagues [42] found that compared with ELBW infants who were born between 1982 and 1989, those who were born between 1990 and 1998 had a 1.75-fold increase in the rate of CP and a 1.3-fold increase in the rate of neurodevelopmental disability. Shankaran and colleagues [43] examined the highest risk group at the threshold of viability. These risks included a birth weight of less than 750 g, a gestational age of less than 24 weeks, and a 1-minute Apgar rating of 3 or less. Among survivors, the overall neurodevelopmental disability rate was 60%. Almost one in three survivors had one of the CP syndromes and almost one in two survivors had cognitive developmental disability. Thus, at the end of the 1990s, US trends were suggesting that increased rates of survival of extremely preterm infants were accompanied by increased rates of CP for infants in the most vulnerable gestation groups. These data highlighted the need for understanding the mechanisms of neuroprotection and neurodevelopmental vulnerability among those who are at the threshold of viability.

An important observation occurred when examining the relationship between the severity of ROP and 5-year motor, self-care, and communicative functional status in the multicenter Cryosurgery for Retinopathy of Prematurity Study [44]. Among the children who had had threshold ROP and had favorable visual status at 5.5 years, self-care functional limitations were found in 25%, motor limitations were found in 5%, and communicative-cognitive limitations were found in 22%. In contrast, children with threshold ROP who had an unfavorable visual status at 5 years had higher rates of self-care (77%), motor (43%), and communicative-cognitive (66%) functional disability. In addition, the children who had no ROP or prethreshold ROP had rates of motor, self-care, and communicative-cognitive functional disabilities of less than 10%. These data suggests that severe ROP is an important marker for the severity of neuromotor, adaptive, and communicative disability at kindergarten entry. In addition, understanding the mechanisms that are involved in extreme prematurity that result in the absence of retinopathy are critically important for preserving central nervous system neuromotor and higher cortical integrity.

Recently, Vohr and colleagues [30] found that among 120 children who had quadriplegia and had an ELBW, 89% had a Bayley MDI of less than 70, 6.7% had hearing impairment, and 5.8% had visual impairment. Among the children who had diplegia, monoplegia, or hemiplegia 61% had cognitive developmental disability, 4.3% had hearing impairment, and 0.6% had visual impairment. Thus, efforts to decrease the rates of CP in ELBW must also examine the vulnerability of associated pathways that have an impact on cognitive and sensory disability.

Future directions

As neonatal care evolves to increase survival at the limits of viability, comprehensive efforts are required to find interventions that decrease parenchymal brain injury and the severity of CP. It is not known how the children of extremely preterm gestation who have hemiplegic and diplegic CP are doing with respect to cognitive, functional, growth, and health status as compared with very preterm and moderately preterm survivors in preschool years. Most importantly, intervention—whether nutritional, pulmonary management, or infection control—should be examined with respect to reducing degrees of gross motor, fine motor, oral motor, and communicative functional impairments. If neonatologists are to move beyond strategies for increasing survival and develop methods for optimizing health, development, and educational outcomes, there must be combined strategies that enhance neuroprotection and support families in optimizing their child's development after discharge.

To accomplish this vision, four major challenges must be addressed. First, explicit hypotheses about inflammatory mediators, disruption of the blood–brain barrier, and mechanisms that impair parenchymal brain integrity must have their impact assessed on emerging developmental processes of feeding skills, hand skills, mobility, and communicative skills [45–47].

Second, robust developmental variables must be defined, a priori, and include severity and functional outcome facets so that the effects of new interventions on severe multiple disability can be measured consistently. It is wrong to equate a child who is unable to walk, say words, feed oneself, and see with a child who is legally blind but able to read large print, run on the playground with peers, and do all of his or her neurodevelopmental self-care tasks. Often, both of these children are categorized as having a major disability.

Third, clinical trials need to analyze the impact of neonatal interventions to decrease parenchymal brain injury (IVH grade 3 or 4, or cystic periventricular leukomalacia), and decrease the severity and prevalence of CP [48]. In particular, it is also important to understand what biomarkers might predict which infants with sequentially normal sonograms go on to have one of the CP syndromes.

Fourth, by understanding the mechanisms whereby short-term neonatal morbidities increase developmental motor disability, additional developmental supports and family interventions after discharge can be promoted. Long-term outcomes in children who have CP are compromised often by adverse family and community factors, such as parental isolation, limited transportation, fragmented medical care, low parental education attainment, inadequate child care, overwhelmed early intervention programs, and family stressors. By combining biomedical risk reduction strategies and explicitly designing, prioritizing, and evaluating our biopsychosocial interventions, progress can be made toward increasing survival, promoting function, and enhancing community participation [56].

Acknowledgments

This research was supported by 1U01 HD37614 entitled "NICHD Family and Child Well Being Network: Child Disability." This article is dedicated to Maggie C. Daley and Shirley Welsh Ryan for their commitment to enhancing quality care for children who have cerebral palsy. Jennifer J. Park provided invaluable editing and technical assistance.

References

[1] Horbar JD, Badger GJ, Carpenter JH, et al. Trends in mortality and morbidity for very low birth weight infants, 1991–1999. Pediatrics 2002;110:143–51.
[2] Lemons JA, Bauer CR, Oh W, et al. Very low birth weight outcomes of the National Institute of Child Health and Human Development Neonatal Research Network. January 1995 through December 1996. Pediatrics 2001;107e:1–8.
[3] Doyle LW. Evaluation of neonatal intensive care for extremely low birthweight infants in Victoria over two decades: I. effectiveness. Pediatrics 2004;113:505–9.

[4] Marlow N, Wolke D, Bracewell MA, et al, EPICure Study Group. Neurologic and developmental disability at six years of age after extremely preterm birth. N Engl J Med 2005;352(1):9–19.

[5] Vohr BR, Allen M. Extreme prematurity—the continuing dilemma. N Engl J Med 2005;352:71–2.

[6] World Health Organization. International classification of functioning disability and health. Geneva (Switzerland): World Health Ortganization; 2001.

[7] National Research Council and Institute of Medicine. children's health, the nation's wealth: assessing and improving child health. Committee on Evaluation of Children's Health. Board on Children, Youth, and Families, Division of Behavioral and Social Sciences and Education. Washington DC: The National Academies Press; 2004.

[8] Stanley F, Blair E, Alberman E. Cerebral palsies: epidemiology and casual pathways. Clinics in Developmental Medicine. No. 151. London: Mackeith Press; 2000.

[9] Blair E, Watson L. Epidemiology of cerebral palsy. Semin Fetal Neonatal Med 2006;11:117–25.

[10] Himmelmann K, Hagberg G, Beckung E, et al. The changing panorama of cerebral palsy in Sweden. IX. Prevalence and origin in the birth-year period 1995–1998. Acta Paediatr 2005; 94(3):287–94.

[11] Hamrick SE, Miller SP, Leonard C, et al. Trends in severe brain injury and neurodevelopmental outcome in premature newborn infants: the role of cystic periventricular leukomalacia. J Pediatr 2004;145(5):593–9.

[12] Surman G, Newdick H, Johnson A. Oxford Register of Early Childhood Impairments Management Group. Cerebral palsy rates among low-birthweight infants fell in the 1990s. Dev Med Child Neurol 2003;45(7):456–62.

[13] Neil JJ, Inder TE. Imaging perinatal brain injury in premature infants. Semin Perinatol 2004; 28(6):433–43.

[14] De Vries LS, Van Haastert IL, Rademaker KJ, et al. Ultrasound abnormalities preceding cerebral palsy in high-risk preterm infants. J Pediatr 2004;144(6):815–20.

[15] Laptook AR, O'Shea TM, Shankaran S, et al, NICHD Neonatal Network. Adverse neurodevelopmental outcomes among extremely low birth weight infants with a normal head ultrasound: prevalence and antecedents. Pediatrics 2005;115(3):673–80.

[16] Mirmiran M, Barnes PD, Keller K, et al. Neonatal brain magnetic resonance imaging before discharge is better than serial cranial ultrasound in predicting cerebral palsy in very low birth weight preterm infants. Pediatrics 2004;114(4):992–8.

[17] Campbell S. The child's development of functional movement. In: Physical therapy for children. Philadelphia: W.B. Saunders Company; 1994. p. 3–37.

[18] Allen MC, Alexander G. Gross motor milestones in preterm infants: correction for degree of prematurity. J Pediatr 1990;116(6):955–9.

[19] Russell DJ, Rosenbaum PL, Avery LM, et al, editors. Gross Motor Function Measure (6MFM-66 & 6MFM-88) user's manual. London: MacKeith Press; 2002. p. 156–8.

[20] Bax M, Goldstein M, Rosenbaum P, et al. Proposed definition and classification of cerebral palsy, April 2005. Dev Med Child Neurol 2005;47(8):571–6.

[21] Folio MR, Fewell RR, editors. Peabody developmental motor scale. 2nd edition. Austin (TX): ProEd; 2000.

[22] Einspieler C, Prechtl HFR, Bos AF, et al. Prechtl's method on the qualitative assessment of general movements in preterm, term and young infants. London: Mac Keith Press; 2004.

[23] Gesell A, Halverson HM, Thompson H, et al. 1940. The first five years of life: a guide to the study of the preschool child. New York: Harper & Row, Publishers; 1940.

[24] Bayley N. Mental growth during the first three years. Genet Psychol 1933;14:1.

[25] Illingworth RS. The development of the infant and young child: normal and abnormal. 8th edition. London: Churchill Livingstone; 1984.

[26] Griffiths R. The abilities of babies. London: University of London Press; 1954.

[27] Neligan G, Prudham D. Norms for four standard developmental milestones by sex, social class and place in family. Devel Med Child Neurol 1969;11:413–22.

[28] Capute AJ, Biehl RF. Functional developmental evaluation: prerequisite to habilitation. Pediatr Clin North Am 1973;20:3–26.

[29] Schmidt B, Asztalos EV, Roberts RS, et al, Trial of Indomethacin Prophylaxis in Preterms (TIPP) Investigators. Impact of bronchopulmonary dysplasia, brain injury, and severe retinopathy on the outcome of extremely low-birth-weight infants at 18 months: results from the trail of indomethacin prophylaxis in preterms. JAMA 2003;289(9):1124–9.

[30] Vohr B, Msall M, Wilson D, et al. Spectrum of gross motor function in extremely low birth weight children with cerebral palsy at 18 months of age. Pediatrics 2005;116(1):123–9.

[31] Vohr B, Wright LL, Poole WK, et al. Neurodevelopmental outcomes of extremely low birth weight infants <32 weeks' gestation between 1993 and 1998. Pediatrics 2005;116(3):635–43.

[32] Stoll BJ, Hansen NI, Adams-Chapman I, et al, National Institute of Child Health and Human Development Neonatal Research. Neurodevelopmental and growth impairment among extremely low-birth-weight infants with neonatal infection. JAMA 2004;292(19):2357–65.

[33] Hintz SR, Kendrick DE, Stoll BJ, et al. Neurodevelopmental and growth outcomes of extremely low birth weight infants after necrotizing enterocolitis. Pediatrics 2005;115(3):696–703.

[34] Wood NS, Marlow N, Costeloe K, et al. Neurologic and developmental disability after extreme preterm birth. N Engl J Med 2000;343:378–84.

[35] Msall M, Tremont MR, Ottenbacher KJ. Functional assessment of preschool children: optimizing developmental and family supports in early intervention. Infants Young Child 2001;14(1): 46–66.

[36] Doyle LW. Evaluation of neonatal intensive care for extremely-low-birth-weight infants. Semin Fetal Neonatal Med 2006;11:139–45.

[37] Jacobs SE, O'Brien KO, Inwood S, et al. Outcome of infants 23–26 weeks' gestation pre and post surfactant. Acta Paediatr 2000;89:959–65.

[38] Mestan KL, Marks JD, Hecox K, et al. neurodevelopmental outcomes of premature infants treated with inhaled nitric oxide. N Engl J Med 2005;353:23–32.

[39] Ment L, Vohr B, Allan W. Outcome of children in the indomethacin intraventricular hemorrhage prevention trial. Pediatrics 2000;105(3 Pt 1):485–91.

[40] Doyle LW, Halliday HL, Ehrenkranz RA, et al. Impact of postnatal systemic corticosteroids on mortality and cerebral palsy in preterm infants: effect modification by risk for chronic lung disease. Pediatrics 2005;115(3):655–61.

[41] Schmidt B, Davis P, Moddemann D, et al. Long-term effects of indomethacin prophylaxis in extremely-low-birth-weight infants. N Engl J Med 2001;344(26):1966–72.

[42] Wilson-Costello D, Friedman H, Minich N, et al. Improved survival rates with increased neurodevelopmental disability for extremely low birth weight infants in the 1990s. Pediatrics 2005;115(4):997–1003.

[43] Shankaran S, Johnson Y, Langer JC, et al. Outcome of extremely-low-birth-weight infants at highest risk: gestational age < or =24 weeks, birth weight < or =750 g, and 1-minute Apgar < or =3. Am J Obstet Gynecol 2004;191(4):1084–91.

[44] Msall M, Phelps DL, DiGaudio KM, et al. Severity of neonatal retinopathy of prematurity is predictive of neurodevelopmental functional outcome at age 5.5 years. Pediatrics 2000;106(5): 998–1005.

[45] Back SA, Rivkees SA. Emerging concepts in periventricular white matter injury. Semin Perinatol 2004;28(6):405–14.

[46] Dammann O, Leviton A. Inflammatory brain damage in preterm newborns—dry numbers, wet lab, and causal inferences. Early Hum Dev 2004;79(1):1–15.

[47] Leviton A, Dammann O. Coagulation, inflammation, and the risk of neonatal white matter damage. Pediatr Res 2004;55(4):541–5.

[48] Murata Y, Itakura A, Matsuzawa K, et al. Possible antenatal and perinatal related factors in development of cystic periventricular leukomalacia. Brain Dev 2005;27(1):17–21.

[49] Mikkola K, Ritari N, Tommiska V, et al. Neurodevelopmental outcome at 5 years of age of a national cohort of extremely low birth weight infants who were born in 1996–1997. Pediatrics 2005;116(6):1391–400.

[50] Aziz K, Vickar DB, Sauve RS. Province-based study of neurologic disability of children weighing 500 through 1249 grams at birth in relation to neonatal cerebral ultrasound findings. Pediatrics 1995;95(6):837–44.

[51] Finnstrom O, Otterblad Olausson P, Sedin G, et al. Neurosensory outcome and growth at three years in extremely low birthweight infants: follow-up results from the Swedish national prospective study. Acta Paediatr 1998;87(10):1055–60.

[52] Fily A, Pierrat V, Delporte V, et al, EPIPAGE Nord-Pas-de-Calais Study Group. Factors associated with neurodevelopmental outcome at 2 years after very preterm birth: the population-based Nord-Pas-de-Calais EPIPAGE cohort. Pediatrics 2006;117(2):357–66.

[53] Shinwell ES, Karplus M, Reich D, et al. Early postnatal dexamethasone treatment and increased incidence of cerebral palsy. Arch Dis Child Fetal Neonatal Ed 2000;83(3):F177–81.

[54] Capute AJ, Accardo PJ. The infant neurodevelopmental assessment: a clinical interpretive manual for CAT-CLAMS in the first two years of life. Curr Probl Pediatr 1996;26:238–57 (part 1); 279–306 (part 2).

[55] Hogan DP, Msall ME. Health and disability indicators for preschool and school age children. In: Brown B, editor. Indicators of child and youth well-being: completing the picture. Rahway, NJ: Lawrence Erlbaum Associates; 2006, in press.

[56] Marlow N. Neurocognitive outcome after very preterm birth. Arch Dis Child Fetal Neonatal Ed 2004;89:F224–8.

ELSEVIER
SAUNDERS

Clin Perinatol 33 (2006) 285–300

CLINICS IN
PERINATOLOGY

Cerebral Palsy and Intrauterine Growth

Stephen Jarvis, MD[a],*, Svetlana V. Glinianaia, MD[b],
Eve Blair, PhD[c]

[a]*Institute of Child Health, School of Clinical Medical Services, University of Newcastle,*
Newcastle upon Tyne NE1 4LP, UK
[b]*School of Population and Health Sciences, University of Newcastle,*
Newcastle upon Tyne NE2 4HH, UK
[c]*Centre for Child Health Research, University of Western Australia, Perth, Western Australia*

Intrauterine growth is the increase over time in fetal size. Because growth velocity (eg, millimeters per week of gestation) is rarely used in pregnancy outcome studies, most of the discussion herein concerns the relative size at birth (eg, weight compared with that expected for gestational age) as an admittedly inadequate [1] surrogate for intrauterine growth.

Infants who are somewhat heavier at birth than is average for their gestational age and gender are at the lowest risk of having cerebral palsy and the lowest risk of perinatal death [2]. This optimum birth weight for best outcomes seems to be about one standard deviation (SD) heavier than the average birth weight for gestational age among healthy infants (Z score=+1). At all gestations, infants who are either smaller or larger than this optimum size have a progressively increased risk of cerebral palsy (Fig. 1) [3]. These findings are based on a large collaborative study of 4307 singleton children with cerebral palsy recorded in population registers across Europe in which gestational ages were largely confirmed by ultrasound dating [3]. They confirm and expand the results from several earlier cohort [4,5] and case-control [6–9] studies.

Several problems arise in the interpretation of the results from these and other reports of the relationship between cerebral palsy and the size-for-gestation.

Work for this article was supported by European Commission fund DGXII-BIOMED2-Contrat NBMH4-983701.

* Corresponding author. Institute of Child Health, School of Clinical Medical Services, University of Newcastle, Newcastle upon Tyne NE1 4LP, UK.

E-mail address: s.n.jarvis@ncl.ac.uk (S. Jarvis).

The influence of gestational age

Judgment of the relative size of infants at birth must take into account gestational age, because this age has a profound effect on the risk for cerebral palsy (Fig. 1) [10]. Low birth weight infants (<2500 g) may have elevated risks of cerebral palsy because they are (1) of optimum weight for gestation but are born too early (eg, preterm only), (2) light for gestational age but born at term (small for gestational age [SGA] only), (3) both preterm and light for gestational age, or (4) heavy for gestational age but delivered very early (one fifth of infants at greater than the 90th centile preterm weigh less than 2500 g).

Thus, significance of birth weight cannot be properly understood without also considering gestational duration [11]. Because many studies of the risk for cerebral palsy use birth weight alone unqualified by the gestational age at birth [12,13], the observed increase in the risk for cerebral palsy associated with low birth weight has dominated the results and often been attributed to intrauterine growth retardation [14]. In fact, one third of infants with cerebral palsy are of above average weight for gestational age, and more than two thirds are heavier than the most common criterion for SGA (10th centile weight for gestational duration) [3].

A related problem in studies of cerebral palsy and intrauterine growth is the bias introduced by the selection of study populations using birth weight cutoffs

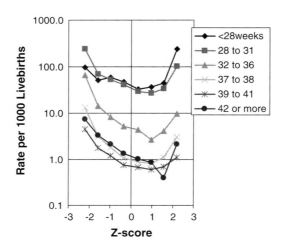

Fig. 1. Prevalence of cerebral palsy by Z score of weight for gestation. Rates at size extremes for very preterm (<32 week) infants are likely to underestimate rates of fetal brain damage on account of very high neonatal mortality, which will be greatest in the most severely growth restricted. Z scores equate to centiles, for example, the 90th centile equals approximately 1.28 SDs above the mean fetal weight using fetal standards. (*Adapted from* Jarvis SN, Glinianaia SV, Torrioli M-G, et al. Cerebral palsy and intrauterine growth in single births: a European collaborative study. Lancet 2003; 362:1107; with permission.)

(eg, <1500 g) [11]. This practice results in an overrepresentation of small-for-dates infants because only they can satisfy the weight criterion at later gestations.

Birth weight for gestational age

When birth weight and gestational age data are both available, a more sophisticated account of relative size can be made using centile charts. Commonly, the attempt is made to define a "high-risk" subset of SGA and a similar high-risk group of large for gestational age (LGA) infants, leaving by exclusion a group who are considered an appropriate size for gestation (AGA). The actual centiles chosen to define these subgroups vary (eg, less than the 10th centile or less than the third centile for SGA). Regardless of the ones used, there are underlying weaknesses in this approach:

- The implications of falling beyond the cut point can be variable. For example, a group defined as below the 10th centile includes infants at 85% and 50% of their expected birth weight, a difference of more than 1 kg for an expected weight over 3 kg. The variability of implications would be compounded if inappropriate centile charts were used [15]. Charts may be out of date. With the average weight of healthy infants at birth increasing by up to 50 g every 10 years [16,17], progressively fewer infants are qualifying as SGA as defined by old growth charts. The centile charts may also have insufficient adjustment for nonpathologic determinants of size for gestation, such as gender, parity, and maternal height [18].
- There is an assumption that SGA or LGA groups consist of "inappropriately" grown infants. For example, SGA infants are often considered to be pathologically small owing to some interference that restricts intrauterine growth rather than simply constitutionally small by virtue of genetic growth potential. Evidence of truly abnormal growth velocity among SGA infants is rarely available, and the identification of a pathologic subset based on abnormal body proportions is still uncertain. There are no discontinuities in risk profiles with changes in the size of infants at any gestation. On the contrary, the relationship of perinatal outcomes to relative birth weight for gestational age is usually continuous and often exponential [3,19–21].
- This continuous relationship can mean that the risk for a poor outcome changes progressively even within the range of what is considered an appropriate birth weight, for example, between the 10th and 90th centile. Because the great majority of births occur in this weight range, the relatively small changes in risks among them can contribute a large proportion of excess neonatal deaths and morbidity associated with variations in intrauterine growth. Many study samples are too small to categorize weight for gestation more precisely than as SGA, AGA, and LGA, and their results are too simplistic and may overestimate the minimum risk of cerebral palsy for the most optimally grown infants.

Suitable growth standards

The size of preterm infants should be compared with that expected of their "healthy" peers. It is now clear that infants born before 37 weeks' gestation are not healthy in this sense but tend to be lighter [22] and slower growing [23] than fetuses of the same post conceptional age, presumably for reasons related to their preterm birth. Because conventional "neonatal" birth weight standards are based on the observed birth weights of infants born at different gestational ages, comparing the weight of preterm infants with cerebral palsy with these standards compares them with other preterm infants who themselves are more likely to be abnormally grown. To avoid this problem, the relative size of infants born before term should be judged using reference standards based on the intrauterine weight for gestational age ("fetal" standards) rather than birth weights. Such fetal standards are derived from ultrasound-based estimates of the weights of healthy infants in utero at known gestational ages [24,25]. The standards can be tailored to allow for other important fetal characteristics, such as sex, ethnicity, and parity, as well as maternal height [26].

Early studies of the risk for cerebral palsy in which the birth weight and gestational age of cases were known used neonatal weight standards to judge the relative size of cerebral palsy cases, often using gestation-of-delivery matched controls [6,8,27,28]. Typically, these studies reported that the risk for cerebral palsy was not elevated for very preterm SGA infants. The authors believe this is because the neonatal growth standards and the controls used were equally biased by the inclusion of an excess of abnormally light preterm infants. As seen in Fig. 1, when fetal growth standards are used, there is a significant elevation of the risk for cerebral palsy for very preterm SGA infants in a similar pattern to that which applies at term. The use of gestation-matched preterm controls can also make it impossible to disentangle the risk of cerebral palsy attributable to factors that are themselves associated with poor growth and preterm delivery. For instance, maternal pre-eclampsia, which is one of the most frequently occurring causes of growth restriction, can also be an indication for elective preterm birth. Although the risk for cerebral palsy in a SGA infant born very preterm owing to pre-eclampsia is lower than that in an infant born equally preterm for some other reason, it is considerably higher than the risk in the healthy term born infant without pre-eclampsia.

Appropriate denominators

Because cerebral palsy is usually not described until well after the neonatal period, the infants used to form the denominator for rates have survived at least the first month of life, the period of highest postnatal mortality. If neonatal deaths are included, they artifactually decrease the estimated rate, because they could not be included in the numerator even if they had cerebral damage that would have resulted in cerebral palsy had they survived. Survival is strongly associated with size at birth [19]. Among very preterm infants who have the highest mortality, this can mean that the risk of cerebral palsy associated with small or very large size will be underestimated unless early deaths are excluded from the denominators [3].

Estimating the risk of cerebral palsy associated with variations in weight for gestation can be done without knowing the denominators, that is, the actual number of unaffected surviving infants in each weight-for-gestation category. Several case-control studies have calculated the odds ratios for cerebral palsy by birth weight for gestation [6–8,28] by using the distribution of birth weight for gestation in controls as an estimate of that in the source population from which the cases were drawn. If it is assumed that the weight distribution within each gestation week is gaussian (a reasonable assumption for term birth weights and for fetal weights), the use of controls is unnecessary. The distribution of weight for gestation of the source population will be adequately represented by the appropriate fetal growth standard. This method was used in the European study from which Fig. 1 is drawn [3]. It has the advantage of avoiding the bias to reduced intrauterine growth inherent in using preterm born controls.

Size versus growth/shape

Weight, at any gestation, is a snapshot of the infant's size. When compared with normative growth charts, a single reading at the 10th centile, especially if the chosen standard is carefully adjusted for factors such as gender, parity, and ethnicity, merely indicates that among 100 infants of this gestational age in the standard population, 10% will be lighter. To assess whether growth is proceeding as expected, two or more readings at least a month apart are required [1]. The difference between these readings should ideally be compared with growth velocity standards (because normal growth velocity also shows constitutional variation between infants). In practice, there are few studies of the true relationship between intrauterine growth and perinatal outcomes. The authors are aware of only three such studies based on sequential ultrasound scanning of high-risk infants who were later followed up and among whom a number with decelerating growth had severe perinatal problems [29] or subsequent intellectual and behavioral impairments [30,31].

In the past, the timing of "growth failure" was imputed from the proportionality of the body parts at birth (ie, the shape of the baby) [32–34]. No one has comprehensively investigated fetal body shape ultrasonically, and doubt remains as to whether it is possible to characterize the growth history of infants in utero from the ratios of body measurements [35]. It is not clear that there is a single pattern of relative growth of different body parts applicable to all fetuses [36]. The discussion that follows is confined to studies of cerebral palsy in which intrauterine growth was judged by variations in size (ie, birth weight for gestational age), and in which either preterm infants were excluded (ie, studies restricted to term births) or fetal growth standards were used to assess the appropriateness of size.

Studies relating the size at birth to the risk for cerebral palsy in term infants

The three case-control studies [6,8,9], two cohort studies [3,5], and one cross-sectional case study [4] exclude from their case material cerebral palsy of known postneonatal origin, whereas one study also excludes nonspastic cases [6]. Only some reports allow the illustration of the relationship among term infants in isolation. Fig. 2 combines the results from these studies [3,5,6,8] using a common metric for relative size—the Z score of birth weight for gestation—and a central reference value to calculate the change in risk associated with smaller or larger infants (ie, average birth weight=Z score of zero).

The results of these studies differing in time, geographic location, and methods are remarkably consistent. Nevertheless, there is a major difference in sample size, with the Western European study being the largest by orders of magnitude; therefore, that study must have the most precise estimates of relative odds. In agreement with the second largest study, the Western European study shows a clear minimum of risk at a Z score of +1 SD.

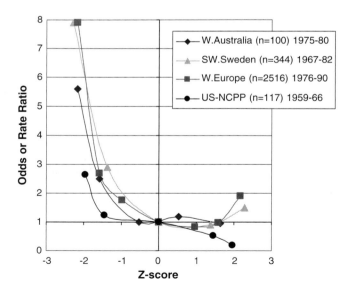

Fig. 2. Risk of cerebral palsy by Z score of weight for gestation (term births only). The studies, from Western Europe and the United States, exclude twins. The range of Z scores in the reference value varies between studies. A wide range (eg, 10th to 90th centiles in the United States) tends to depress the risks associated with extreme size categories. (*Data from* Refs. [3,5,6,8].)

Does the relationship between cerebral palsy and intrauterine size vary by the type and severity of cerebral palsy or by characteristics of the fetus?

With the possible exception of preterm born dyskinetic cases, Figs. 3a and b show that the reversed J-shaped relationship with an optimum weight for gestational age at about +1 SD persists for every type of cerebral palsy irrespective of whether cases are born at term ($\geq$37 completed weeks) or not. When all gestational ages are combined, these increases in risk to either side of optimum weight are statistically significant for each type separately. This finding broadly confirms the earlier observation of similar relationships in the two case-control studies of Swedish children with cerebral palsy that had sufficient numbers for analysis by type [8,28].

The severity of cerebral palsy as judged by difficulty in walking and intellectual deficit is related to the degree of "size" deviation (Fig. 4) [37]. Using the combined criterion of no independent walking and an Intelligence Quotient (IQ) of less than 50 to define severe cerebral palsy, the probability that cases of cerebral palsy will be in this severe group is significantly elevated to either side of the reference band. For a Z score less than 0.67, the odds ratio equals 1.36 and the 95% confidence interval (CI), 1.05 to 1.78; for a Z score of 1.28 or greater, the odds ratio equals 1.44 and the 95% CI, 1.02 to 2.05. The patterns of risk increase for more severe forms of cerebral palsy at nonoptimal sizes were seen in unilateral and bilateral spastic cases, for term and preterm births, and rather more obviously for males than females [37]. Not only the frequency of cerebral palsy

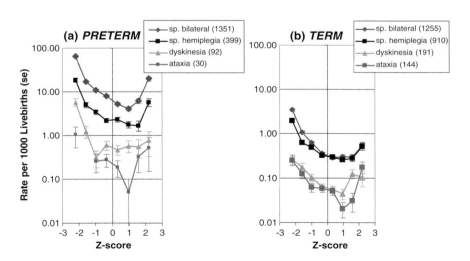

Fig. 3. Prevalence of cerebral palsy by type of disorder in (*a*) preterm and (*b*) term infants. Error bars show standard errors. Fetal standards are used to assign Z scores. A small number of German cases of spastic bilateral cerebral palsy increase the total numerator from 4307 (Fig. 1) to 4372. (*Adapted from* Jarvis SN, Glinianaia SV, Torrioli M-G, et al. Cerebral palsy and intrauterine growth in single births: a European collaborative study. Lancet 2003;362:1108; with permission.)

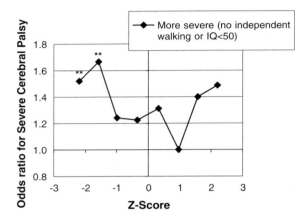

Fig. 4. Probability of more severe versus milder cerebral palsy by Z score of weight for gestation. Odds ratios (**$P<.01$) are by reference to Z score band 0.67 to <1.28 (approximately 75th to 90th fetal centiles). Analysis based on a subset of 3122 Western European cases with sufficient data to assign severity. (*Data from* Jarvis SN, Glinianaia SV, Arnaud C, et al. Case gender and severity in cerebral palsy varies with intrauterine growth. Arch Dis Child 2005;90:474–9.)

but also the relative severity of the cases increases away from the same optimum weight for gestational age.

The gender of the fetus also seems to influence the relationship between cerebral palsy and intrauterine growth [37]. Fig. 5 shows that at every Z score less than 0.67 (ie, below the 75th weight centile), the rate for males is statistically significantly greater than that for females. At a Z score of +1.3 (about the 90th centile),

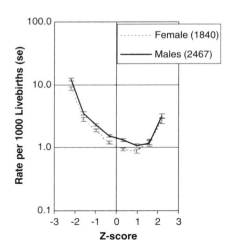

Fig. 5. Differences in gender-specific prevalence of cerebral palsy by Z score of weight for gestation. Analysis using data set from the same study as in Figs. 1 and 3. Cases of each gender are related to their own fetal size standard. Z score of zero represents a heavier absolute male birth weight than that for females.

the difference disappears. Inspection of the statistically nonsignificant results from Western Australia [6] also suggests a higher risk in males who are SGA that disappears or even reverses for those heavier than the 90% weight for gestation centile.

What are the known "causes" of intrauterine growth disturbances? Are these same risk factors associated with cerebral palsy? If so, is growth disturbance part of the causal pathway?

Numerous studies have attempted to address these questions. The subject has been reviewed fully in two recent reports [14,38]. The authors have been able to find few new and relevant publications. Table 1 summarizes the results of studies that satisfy the inclusion criteria noted previously [3,6,8,14,20,38–46]. Many

Table 1

Risk factors associated with abnormalities of size for gestation in term or near-term births and their association with risk of cerebral palsy

Factor (X) associated with aberrant size at birth	Is X a risk factor for cerebral palsy	Is risk of cerebral palsy with X primarily in LGA/SGA?	References
Congenital anomalies[a]	Yes	No	[6,8]
TORCH infections	Yes	No evidence	[6,8]
Chromosomal defects	Yes	Not known	[14]
Twinning in 3rd trimester	Yes	Possibly in VPTB (LGA)	[38]
Placental[a] and cord anomalies	Yes	No evidence	[6,39]
Pre-eclamptic toxemia[a]	Yes	No	[6,40]
Bacterial genital tract infection	Yes	No evidence	[6]
Preterm birth[a]	Yes	?No	[3,20]
Maternal starvation	No		[38]
Maternal alcohol abuse	Yes	Not known	[38]
Maternal smoking	NK		[14]
Maternal lung/cyanotic heart disease	NK		[14]
Maternal renal/malabsorption disease	NK		[14]
Maternal diabetes (including gestational)[a]	?Yes	Not known	[41–43]
Small maternal size (or low birth weight)	NK		[44,45]
Socioeconomic deprivation	Yes	No	[46]
Neonatal hypothermia	Yes	Little or no contribution	[6]
Neonatal hypoglycemia	Yes	Little or no contribution	[6]
Intrapartum stress	Yes	No	[38]
Clinical signs of birth asphyxia/hypoxia	Yes	No evidence	[6,8]

Abbreviations: TORCH, toxoplasmosis, other infection, rubella, cytomegalovirus, herpes; VPTB, very pre-term birth (<32 weeks gestational age).

[a] Indicates a risk factor also associated with large size at birth. Otherwise, these are all risk factors for small size.

studies are small and underpowered. The finding of "no evidence" in the third column indicates that no evidence of an association was found in a small study but does not rule out the possibility of a clinically significant association.

Several of the following causal mechanisms could result in a concentration of cerebral palsy at the extremes of growth, where $\rightarrow$ denotes causation, although mechanism B tends to be the default assumption in much of the literature with intrapartum events as the putative cause:

A. Risk factor $\rightarrow$ abnormal growth $\rightarrow$ cerebral palsy
B. Abnormal growth $\rightarrow$ risk factor $\rightarrow$ cerebral palsy
C. Risk factor $\rightarrow$ cerebral palsy $\rightarrow$ abnormal growth
               $\rightarrow$ abnormal growth
D. Risk factor
          $\rightarrow$ cerebral palsy

If the excess risk for cerebral palsy associated with a factor "X" (Table 1) was not concentrated at the growth extreme associated with X, this "cause" of cerebral palsy is likely to be operating independently of aberrant growth, suggesting mechanism D. For instance, although birth at less than 32 weeks' gestation is associated with relatively small size at birth and also elevates the risk for cerebral palsy by 50 times when compared with the risk for births at 39 to 41 weeks, the latter applies more or less equally at each size centile (see Fig. 1). Even mechanism D may show a concentration of cerebral palsy at the extremes of growth if both causal paths (to abnormal growth and to cerebral palsy) were dose dependent, that is, the more severe the risk factor, the higher the risk of cerebral palsy and the more severe the degree of growth abnormality.

Despite a paucity of evidence, Table 1 indicates that the risk of cerebral palsy with factors associated with growth restriction is not concentrated in infants with growth anomaly. In fact, the risk of cerebral palsy is lower in SGA than in AGA infants exposed to twinning [38] or evidence of birth asphyxia [6,8]. This observation suggests an alternative causal mechanism. If growth restriction can represent a beneficial adaptive mechanism in the presence of a suboptimal exposure, the failure to make the appropriate adaptation may be responsible for the increase in risk of cerebral palsy associated with that exposure. Testing this hypothesis will require the ability to measure the severity of an exposure associated with growth anomaly independently of the degree of growth anomaly observed.

Implications

Do studies of abnormal growth or size give information about the timing of any intrauterine events associated with cerebral palsy?

If the increased risk of cerebral palsy associated with growth anomaly involved a single pathway, the striking pattern in Fig. 1 could be interpreted to mean that the growth disturbance associated with cerebral palsy has already occurred by 28 weeks of pregnancy. Nevertheless, there are likely to be many possible routes to cerebral palsy associated with growth anomaly, summarized diagrammatically in mechanisms A to D. In mechanisms A and B, cerebral palsy is the direct or indirect consequence of the growth anomaly; therefore, the brain-damaging event would have to have occurred after the onset of growth deviation, neonatal hypoglycemia being a biologically plausible example. Because it takes weeks for growth deviation to become clinically discernible, mechanisms C and D would imply that the brain-damaging event occurred at least weeks before delivery.

Can abnormal growth, per se, cause cerebral palsy?

The real conundrum is whether cerebral palsy is a consequence (mechanisms A or B) or a cause (mechanism C) of growth deviation or simply an associated phenomenon (mechanism D). When the focus was entirely on the high risk for cerebral palsy in SGA infants, there was an understandable tendency to characterize the process as due to intrauterine growth restriction [14]. This causation was usually attributed to a constraint in fetal nutritional or oxygen supply with an effect on the fetal brain either directly from anoxia/hypoglycemia or indirectly by increased vulnerability to intrapartum stress.

The recognition that larger infants are at higher risk for cerebral palsy (and for other poor perinatal outcomes) has been mechanistically attributed to their disproportionate size in relation to the mother and to the increased risk of traumatic delivery. Nevertheless, as can be seen in Fig. 1, this excess risk applies equally to preterm infants who are overweight for their gestational age but actually of very small size relative to the mother. It has been proposed that the risk for relatively large infants could result from the association of cerebral palsy with specific, albeit, rare causes of megalencephaly [47]. The alternative attribution of high risk in this heavy infant group to maternal hyperglycemia and its degree of control does not seem to offer an obvious biologic route to fetal brain damage.

By way of contrast, the observation that the relationship of the risk for cerebral palsy with intrauterine size is continuous rather than confined to a clear "pathological" subset of SGA infants, and that this continuity extends beyond an optimum to encompass a progressive increase in the risk for abnormally large infants might suggest an alternative explanation. It does not seem implausible that the brain abnormalities underlying cerebral palsy occur before growth becomes disturbed. Several strong candidates for the causes of cerebral palsy, such as inherited clotting disorders [48], thyroid disturbance in the mother [49], vanishing twin [50] or twin/twin transfusions, and intrauterine infections [51], may exert their effects antenatally without any necessary pre-existing growth abnormality. As seen in Table 1, there is little evidence to refute this suggestion. On the contrary, once an insult to the developing brain or other organs has occurred, the control of fetal growth might be disturbed in a way that could err in either direction (mechanism C). The subsequent observation that these growth-disturbed infants have an excess of apparently noxious intrapartum factors in the chain of associated events may reflect their already compromised status [14].

This thesis that growth disturbances are a generic result of fetal insult is consistent with the almost identical association of intrauterine growth disturbances with perinatal mortality [19]. Furthermore, the type of cerebral palsy seems to have little influence on the relationship with size at birth.

Is there something about the intrauterine growth of male infants that might make them more susceptible to cerebral palsy?

If relative maturity of the fetus in utero is a form of "growth," the short answer to this question might be that male infants are up to a month less mature at term (and presumably also proportionately less mature at earlier gestations) than their female counterparts [52,53]. This maturity difference is specifically true for cerebral anatomy (lateralization [54] and myelination [55]) and can be measured as differences of in utero behavioral adaptation to evoked responses [52]. Such immaturity might make male brains more vulnerable to insult at a variety of stages including intrapartum stressors.

Fig. 5 raises the intriguing possibility that the optimum size at birth for males is further from their population mean weight than is true for females. The rate of cerebral palsy in males even at the 90th to 97th weight centiles is lower (relative risk, 0.82; 95%CI, 0.67–1.01) than for males of "normal" birth weight (25th to 75th centiles), whereas for females, the reverse is true (Fig. 5). As male infants are significantly heavier than females, being further from optimum birth weight may arise owing to maternal constraint, a limit to intrauterine growth rate created by the limits of maternal resources which are reached earlier for the male infant than for the smaller female infant [44].

What are the implications for obstetricians?

The focus should arguably move to a detailed assessment of the health of fetuses in utero. Estimates of fetal size or preferably of the rate of change in fetal size may give important clues to the health of the fetus. If the brain damage associated with cerebral palsy precedes growth changes (mechanism C), recognition of growth restriction occurs too late for preventative intervention. With mechanism D, growth abnormality may be the first, albeit, crude signal that in utero pathology is occurring. This finding may indicate the need for further investigation with a view to potential in utero treatment (eg, of infections) or delivery in optimal circumstances. If the risk for cerebral palsy is elevated as a consequence of growth deviation (mechanisms A or B), underlying causes of growth abnormality may be pursued (placental compromise, gestational diabetes) or early delivery considered before fetal brain damage occurs.

These suggestions may be more pertinent in male infants, in twins, in situations in which a single measure of size is well away from the optimal for that gestation, and when other known or significant risk factors for cerebral palsy are present. The latter include Leiden V consanguinity [48], a maternal history of thyroid disease [49], maternal infection [51], or familial twinning [50].

Whether any wider obstetric public health measures could be justified is open to question. There is little convincing evidence that intrauterine growth can be enhanced in developed countries by macronutrient supplementation during pregnancy, and, with a few exceptions (eg, folate levels), not enough is known about the role of micronutrition in pregnancy. A woman's ability to sustain intrauterine growth seems to be determined by her socioeconomic circumstances and nutritional experience throughout childhood, mediated perhaps by her own birth weight and childhood growth [45,56]. More urgent public health interventions could be made in an attempt to increase the fitness of future rather than contemporary mothers.

What research is needed?

Research is needed to identify which causal mechanisms are responsible for the observed association between cerebral palsy and intrauterine growth anomaly. Cohorts of fetuses who have been subject to sequential (at least two) assessments of intrauterine size and with an accurately timed length of gestation should be observed in an attempt to characterize when in pregnancy the growth deviation associated with cerebral palsy or early brain lesions occurs. Because the outcome is rare, this would be easier in high-risk cohorts. There is some advantage to studying larger representative cohorts in which growth velocity patterns associated with optimal perinatal outcomes could be identified. The risks associated with observed fetal growth could be judged not in relation to a normative but to an optimal growth pattern. This investigation would be facilitated by the reliable prenatal identification of poor outcomes such as cerebral palsy, but this goal remains elusive at the population level.

Currently, most of the events that relate cerebral palsy to intrauterine growth are still hidden, although only a few centimeters away from view.

Acknowledgments

Figs. 1, 3–5, and associated analyses are based on data from the European Collaboration of Cerebral Palsy registers (SCPE). SCPE participants include C. Cans, J. Fauconnier (RHEOP, Grenoble, France), C. Arnaud (INSERM, Toulouse, France), J. Chalmers (ISDSHS, Edinburgh, United Kingdom), V. McManus (Lavanagh Centre, Cork, Ireland), J. Parkes, H. Dolk (Belfast, United Kingdom), G. Hagberg, B. Hagberg, P. Uvebrant (Gotenborg University, Gotenborg, Sweden), O. Hensey, V. Dowding (Central Remedial Clinic, Dublin, Ireland), S. Jarvis, A. Colver, (University of Newcastle, Newcastle, United Kingdom), A. Johnson, G. Surman (NPEU, Oxford,United Kindgom), I. Krägeloh-Mann, R. Michaelis

(Tubingen University, Tubingen, Germany), P.O.D. Pharoah, M.J. Platt (University of Liverpool, Liverpool, United Kingdom), M. Topp, P. Udall (DIKE, Copenhagen, Denmark), MG. Torrioli, M. Miceli (CITCPR, Rome, Italy), M. Wichers (Groot Klimmendal RC, Arnhem, Netherlands).

References

[1] Altman D, Hytten F. Assessment of fetal size and fetal growth. In: Chalmers I, Enkin M, Keirse J, editors. Effective care in pregnancy and childbirth. Oxford: OUP; 1989. p. 411–8.

[2] Wilcox AJ, Russell I. Birthweight and perinatal mortality. II. On weight specific mortality. Int J Epidemiol 1983;12(3):319–25.

[3] Jarvis SN, Glinianaia SV, Torrioli M-G, et al. Cerebral palsy and intrauterine growth in single births: a European collaborative study. Lancet 2003;362:1106–11.

[4] Liu J, Li Z, Lin Q, et al. Cerebral palsy and multiple births in China. Int J Epidemiol 2000;29: 292–9.

[5] Ellenberg JH, Nelson KB. Birthweight and gestational age in children with cerebral palsy or seizure disorders. Am J Dis Child 1979;133:1044–8.

[6] Blair E, Stanley F. Intrauterine growth and spastic cerebral palsy. I. Association with birthweight for gestational age. Am J Obstet Gynecol 1990;162(1):229–37.

[7] Topp M, Langhoff-Roos J, Uldall P, et al. Intrauterine growth and gestational age in preterm infants with cerebral palsy. Early Hum Dev 1996;44:27–36.

[8] Uvebrant P, Hagberg G. Intrauterine growth in children with cerebral palsy. Acta Paediatr 1992;81:407–12.

[9] Palmer L, Petterson B, Blair E, et al. Family patterns of gestational age at delivery and growth in utero in moderate and severe cerebral palsy. Dev Med Child Neurol 1994;36:1108–19.

[10] Drummond PM, Colver AF. Analysis by gestational age of cerebral palsy in singleton births in northeast England 1970–1994. Paediatr Perinat Epidemiol 2002;16:172–80.

[11] Blair E. The undesirable consequences of controlling for birthweight in perinatal epidemiologic studies. J Epidemiol Comm Health 1996;50:559–63.

[12] Pharoah POD, Cooke T, Johnson MA, et al. Epidemiology of cerebral palsy in England and Scotland 1984–9. Arch Dis Child Fetal Neonatal Ed 1998;79:F21–5.

[13] Colver A, Gibson M, Hey EN, et al. Increasing rates of cerebral palsy across the severity spectrum in North East England 1964–1993. Arch Dis Child Fetal Neonatal Ed 2000;83(1): F7–13.

[14] Stanley F, Blair E, Alberman E. Cerebral palsies: epidemiology and causal pathways. Cambridge: Cambridge University Press; 2000.

[15] Hemming K, Hutton J, Glinianaia S, et al. Differences between European birth weight standards: impact on small for gestational age classification. Dev Med Child Neurol, in press.

[16] Bonellie SR, Raab GM. Why are babies getting heavier? Comparison of Scottish births from 1980 to 1992. BMJ 1997;315:1205.

[17] Skjaerven R, Gjessing HK, Bakketeig LS. Birthweight by gestational age in Norway. Acta Obstet Gynecol Scand 2000;79:440–9.

[18] Gardosi J, Chang A, Kalyan B, et al. Customised antenatal growth charts. Lancet 1992;339: 283–7.

[19] Wilcox AJ, Skjaerven R. Birth weight and perinatal mortality: the effect of gestational age. Am J Public Health 1992;82(3):378–82.

[20] Lackman F, Capewell V, Richardson B, et al. The risks of spontaneous delivery and perinatal mortality in relation to size at birth according to fetal versus neonatal growth standards. Am J Obstet Gynecol 2001;184:946–53.

[21] Patterson R, Prihoda T, Gibbs C, et al. Analysis of birth weight percentile as a predictor of perinatal outcome. Obstet Gynecol 1986;68:459–63.

[22] Gardosi J. Customized fetal growth standards: rationale and clinical application. Semin Perinatol 2004;28(1):33–40.

[23] Hediger ML, Scholl TO, Schall JI, et al. Fetal growth and the etiology of preterm delivery. Obstet Gynecol 1995;85(2):175–82.

[24] Hadlock F, Harrist R, Martinez-Poyer J. In utero analysis of fetal growth: a sonographic weight standard. Radiology 1991;181:129–33.

[25] Marsal K, Persson P-H, Larsen T, et al. Intrauterine growth curves based on ultrasonically estimated fetal weights. Acta Paediatr 1996;85:843–8.

[26] Gardosi J, Mongelli M, Wilcox M, et al. An adjustable fetal weight standard. Ultrasound Obstet Gynecol 1995;6:168–74.

[27] Foley J. Birth-weight ratio and cerebral palsy. Early Hum Dev 1995;40(2):145–56.

[28] Kyllerman M, Bager B, Bensch J, et al. Dyskinetic cerebral palsy. I. Clinical categories, associated neurological abnormalities and incidences. Acta Paediatr Scand 1982;71:543–50.

[29] Benso L, Aicardi G, Fabris C, et al. What longitudinal studies can tell us about fetal growth. In: Johnston F, Zemel B, Eveleth P, editors. Human growth in context. London: Smith-Gordon; 1999. p. 41–50.

[30] Fancourt R, Campbell S, Harvey D, et al. Follow up study of small-for-dates babies. BMJ 1976;1:1435–7.

[31] Parkinson C, Wallis S, Harvey D. School achievement and behaviour of children who were small-for-dates at birth. Dev Med Child Neurol 1981;23:41–50.

[32] Gould J. The low birthweight infant. In: Falkner F, Tanner J, editors. Human growth: a comprehensive treatise, Vol. I. Developmental biology, prenatal growth. New York and London: Plenum Press; 1986.

[33] Kramer MS, Olivier M, McLean F, et al. Impact of intrauterine growth retardation and body proportionality on fetal and neonatal outcome. Pediatrics 1990;86(5):707–13.

[34] Villar J, Belizan JM. The timing factor in the pathophysiology of the intrauterine growth retardation syndrome. Obstet Gynecol Surv 1982;37(8):499–506.

[35] Vik T, Vatten L, Jacobsen G, et al. Prenatal growth in symmetric and asymmetric small-for-gestational-age infants. Early Hum Dev 1997;48(1–2):167–76.

[36] Lampl M, Jeanty P. Timing is everything: a reconsideration of fetal growth velocity patterns identifies the importance of individual and sex differences. Am J Human Biol 2003;15(5): 667–80.

[37] Jarvis SN, Glinianaia SV, Arnaud C, et al. Case gender and severity in cerebral palsy varies with intrauterine growth. Arch Dis Child 2005;90:474–9.

[38] Blair E. Paediatric implications of IUGR with special reference to cerebral palsy. In: Kingdom J, Baker P, editors. Inrauterine growth restriction: aetiology and management. London: Springer-Verlag; 2000.

[39] Wolstenholme J, Rooney DE, Davison EV. Confined placental mosaicism, intrauterine growth retardation and adverse pregnancy outcome. Prenat Diagn 1994;14:345–61.

[40] Xiong X, Demianczuk NN, Buekens P, et al. Association of preeclampsia with high birth weight for age. Am J Obstet Gynecol 2000;183(1):148–55.

[41] Ircha G, Zawodniak-Szalapska M, Cypryk K, et al. Prospective neurological analysis of development of children of mothers with IDDM. Ginekol Pol 1999;70(10):795–9.

[42] McMahon MJ, Ananth C, Liston R. Gestational diabetes mellitus: risk factors, complications and infant outcomes. J Reprod Med 1998;43:372–8.

[43] Pedersen JF, Molsted-Pedersen L. Early growth retardation in diabetic pregnancy. BMJ 1979; 1(6155):18–9.

[44] Ounsted M, Ounsted C. Maternal regulation of intrauterine growth. Nature 1966;212:995–7.

[45] Martin R, Davey-Smith G, Frankel S, et al. Parents growth in childhood and the birthweight of their offspring. Epidemiology 2004;15:308–16.

[46] Dolk H, Pattenden S, Johnson A. Cerebral palsy, low birthweight and socio-economic deprivation: inequalities in a major cause of childhood disability. Paediatr Perinat Epidemiol 2001; 15:359–63.

[47] Petersen MC, Palmer FB. Birthweight and risk for cerebral palsy. Lancet 2003;362(9390): 1089–90.

[48] Thorarensen O, Ryan S, Hunter J, et al. Factor V Leiden mutation: an unrecognised cause of hemiplegic cerebral palsy, neonatal stroke and placental thrombosis. Ann Neurol 1997;42: 372–5.

[49] Nelson KB, Ellenberg JH. Antecedents of cerebral palsy: multivariate analysis of risk. N Engl J Med 1986;315:81–6.

[50] Pharoah POD, Cooke T. A hypothesis for the etiology of spastic cerebral palsy: the vanishing twin. Dev Med Child Neurol 1997;39:292–6.

[51] Grether JK, Nelson KB. Maternal infection and cerebral palsy in infants of normal birthweight. JAMA 1997;278:207–11.

[52] Leader LR, Baille P, Martin B, et al. The assessment and significance of habituation to a repeated stimulus by the human fetus. Early Hum Dev 1982;7(3):211–9.

[53] Birkbeck JA. Metrical growth and skeletal development of the human fetus. In: Roberts DF, Thomson AM, editors. The biology of human fetal growth. Symposia of the Society for the Study of Human Biology, Vol. 15. London: Taylor and Francis; 1976. p. 39–68.

[54] Taylor DC. Differential rates of cerebral maturation between sexes and between hemispheres: evidence from epilepsy. Lancet 1969;2(7612):140–2.

[55] Geschwind N, Galaburda A. Cerebral lateralization: biological mechanisms, associations and pathology. Arch Neurol 1985;42:428–59.

[56] Reading R, Jarvis S, Openshaw S. Measurement of social inequalities in health and use of health services among children in Northumberland. Arch Dis Child 1993;68:626–31.

ELSEVIER
SAUNDERS

CLINICS IN
PERINATOLOGY

Clin Perinatol 33 (2006) 301–313

Risk of Cerebral Palsy in Multiple Pregnancies

Peter O.D. Pharoah, MD, MSc, FRCP, FRCPCH, FFPHM

Department of Public Health, FSID Unit of Perinatal and Paediatric Epidemiology,
Muspratt Building, University of Liverpool, Liverpool L69 3GB, United Kingdom

It is pertinent to appreciate that when considering the risk of cerebral palsy (CP) in multiple pregnancies, the syndrome is not a single nosologic entity and various pathologic processes may give rise to the clinical features of the syndrome. Some of the risk factors associated with these pathologic processes occur more commonly in multiple than in singleton pregnancies. Some risk factors may be peculiar to multiple pregnancies, however, particularly monochorionic (MC) and monozygotic (MZ) multiple pregnancies.

The article by Little [1] with the earliest clinical description of CP in 1862 was entitled "On the incidence of abnormal parturition, difficult labor, premature birth and asphyxia neonatorum on the mental and physical condition of the child, especially in relation to deformities." Inherent in the title are risk factors that are more prevalent in multiple than singleton pregnancies.

For many years, peripartum birth injury or hypoxic-ischemic cerebral impairments were considered to be the main cause of CP. This presumed cause was appealing because it was considered that with improved obstetric and neonatal care, early detection of fetal distress, and pre-emptive induction of labor or Caesarean section, there would be a significant reduction in the prevalence of CP. These hopes were not fulfilled, and although perinatal mortality rates fell significantly, there was no concurrent decline in CP rates among term infants [2]. Some studies reported an increase in the prevalence among very low birth weight infants [3–5], which led to a reappraisal of possible causes of CP [6–9].

The timing of the insult that leads to CP may be conveniently divided into prepartum, peripartum, and postnatal periods. CP sustained from a postnatal

---

Please note that article originally appeared in Obstetrics and Gynecology Clinics of North America, Vol 32, Issue 1.

E-mail address: p.o.d.pharoah@liverpool.ac.uk

insult also has been termed acquired [10–12] or late impairment CP [13]. This group comprises approximately 10% of all cases of CP [14,15], and the major causes are head injury, cerebral infections, hypoxia, and gastroenteritis with severe dehydration. Multiple compared with singleton gestations are not especially at risk in this category of CP and are not considered further.

At one time, peripartum sustained cerebral impairment as a result of birth asphyxia was considered to be most frequent cause of CP. The failure of CP prevalence to decrease with falling perinatal mortality rates [2], the lack of association of CP with indicators of birth asphyxia [16], and poor obstetric care and the positive association with adverse antenatal events [17] have relegated birth asphyxia to a minor role. Undoubtedly, severe birth asphyxia may cause CP. Studies based on the National Collaborative Perinatal Project and the Western Australian CP register estimated that 3% to 13% and 8%, respectively, of CP was attributable to birth asphyxia [16,18]. In estimating what proportion of CP may be attributable to birth asphyxia, the problems lie in the defining criteria and the fact that these criteria, such as markers of fetal distress and low Apgar scores, may be the result rather than the cause of CP.

Multiple compared with singleton gestations are not at especially increased risk of birth asphyxial events that result in CP. These events, together with postnatal causes, account for approximately 20% of all cases of CP. This leaves approximately 80% of CP that is sustained prepartum or as a result of hypoxic-ischemic damage attributable to difficulties in maintaining physiologic normality in blood pressure and oxygenation in extremely preterm infants. The important role played by prepartum risk factors is supported by the observation that a high proportion of children with CP showed intrauterine growth restriction [19,20] and a higher proportion of coincident congenital anomalies and other dysmorphic features than controls [16,21]. In this group, clinically important and etiologically significant differences are found between singleton and multiple births, which is the focus of the rest of this article.

Multiple versus singleton birth differences in crude cerebral palsy prevalence

The greater risk of CP in multiple compared with singleton gestations was recognized by Freud more than a century ago [22]. A review of case series reports found that twins comprised 5% to 10% of CP but only 1.6% of all births [23], which indicated a twin:singleton relative risk of approximately 5. The development of population-based registers of CP has enabled prevalence comparisons to be made for multiple and singleton births. Combined data from two registries [24,25] showed relative risks for twins and triplets compared with singletons to be 4.9 and 12.7, respectively, and a large collaborative report based on five population-based studies found that twins were at a fourfold increased risk of CP compared with twins [26].

Risk factors for cerebral palsy in multiple and singleton gestations

One important risk factor for CP in multiple and singleton births is birth weight, with a sharp rise in prevalence of CP with decreasing birth weight [27]. Combined data from three population-based registries show that the relative risks of CP in birth weight groups of 1000 g, 1000 to 1499 g, and 1500 to 2499 g compared with 2500 g or more are 66.5, 57.4, and 8.9, respectively [28]. The shift to the left in the birth weight frequency distribution of multiple births plays a significant role in the higher prevalence of CP in multiple compared with singleton births. Fig. 1, drawn from 1993 to 2000 national data for England and Wales, shows the birth weight frequency distribution for all live births by multiplicity of birth. To subdivide twins into MZ and DZ groups, Weinberg's rule has been applied [29]. This rule assumes that all unlike sex twin are DZ and that the same number of like-sex twins are DZ. The total number of DZ twins is twice the number of unlike sex twins, and the total number of MZ twins is all twins minus the number of unlike sex pairs.

Infants of birth weight less than 1500 g comprise 0.9% of singleton, 9.4% of twins, 32.2% of triplets, and 73.3% of quadruplet live births [30]. It is pertinent also that the birth weight frequency distribution of MZ twins is shifted to the left of DZ twins. In twins, the lower the birth weight, the greater the proportion that is MZ, and there is a highly significant statistical trend in the association of birth weight with zygosity. In twins of birth weight less than 1500 g, 41% are MZ compared with infants who weigh 2500 g or more, in which 28% are MZ.

Because birth weight is an important confounder, birth weight–specific rather than crude prevalence should be examined when comparing CP prevalence in

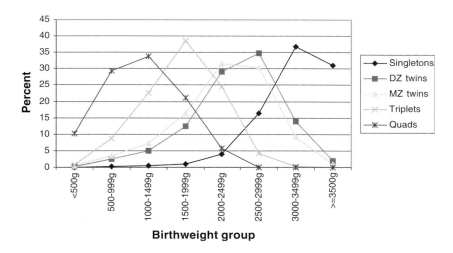

Fig. 1. Birth weight frequency distribution of singletons and multiples.

Table 1
Birth weight–specific prevalence of cerebral palsy in singletons and multiples

Birthweight		Singletons	Twins	Triplets
< 1500g	No. CP	230	56	7
	No. infant survivors	3810	934	179
	CP prevalence/1000	60.4	60.0	39.1
	(95% CI)	(53.2–68.4)	(46.8–77.1)	(19.1–78.5)
1500–2499 g	No. CP	271	58	5
	No. infant survivors	25487	5492	284
	CP prevalence/1000	10.6	10.6	17.6
	(95% CI)	(9.4–12.0)	(8.2–13.6)	(7.5–40.5)
≥ 2500 g	No. CP	849	33	0
	No. infant survivors	569932	6794	40
	CP prevalence/1000	1.5	4.9	0
	(95% CI)	(1.4–1.6)	(3.5–6.8)	

Data from Pharoah POD, Cooke T. Cerebral palsy and multiple births. Arch Dis Child Fetal Neonatal Ed 1996;75:F174–7; Watson L, Stanley F. Report of the Western Australian Cerebral Palsy Register. Perth: TVW Telethon Institute for Child Health Research; 1999. (*Data from* Refs. [23,24].)

singleton and multiple gestations (Table 1). For infants of low birth weight (< 2500 g), there is no significant increase in risk, but for infants of birth weight 2500 g or more there is a highly statistically significant three- to fourfold increase in risk of CP in twins compared with singletons. There are two major components to the difference in crude CP prevalence between multiple and singleton pregnancies: (1) the greater proportion of multiples that is preterm or very low birth weight and (2) some other factor that is peculiar to the process of multiple gestation.

Twinning, zygosity, chorionicity, and cerebral palsy

It has long been recognized that fetal death of a twin is frequently associated with severe morbidity in the surviving co-twin. There are various central nervous system abnormalities, including polymicrogyria [31–34], multicystic encephalopathy or porencephaly [35,36], ventriculomegaly or hydranencephaly [37–39], cortical atrophy [40], and cerebral infarction [41]. Clinically these neurologic pathologies are usually manifest as CP that may vary greatly in its severity, ranging from some minimal limitation of motor function to severe quadriparesis. Not only may the severity of the motor disability vary but also it may be accompanied by a variable degree of learning or cortical visual disability. In almost all these case reports, the common denominator has been that the gestation was MC.

The high risk in the surviving twin whose co-twin died in utero also has been reported in population-based studies of CP. This risk is approximately 1:10 compared with 1:400 of all births [24,42]. Based on an analysis of two national surveys and a regional survey, birth weight–specific CP prevalence when both twins survive or when only one twin survives and the co-twin is a fetal or infant death is shown in Table 2 [43–46]. Because neither zygosity nor chorionicity was recorded, only like- and unlike-sex twins could be compared. Several salient points may be made from this table. When one twin dies in utero, the CP prevalence in the surviving co-twin is high, regardless of birth weight group and is higher in like- than unlike-sex twins (Table 2). When both twins are live births and one dies in infancy, the CP prevalence is even greater than if the twin had died in utero. Low birth weight twins in this group are at particularly high risk and like-sex twins are at greater risk than unlike-sex twins (Table 2). When both twins survive, like-sex twins are at greater risk than unlike-sex twins, particularly among larger infants (Table 2). The combined data (Table 2) confirms that birth weight is an important factor, but twins of like sex are independently at greater risk than those of unlike sex. These data support the observation that monozygosity—and specifically monochorionicity—plays a significant role in the pathogenesis of CP.

The case reports of CP in the surviving twin associated with late fetal death of the co-twin led to the assumption that only late and not early fetal death

Table 2
Birth weight–specific cerebral palsy prevalence in twins

	Like sex		Unlike sex	
Birth weight	Cerebral palsy/number responders	Cerebral palsy prevalence/1000 infant survivors	Cerebral palsy/number responders	Cerebral palsy prevalence/1000 infant survivors
Cerebral palsy in surviving twin of co-twin fetal death[a]				
< 1500 g	15/91	164.8	3/29	103.4
≥ 1500g	20/246	81.3	2/104	19.2
All	35/337	103.9	5/133	37.6
Cerebral palsy in surviving twin of co-twin infant death[b]				
< 1500 g	44/207	212.6	12/87	137.9
≥ 1500g	8/187	42.8	0/75	0
All	52/394	132.0	12/162	74.1
Cerebral palsy: both twins survive infancy[c]				
< 1500 g	52/984	52.8	17/393	43.3
≥ 1500g	54/12037	4.5	13/5841	2.2
All	106/13021	8.1	30/6234	4.8
Combined cerebral palsy birth weight–specific prevalence[d]				
< 1500 g	111/1282	86.6	32/509	62.9
≥ 1500g	82/12470	4.5	15/6020	2.5
All	193/13752	14.0	47/6529	7.2

[a] Like versus unlike sex, Mantel-Haenszel weighted relative risk 2.60 (95% CI 1.06–6.39).
[b] Like versus unlike sex, Mantel-Haenszel weighted relative risk 1.77 (95% CI 1.01–3.25).
[c] Like versus unlike sex, Mantel-Haenszel weighted relative risk 1.29 (95% CI 0.71–2.21).
[d] Like versus unlike sex, Mantel-Haenszel weighted relative risk 1.76 (95% CI 1.29–2.41).
From Keith LG, Blickstein I, editors. Multiple Pregnancy. (Table 3, Chapter 69). Stamford (CT): Thomson Publishing Services; 2005; with permission.

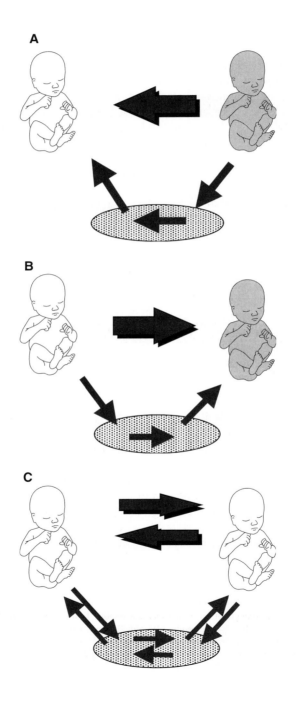

had adverse consequences for the co-twin. This information promulgated the recommendation that early obstetric intervention after fetal death of a twin could prevent neurologic impairment in the co-twin [35], although other researchers questioned the appropriateness of the recommendation [36,47–50]. Subsequently, it became clear that second-trimester demise of a twin also could be complicated by serious morbidity in the co-twin [33,37,41].

The use of ultrasonographic examination in early gestation has established the "vanishing" twin phenomenon, in which first-trimester loss of a twin occurs in 13% to 78% of multiple pregnancies [51]. The prognosis for the surviving twin after such early loss of the co-twin has been considered good, unlike the effect of later fetal death [52]. There have been reports of adverse effects in the surviving twin even after first-trimester loss of the co-twin, however [31,38], and it has been hypothesized that the cause of CP in apparently singleton gestations may be attributable to a vanishing twin [53].

Because monochorionicity is a key feature in the high risk of CP in multiple compared with singleton gestations, early first-trimester recognition of MC gestation with a vanishing twin must be quantified to determine whether it is of etiologic relevance to CP in apparently singleton infants. This determination may require transvaginal rather than transabdominal ultrasound examination soon after conception is recognized. One selected series with a disproportionate number of dichorionic gestations as a result of in vitro fertilization, observed nine MC gestations, of which five delivered twins, one delivered a singleton, and three aborted both fetuses [54]. Although early loss of one twin in an MC gestation is uncommon, it remains tenable that a vanishing twin in an MC gestation could account for some cases of CP.

Also of relevance in pathogenesis of CP in apparently singleton infants is the failure to recognize or register a second-trimester fetal demise that usually presents as a fetus papyraceus. The World Health Organization definition of fetal death is "death before the complete expulsion or extraction from its mother of a product of conception irrespective of the duration of the pregnancy." For countries that subscribe to this definition, the requirement is for a fetus papyraceus to be registered as a stillbirth regardless of the gestational age at which fetal demise occurred. In the United States, the definition promulgated by the World Health Organization but revised in the 1992 Revision of the Model State Vital Statistics Act and Regulations is recommended. The Model State Vital Statistics Act recommends reporting the death of a fetus of 350 g or more or, if weight is unknown, of 20 complete weeks' gestation or more. The implication for a fetus papyraceus varies. It should be reported in all areas that require fetal

---

Fig. 2. Mechanisms of fetal damage in MC twins. (*A*) Embolic theory: thromboplastin-like material or emboli are transferred through an open placental anastomosis to the survivor. (*B*) Ischemic theory: blood is shunted into the low-resistance circulation of the dead fetus. (*C*) Hemodynamic instability theory: bidirectional shunting leads to ischemic damage that affects either or both fetuses. *From* Keith LG, Blickstein I, editors. Multiple Pregnancy. (Chapter 69, Fig. 1). Stamford (CT): Thomson Publishing Services; 2005; with permission.

deaths to be reported, which would capture a fetus papyraceus because the key feature is the gestational age at delivery and not the presumed gestational age at death. Because not all areas specify how gestational age is calculated, there is variability in interpreting whether the fetus papyraceus should be registered. A similar variability in interpretation exists in the United Kingdom, where the legal responsibility for registering a stillbirth lies with the parents. Obstetricians may not inform a mother that a fetus papyraceus is present so that only the singleton survivor gets registered [55–59]. In a population-based register, of 18 cases of CP in which the obstetric records of the mother had recorded a twin gestation, 6 cases had been registered as only singletons. In all 6 cases, the twin death was a fetus papyraceus or a small, severely macerated fetus of which the mother had not been aware [56].

The variability in the interpretation of the definition of fetal death is surely not confined to the United States and United Kingdom, yet it is of immense significance to the origin of CP and to estimates of the comparative risk of CP in multiple and singleton gestations. Clarification and application of an internationally accepted definition of fetal death are necessary. Registering the presumed gestational age of fetal demise and the gestational age of expulsion regardless of birth weight must be considered.

Pathogenic mechanisms in cerebral palsy

Monochorionicity, with its placental vascular anastomoses, is a common component when there is fetal demise of one twin and CP in the co-twin. Benirschke [60] observed numerous fibrin thrombi occluding blood vessels, which resulted in renal cortical necrosis and cerebral infarction in one case. He proposed that thromboplastin-rich material or thromboemboli were transfused from the dead twin, which led to disseminated intravascular coagulation in the co-twin (Fig. 2A). Although disseminated intravascular coagulation occasionally has been reported after demise of one twin [61–63], it is not always the case, and other pathogenic mechanisms must be considered [37,47,64].

An alternative explanation for the pathogenesis of CP is that the dead fetus has a low vascular resistance with acute twin-twin transfusion and exsanguination of the surviving fetus, which results in ischemic cerebral impairment (Fig. 2B) [65,66].

The mechanisms illustrated in Fig. 2A and B entail fetal demise of one twin. As shown in Table 2, however, there is a high prevalence of CP even when both twins survive. It is particularly notable when both are born alive but one dies in infancy (Table 2). In this group, like-sex twins with a birth weight of 1500 g or more are at risk of CP that is unlikely to be attributable to preterm delivery. Another proposed pathogenic mechanism is that hemodynamic instability with to-and-fro shunting of blood between fetuses may affect either or both fetuses. The severity of damage sustained by the fetuses varies from fetal death to normal survival and may differ between fetuses (Fig. 2C) [67–70]. In these cases, it is the MC placentation per se that lies behind the damage to either or both fetuses.

MC gestations face a double jeopardy for CP. There are problems associated with the twin-twin transfusion effects as a result of placental vascular anastomoses (Fig. 2), and there is a preponderance of preterm infants among MZ compared with DZ gestations (see Fig. 1). A further risk is that the MC subset of MZ gestations is at greatest risk of preterm delivery. The prevalence of birth weight less than the fifth percentile in both twins was 7.5% in MC compared with 1.7% in DC twins [71].

Cerebral palsy and assisted reproductive technology

Inevitably, the rise in incidence of multiple gestations as a result of assisted reproductive technology (ART) has raised concerns over the implication it has for the prevalence of CP [72,73]. Researchers have estimated that there may be approximately an 8% increase in the prevalence of CP in the United States solely because of the increase in multiple births from ART [74]. To the extent that multiple gestations are associated with an increase in prevalence of preterm infants, fetuses conceived with ART—as with spontaneous conceptions—are at increased risk of CP. The extent of MC placentation as a cause of CP in ART gestations is more difficult to estimate. Primarily, ART gestations are DZ and are not at risk because of monochorionicity. Researchers recognize, however, that MZ division occurs more frequently in ART than in spontaneous conceptions. It has been estimated that after artificial induction of ovulation, MZ splitting occurred in 1.2% of cases as compared with 0.45% in spontaneous ovulation, with MZ having occurred in 13 of 126 cases (10.3%) [75]. Among gestations achieved with various ART methods, 7 of 71 (9.9%) were MZ gestations [76]. An analysis of national data that examined the increasing trend in MZ gestations estimated that 15.7% of ART gestations were MZ [77]. The determination of the increased risk of CP in ART gestations ideally requires a large scale follow-up study.

Summary

Multiple compared with singleton gestations are at five- to tenfold increased risk of CP. A major component of the increased risk in CP is associated with the higher proportion of multiple gestation fetuses that are born preterm with cerebral impairment from periventricular hemorrhage or leukomalacia. A greatly increased risk of CP is also associated with MC placentation. It is particularly notable in the surviving twin with fetal or early infant death of the co-twin. The failure to register or record early loss of a vanishing twin or later fetal demise as a fetus papyraceus may lead to a significant underestimate of the risk of CP in multiple gestations and an overestimate of the risk in apparently singleton infants.

The increased risk associated with MC placentation has been variously ascribed to transfer of thromboplastin or thromboemboli from the dead to the surviving fetus, exsanguination of the surviving fetus into the low pressure reservoir of the dead fetus, or hemodynamic instability with bidirectional shunting of blood between the two fetuses. An increased risk of CP in ART gestations is to be expected because of the higher proportion of preterm births. The increase in risk of CP associated with MC placentation will not be observed except for the minority of ART gestations that undergo MZ splitting.

References

[1] Little WJ. On the incidence of abnormal parturition, difficult labour, premature birth and asphyxia neonatorum on the mental and physical condition of the child, especially in relation to deformities. Transactions of the Obstetrical Society of London 1862;3:293–344.

[2] Stanley FJ, Watson L. Trends in perinatal mortality and cerebral palsy in Western Australia 1967 to 1985. BMJ 1992;304:1658–63.

[3] Dowding VM, Barry C. Cerebral palsy: changing patterns of birth weight and gestational age (1976/81). Irish Med J 1988;81:25–9.

[4] Pharoah POD, Cooke T, Cooke RWI, et al. Birth weight specific trends in CP. Arch Dis Child 1990;65:602–6.

[5] Bhushan V, Paneth N, Kiely JL. Impact of improved survival of very low birth weight infants on recent secular changes in the prevalence of cerebral palsy. Pediatrics 1993;91:1094–100.

[6] Illingworth RS. Why blame the obstetrician? BMJ 1979;278:797–801.

[7] Naeye RL, Peters EC, Bartholomew M, et al. Origins of cerebral palsy. Am J Dis Child 1989; 143:1154–61.

[8] Torfs CP, van den Berg B, Oechsli FW, et al. Prenatal and perinatal factors in the etiology of cerebral palsy. J Pediatr 1990;116:615–9.

[9] Bedrick ED. Perinatal asphyxia and cerebral palsy: fact, fiction, or legal prediction? Am J Dis Child 1989;143:1139–40.

[10] Swinyard CA, Swensen J, Greenspan L. An institutional survey of 143 cases of acquired cerebral palsy. Dev Med Child Neurol 1963;5:615–25.

[11] Arens LJ, Molteno CD. A comparative study of postnatally-acquired cerebral palsy in Cape Town. Dev Med Child Neurol 1989;31:246–54.

[12] Pharoah POD, Cooke T, Rosenbloom L. Acquired cerebral palsy. Arch Dis Child 1989; 64:1013–6.

[13] Maudsley G, Hutton JL, Pharoah POD. Causes of death in cerebral palsy: a descriptive study. Arch Dis Child 1999;81:390–4.

[14] Paneth N, Kiely J. The frequency of cerebral palsy: a review of population studies in industrialised nations since 1950. Clinics in Developmental Medicine 1984;87:46–56.

[15] Stanley F, Blair E. Postnatal risk factors in the cerebral palsies. Clinics in Developmental Medicine 1984;87:135–49.

[16] Nelson KB, Ellenberg JH. Antecedents of cerebral palsy: multivariate analysis of risk. N Engl J Med 1986;315:81–6.

[17] Niswander K, Henson G, Elborne D, et al. Adverse outcome of pregnancy and the quality of obstetric care. Lancet 1984;324:827–32.

[18] Blair E, Stanley F. Intrapartum asphyxia: a rare cause of cerebral palsy. J Pediatr 1988;112: 515–9.

[19] Freud S. Infantile cerebrallahumung: Nothnagels specielle pathologie und therapie. [Infantile cerebral paralysis. Translation by Russin LA. Miami: University of Miami Press, 1968.] Vienna: A. Holder; 1897.

[20] Alberman E. Birthweight and length of gestation in cerebral palsy. Dev Med Child Neurol 1964;5:388–94.

[21] Croen LA, Grether JK, Curry CJ, et al. Congenital abnormalities among children with cerebral palsy: More evidence for prenatal antecedents. J Pediatr 2001;138:804–10.

[22] Pharoah POD, Cooke T, Rosenbloom L, et al. Effects of birthweight, gestational age and maternal obstetric history on birth prevalence of cerebral palsy. Arch Dis Child 1987;62:1035–40.

[23] Javier LF, Root L, Tassanawipas A, et al. Cerebral palsy in twins. Dev Med Child Neurol 1992;34:1053–63.

[24] Pharoah POD, Cooke T. Cerebral palsy and multiple births. Arch Dis Child Fetal Neonatal Ed 1996;75:F174–7.

[25] Watson L, Stanley F. Report of the Western Australian Cerebral Palsy Register. Perth: Telethon Institute for Child Health Research; 1999.

[26] Scher AI, Petterson B, Blair E, et al. The risk of mortality or cerebral palsy in twins: a collaborative population-based study. Pediatr Res 2002;52:671–81.

[27] Stanley F, Alberman E. Birthweight, gestational age and the cerebral palsies. Clinics in Developmental Medicine 1984;87:57–68.

[28] Pharoah POD, Cooke T, Johnson MA, et al. Epidemiology of cerebral palsy in England and Scotland, 1984–9. Arch Dis Child Fetal Neonatal Ed 1998;79:F21–5.

[29] Weinberg W. Beiträge zur physiologie und pathologie der mehrlingsgeburten beim menschen. Pflugers Arch Gesamte Physiol Menschen Tiere 1902;88:346–430.

[30] Office for National Statistics. Mortality statistics: childhood, infant and perinatal. Series DH3, Nos. 27–33. London: HMSO; 1996–2002.

[31] Baker EM, Khorasgani MG, Gardner-Medwin D, et al. Arthrogryposis multiplex congenita and bilateral parietal polymicrogyria in association with the intrauterine death of a twin. Neuroped 1996;27:54–6.

[32] Bordarier C, Robain O. Microgyric and necrotic cortical lesions in twin fetuses: original cerebral damage consecutive to twinning? Brain Dev 1992;14:174–8.

[33] Van Bogaert P, Donner C, David P, et al. Congenital bilateral perisylvian syndrome in a monozygotic twin with intra-uterine death of the co-twin. Dev Med Child Neurol 1996;38:166–71.

[34] Larroche JC, Girard N, Narcy F, et al. Abnormal cortical plate (polymicrogyria), heterotopias and brain damage in monozygous twins. Biol Neonate 1994;65:343–52.

[35] D'Alton ME, Newton ER, Cetrulo CL. Intrauterine fetal demise in multiple gestation. Acta Genet Med Gemellol 1984;33:43–9.

[36] Fusi L, Gordon H. Twin pregnancy complicated by single intrauterine death: problems and outcome with conservative management. Br J Obstet Gynaecol 1990;97:511–6.

[37] Anderson RL, Golbus MS, Curry CJR, et al. Central nervous system damage and other anomalies in surviving fetus following second trimester antenatal death of co-twin. Prenat Diag 1990;10:513–8.

[38] Hoyme EH, Higginbottom MC, Jones KL. Vascular etiology of disruptive structural defects in monozygotic twins. Pediatrics 1981;67:288–91.

[39] Jung JH, Graham JM, Schultz N, et al. Congenital hydranencephaly/porencephaly due to vascular disruption in monozygotic twins. Pediatrics 1984;73:467–9.

[40] Ishimatsu J, Hori D, Hamada MT, et al. Twin pregnancies complicated by the death of one fetus in the second or third trimester. J Matern Fetal Investig 1994;4:141–5.

[41] Weig SG, Marshall PC, Abroms IF, et al. Patterns of cerebral injury and clinical presentation in the vascular disruptive syndrome of monozygotic twins. Pediatr Neurol 1995;13:279–85.

[42] Grether JK, Nelson KB, Cummins CK. Twinning and cerebral palsy: experience in four Northern Californian counties, births 1983 through 1985. Pediatrics 1993;92:854–8.

[43] Pharoah POD, Adi Y. Consequences of in-utero death in a twin pregnancy. Lancet 2000; 355:1597–602.

[44] Pharoah POD. Cerebral palsy in the surviving twin associated with infant death of the co-twin. Arch Dis Child Fetal Neonatal Ed 2001;84:F111–6.

[45] Pharoah POD, Price TS, Plomin R. Cerebral palsy in twins: a national study. Arch Dis Child Fetal Neonatal Ed 2002;87:F122–4.

[46] Glinianaia SV, Pharoah POD, Wright C, et al. Fetal or infant death in twin pregnancy: neurodevelopmental consequence for the survivor. Arch Dis Child Fetal Neonatal Ed 2002; 86:F9–15.

[47] Hanna JH, Hill JM. Single intrauterine fetal demise in a multiple gestation. Obstet Gynecol 1984;63:126–30.

[48] Kilby MD, Govind A, O'Brien PMS. Outcome of twin pregnancies complicated by a single intrauterine death: a comparison with viable twin pregnancies. Obstet Gynecol 1994;84:107–9.

[49] Santema JG, Swaak AM, Wallenburg HCS. Expectant management of twin pregnancy with single fetal death. Br J Obstet Gynaecol 1995;102:26–30.

[50] Zorlu CG, Yalçin HR, Çağlar T, et al. Conservative management of twin pregnancies with one dead fetus: is it safe? Acta Obstet Gynecol Scand 1997;76:128–30.

[51] Landy HJ, Keith L, Keith D. The vanishing twin. Acta Genet Med Gemellol 1982;31:179–84.

[52] Landy HJ, Keith LG. The vanishing twin: a review. Hum Reprod Update 1998;4:177–83.

[53] Pharoah POD, Cooke RWI. A hypothesis for the aetiology of spastic cerebral palsy: the vanishing twin. Dev Med Child Neurol 1997;39:292–6.

[54] Benson CB, Doubilet PM, Laks MP. Outcome of twin gestations following sonographic demonstration of two heart beats in the first trimester. Ultrasound Obstet Gynecol 1993;3:343–5.

[55] Heys RF. Selective abortion. BMJ 1996;313:1004.

[56] Pharoah POD, Cooke RWI. Registering a fetus papyraceus. BMJ 1997;314:441–2.

[57] Heys RF. Regulations on registration of a fetus papyraceus need to be revised. BMJ 1997; 314:1352–3.

[58] Griffiths M. Health professionals can exercise discretion. BMJ 1997;314:442.

[59] Gompels MJ, Davies D. Fetus papyraceus is being increasingly registered in Wessex. BMJ 1999;319:1271.

[60] Benirschke K. Twin placenta in perinatal mortality. N Y State J Med 1961;61:1499–508.

[61] Romero R, Duffy TP, Berkowitz RL, et al. Prolongation of a preterm pregnancy complicated by death of a single twin in utero and disseminated intravascular coagulation. N Engl J Med 1984;310:772–4.

[62] Coleman BG, Grumbach K, Arger PH, et al. Twin gestations: monitoring complications and anomalies with US. Radiology 1987;165:449–53.

[63] Skelly H, Marivate M, Norman R, et al. Consumptive coagulopathy following fetal death in a triplet pregnancy. Am J Obstet Gynecol 1982;142:595–6.

[64] Petersen IR, Nyholm HCJ. Multiple pregnancies with single intrauterine demise. Acta Obstet Gynecol Scand 1999;78:202–6.

[65] Golbus MS, Cunningham N, Goldberg JD, et al. Selective termination of multiple gestations. Am J Med Genet 1988;31:339–48.

[66] Fusi L, McParland P, Fisk N, et al. Acute twin-twin transfusion: a possible mechanism for brain-damaged survivors after intrauterine death of a monochorionic twin. Obstet Gynecol 1991;78:517–20.

[67] Bejar R, Vigliocco G, Gramajo H, et al. Antenatal origin of neurologic damage in newborn infants. II. Multiple gestations. Am J Obstet Gynecol 1990;162:1230–6.

[68] Larroche JC, Droulle P, Delezoide AL, et al. Brain damage in monozygous twins. Biol Neonate 1990;57:261–78.

[69] Gonen R. The origin of brain lesions in survivors of twin gestations complicated by fetal death. Am J Obstet Gynecol 1991;161:1897–8.

[70] Grafe MR. Antenatal cerebral necrosis in monochorionic twins. Pediatr Pathol 1993;13:15–9.

[71] Sebire NJ, Snijders RJM, Hughes K, et al. The hidden mortality of monochorionic twin pregnancies. Br J Obstet Gynaecol 1997;104:1203–7.

[72] Imaizumi Y. A comparative study of twinning and triplet rates in 17 countries. Acta Genet Med Gemellol 1998;47:101–14.

[73] Kiely JL, Kiely M. Epidemiological trends in multiple births in the United States, 1971–1998. Twin Res 2001;4:131–3.

[74] Kiely JL, Kiely M, Blickstein I. Contribution in the rise in multiple births to the potential increase in CP [abstract]. Pediatr Res 2000;47:314A.

[75] Derom C, Vlietinck R, Derom R, et al. Increased monozygotic twinning rate after ovulation induction. Lancet 1987;i:1236–8.

[76] Wenstrom KD, Syrop CH, Hammitt DG, et al. Increased risk of monochorionic twinning associated with assisted reproduction. Fertil Steril 1993;60:510–4.

[77] Platt MJ, Marshall A, Pharoah POD. The effects of assisted reproduction on the trends and zygosity of multiple births in England and Wales 1974–99. Twin Res 2001;4:417–21.

ELSEVIER
SAUNDERS

CLINICS IN
PERINATOLOGY

Clin Perinatol 33 (2006) 315–333

Perinatal Infections and Cerebral Palsy

Marcus C. Hermansen, MD[a,b,*],
Mary Goetz Hermansen, CRNP[b]

[a]Department of Pediatrics, Dartmouth Medical School, One Medical Center Drive,
Lebanon, NH 03756-0001, USA
[b]Southern New Hampshire Medical Center, 8 Prospect Street, P.O. Box 2014,
Nashua, NH 03061-2014, USA

Infections of the mother, the intrauterine environment, the fetus, and the neonate can cause cerebral palsy through a variety of mechanisms. Each of these processes is reviewed. The recently proposed theory of cytokine-induced white matter brain injury and the systemic inflammatory response syndrome (SIRS) with multiple organ dysfunction syndrome (MODS) is evaluated critically.

Transplacental fetal infections

A myriad of viral, bacterial, and protozoan transplacental infections causes permanent central nervous system (CNS) damage to the fetus. In addition to the classical TORCH infections (toxoplasmosis, rubella, cytomegalovirus [CMV], herpes simplex, syphilis), HIV, varicella-zoster virus, and lymphocytic choriomeningitis virus have been documented to cause neuralgic sequelae, including cerebral palsy. These transplacental, congenital infections may account for as many as 5% to 10% of the cases of cerebral palsy [1]. A comprehensive review of each of these infections is beyond the scope of this article, although toxoplasmosis, CMV, and herpes deserve discussion.

The prevalence of toxoplasmosis infection during pregnancy is approximately 1 per 1000; approximately 3000 infants are born with congenital toxoplasmosis annually in the United States [2]. Antimicrobial treatment of infants who have

* Corresponding author. Southern New Hampshire Medical Center, 8 Prospect Street, P.O. Box 2014, Nashua, NH 03061-2014.
E-mail address: marcus.hermansen@snhmc.org (M.C. Hermansen).

0095-5108/06/$ – see front matter © 2006 Elsevier Inc. All rights reserved.
doi:10.1016/j.clp.2006.03.002
perinatology.theclinics.com

congenital toxoplasmosis during the first year of life dramatically reduces the risk of adverse neurologic outcomes. Before the current treatment regimens were established the risk of seizures, mental retardation, and motor abnormalities were each approximately 75%. After implementation of the current treatment regimens, the risks have been reduced to approximately 30% for each neurodevelopmental handicap [3,4].

Congenital CMV may occur in as many as 1 in 1000 live births [5] and is the most common viral infection that is associated with cerebral palsy [6]. Up to 7% of all cases of cerebral palsy may be attributable to congenital CMV infection [7]. More than 90% of infants who have congenital CMV are asymptomatic at birth, yet approximately 10% to 15% of these asymptomatic infants will demonstrate developmental abnormalities, most commonly sensorineural hearing loss or learning difficulties. Almost no infant who is born with asymptomatic CMV develops cerebral palsy; however, approximately 80% to 90% of the infants who have symptomatic CMV have some form of severe neurologic disability. The presence of chorioretinitis, microcephaly, and early neurologic abnormalities in the newborn period are associated highly with adverse neurodevelopmental outcomes [8]; the risk for cerebral palsy among survivors of symptomatic CMV infection ranges from 12% [9] to 50% [10].

The prevalence of neonatal herpes simplex virus infection has been estimated to be between 1 per 5000 to 1 per 26,000 live born infants, with 400 to 1000 cases occurring annually in the United States [11]. Neonatal herpes simplex infection presents as one of three distinct syndromes: localized (skin, eye, and mouth) infection, CNS involvement, or disseminated disease. If treatment is initiated at the time the infection is localized to the skin, eye, or mouth, mortality and neurodevelopmental morbidity is extremely uncommon [12]. Treatment of infants who had established CNS involvement or disseminated disease reduced mortality [13]; however, as many as 50% of the survivors demonstrate neurodevelopmental abnormalities, including microcephaly, hydranencephaly, porencephalic cysts, blindness, learning disabilities, and cerebral palsy [12].

Maternal colonization and infection

Maternal colonization and infection can result in cerebral palsy by causing preterm birth, by causing overwhelming sepsis in the fetus or newborn, or by causing placental insufficiency and birth asphyxia. Recently, it also was proposed that proinflammatory cytokines may cause fetal white matter injury directly. Each of these processes is reviewed.

Maternal infections and preterm birth

Approximately half of all cases of cerebral palsy occur in preterm infants [14]. Accordingly, any condition that increases the incidence of prematurity is expected to increase the incidence of cerebral palsy. There is strong evidence that maternal infection and inflammation is a common cause of preterm birth. Approximately 25% of all preterm births are associated with maternal infections, and the risk increases as gestation decreases [15,16]. At 23 to 26 weeks' gestation as many as 45% of women in preterm labor have positive amniotic fluid cultures [16]. Undoubtedly, maternal infections are the cause of a substantial number of cases of cerebral palsy based solely upon their impact on the rate of prematurity.

Intra-amniotic infections

Intra-amniotic infections (IAIs; also referred to as "clinical chorioamnionitis" and sometimes simply as "chorioamnionitis") are symptomatic maternal infections that are diagnosed by a combination of maternal fever, leukocytosis, maternal tachycardia, fetal tachycardia, uterine tenderness, and foul odor of the amniotic fluid [17]. IAIs occur in 50% of preterm births that occur before 30 weeks' gestation [18]. Although one may expect to find histologic chorioamnionitis associated with IAIs, Smulian and colleagues [19] reviewed 139 pregnancies with a diagnosis of clinical chorioamnionitis, and found evidence of histologic chorioamnionitis in only 62% of the cases. It is possible that some patients who are diagnosed with clinical chorioamnionitis are exhibiting clinical symptoms that are due to noninfectious processes, such as epidural anesthesia or placental abruption.

There is a strong association between IAIs, preterm rupture of the fetal membranes, and preterm birth. As early as 1950 Knox and Hoerner [20] concluded that "infection in the female reproductive tract can cause premature rupture of the membranes and induce premature labor." IAI is present in 40% of women who are admitted with contractions and preterm, premature rupture of the membranes (PPROMs), and in 75% of women who start labor after admission for PPROMs [17]. Among women who have PPROMs, the likelihood of IAI increases as gestation decreases [18]. Thus, IAI not only increases the risk for preterm births, but increases the risk most dramatically in the extremely preterm births, those who are at the highest risk for neurodevelopmental disabilities.

The detailed mechanisms by which IAIs cause preterm labor are complex, incompletely understood, and beyond the scope of this article; however, it is known that IAIs initiate an immune response that results in an increased production of cytokines, prostaglandins, and metalloproteinases. These products then cause cervical softening, rupture of the fetal membranes, uterine contractions, and ultimately, preterm birth [21,22].

Not only does IAI result in increased preterm births, but preterm infants who are born following IAIs have more complicated courses than do preterm infants who were born without IAIs. Dammann and Leviton [23,24] found an increased risk for intraventricular hemorrhage and white matter disease in preterm infants who were born following IAIs. Zupan and associates [25] found an increased risk for periventricular leukomalacia (PVL) associated with premature rupture of the fetal membranes and IAIs. Perlman and colleagues [26] found that cystic PVL was associated with two risk factors—prolonged rupture of the fetal membranes (odds ratio, 6.6) and IAI (odds ratio, 6.8). Alexander and colleagues [27] found an increased risk for intraventricular hemorrhage, PVL, and seizures (odds ratio, 2.8, 3.4, and 2.9, respectively) in preterm infants who were born following IAIs. In a recent meta-analysis, Wu and Colford [28] found a relative risk of 1.9 for cerebral palsy in preterm newborns who were born following IAIs.

Histologic chorioamnionitis without intra-amniotic infection

Histologic chorioamnionitis may occur without signs and symptoms of IAI, but with histologic inflammation of the placental (placentitis) or fetal membranes (chorioamnionitis). Although histologic chorioamnionitis theoretically is a non-specific maternal response to a variety of stimuli, most cases are associated with infections. Micro-organisms have been isolated in approximately 75% of placentas that show evidence of histologic chorioamnionitis [19,29–32]. These studies may underestimate the incidence of infection because of the suboptimal microbiological culture techniques for fastidious organisms, such as *Mycoplasma* spp, or because of the administration of intrapartum antibiotics [33].

Surprisingly, few women who have histologic chorioamnionitis develop clinical findings of IAI. Of all women who have histologic chorioamnionitis or with bacteria documented in the fetal membranes, only 5% to 10% demonstrate findings of IAI [34]. Still, histologic chorioamnionitis without IAI is associated with preterm birth. Hillier and colleagues [35] found that premature delivery was related to the recovery of organisms from the fetal membranes (odds ratio, 3.8) and to the presence of histologic chorioamnionitis (odds ratio, 5.0). The proportion of placentas with evidence of infection was highest among those who delivered at the lowest gestational age.

Preterm infants who are born following histologic chorioamnionitis have an increased risk for intraventricular hemorrhage [36–38], periventricular echodensities [38], PVL [28], and cerebral palsy [39]. In Wu and Colford's [28] meta-analysis, the relative risk of cerebral palsy associated with histologic chorioamnionitis was 1.6, although this finding did not reach statistical significance.

Microbial invasion of the amniotic cavity without rupture of the fetal membranes

IAI and histologic chorioamnionitis usually occur following rupture of the fetal membranes [40]; however rupture of the membranes is not a prerequisite for infection of the amniotic cavity. Romero and Chaiworapongsa [41] reviewed 33 studies and concluded that approximately 13% of women in preterm labor with intact membranes had positive amniotic fluid cultures. The most common organisms that are found in the amniotic fluid of women with intact membranes are *Ureaplasma urealyticum*, *Fusobacterium* sp, and *Mycoplasma hominis* [42]. The women with positive amniotic fluid cultures, intact fetal membranes, and preterm labor usually do not develop clinical findings of IAI. When compared with women with negative cultures, they are more likely to develop IAIs (37% versus 9%), be refractory to tocolysis (85% versus 16%), and have spontaneous rupture of the fetal membranes (40% versus 4%) [43].

Bacterial vaginosis

Bacterial vaginosis is caused by an alteration of the normal vaginal flora and is associated strongly with an increased risk for preterm birth [43–46]. Bacterial vaginosis may occur in up to 20% of all pregnancies and carries a twofold to sixfold increased risk for preterm birth [45,47]. Additionally, there is a strong association between the presence of bacterial vaginosis and the subsequent development of chorioamnionitis [48–50].

Goldenberg and colleagues [22] recently estimated that bacterial vaginosis was responsible for 80,000 preterm births annually in the United States. Approximately 4000 of these infants suffer permanent neurologic disabilities, which suggests that bacterial vaginosis is one of the more common causes of cerebral palsy. Randomized controlled trials have shown inconsistent degrees of effectiveness of antibiotics in the treatment of bacterial vaginosis and the prevention of preterm births [51,52].

Nongenital tract infections

Nongenital tract infections also increase the risk for premature births. A meta-analysis by Romero and colleagues [53] found a strong association between urinary tract infections and preterm birth. Other serious maternal infections, including appendicitis and pneumonia [22], increase the risk for preterm birth but are uncommon in the United States today. Maternal periodontal disease probably is the most common nongenital infection that causes prematurity [54]. The births of as many as 18% of all preterm low birth weight infants may be attributable to periodontal disease [55]. Three recent studies suggested that treatment of periodontal disease during the pregnancy could reduce preterm births substantially, and presumably reduce the incidence of the associated neurodevelopmental sequelae [56–58].

Intra-amniotic infection and cytokine-induced brain damage in the preterm newborn

A substantial mass of evidence has accumulated to support the hypothesis that intrauterine infection with a fetal inflammatory response results in production of proinflammatory cytokines, and that these cytokines disrupt oligodendrocyte development in the preterm fetal brain [59–61]. This leads to reduced myelination, white matter injury, PVL, and ultimately, cerebral palsy. Dammann and Leviton [62,63] proposed development of clinical strategies to modify this cytokine-induced white matter injury.

Laboratory evidence supports the possibility of direct cytokine-induced white matter injury [61,63]. Cytokines can have a direct toxic effect by increasing production of nitric oxide synthase, cyclooxygenase, free radicals, and excitatory amino acid release [64,65]. Intraperitoneal injections of cytokines in various animal models produced astrogliosis and white matter encephalomyelitis [66].

Clinical evidence from newborns supports the hypothesis that an inflammatory-induced cytokine release is directly responsible for a significant proportion of white matter damage in small preterm infants. An increased risk for brain injury is associated with elevated cytokine levels. Yoon and colleagues found a fourfold to sixfold increased risk for brain white matter damages associated with elevated interleukin (IL)-1β from amniotic fluid [66] and from umbilical cord blood [67]. Yoon and colleagues [68] performed immunohistochemical staining for cytokines from brain sections of 17 infants who had documented PVL and 17 controls who did not have PVL. Cytokines were documented in 88% of the specimens from infants who had PVL, but in only 18% of the infants who did not have PVL. Yoon and colleagues also found a sixfold risk for cerebral palsy among preterm infants who were born with evidence of a fetal inflammatory response (funisitis) [69] or with elevated amniotic cytokine levels [70].

Finally, it is important to remember that not all cases of PVL in the small preterm neonate are from cytokine-induced damage. Hypocarbia [71] and hypotension [72] that are unrelated to infection also have been implicated as causes of PVL, presumably by reducing cerebral blood flow, which thereby, causes brain ischemia.

Maternal infections and cerebral palsy in the term newborn

There is an increased risk for cerebral palsy in term infants who are born following maternal infection. Grether and Nelson [73] found evidence of maternal infection in 37% of term newborns that developed spastic quadriplegic cerebral palsy, but in only 3% of control term infants. Neufeld and colleagues [74] found a twofold risk for cerebral palsy in term infants who were born after maternal infection. Wu and associates [75] reported that chorioamnionitis at 36 weeks' gestation or longer was associated with a fourfold increased risk for cerebral palsy. Wu and Colford's [28] meta-analysis found that among full-term infants, there was a positive association between clinical chorioamnionitis and cerebral palsy with a relative risk of 4.7.

Although studies consistently indicate an association between maternal infection at term and cerebral palsy, there are different pathophysiologic mechanisms by which the infection causes brain injury. The fetus or newborn may be born infected and suffer septic shock, meningitis, or pneumonia with pulmonary hypertension. The fetus may be born asphyxiated after placental dysfunction, and theoretically, the proinflammatory cytokines may cause brain damage directly, as in the preterm newborn.

Neonatal sepsis following maternal colonization and infection

Since its emergence in the 1970s, group B beta streptococcus (GBS) is the most common bacteria that causes early-onset neonatal sepsis. The rate of GBS colonization in pregnant women usually was found to be 15% to 25%. The neonate can acquire the organism from his or her GBS-colonized mother through vertical transmission from the lower genital tract or from acquisition during passage through the birth canal. If intrapartum antibiotics are not given, approximately 50% of newborns become colonized with GBS [76]; however, neonatal sepsis develops in only 1% to 3% of colonized newborns [77]. The risk factors that predispose a neonate to become infected are prematurity [78], lack of maternal anti-GBS IgG protection [79], prolonged rupture of the fetal membranes, and a high inoculum of the organism in the maternal anogenital tract.

The prevalence of neonatal GBS was approximately 1.4 per 1000 live births before the widespread acceptance of intrapartum antibiotics for the prevention of early-onset GBS sepsis [80]. Over the past 15 years, however, through the efforts of the Centers for Disease Control and Prevention, the American Academy of Pediatrics, and the American College of Obstetricians, guidelines have been established for antenatal screening for GBS and intrapartum antibiotic therapy [81]. With the widespread implementation of these protocols, the incidence of early-onset GBS infection has declined by more than 80% [82]. Neonatal mortality from early-onset sepsis has decreased from 25 per 100,000 live births in 1985 to 1991 to 15 per 100,000 live births in 1995 to 1998 [83]. There are no data available to demonstrate a similar decrease in the incidence of cerebral palsy among the survivors of early-onset GBS infection, although such a decrease should be expected. With current management strategies, neonatal GBS infection is a rare cause of cerebral palsy.

Intra-amniotic infection, chorioamnionitis, placental dysfunction, and birth asphyxia

IAI is the most common antecedent to birth depression, low Apgar scores, and neonatal hypoxic-ischemic encephalopathy in term newborns [73,84–86]. IAI and chorioamnionitis have been associated with an increased risk for neonatal seizures, meconium aspiration syndrome, multiorgan dysfunction, neonatal encephalopathy, and a clinical diagnosis of hypoxic-ischemic encephalopathy [86].

Maberry and colleagues [87] compared the course of 123 newborns who were exposed to IAI with 6769 newborns who were not exposed to IAI. The infants who were born following IAI were significantly more likely to have low 1-minute (20% versus 5%) and 5-minute (3% versus 1%) Apgar scores. Although more infants who were born after IAI were acidemic (15% versus 10%), the result did not reach statistical significance.

Grether and Nelson [73] compared 46 children of normal birth weight who had disabling, unexplained spastic cerebral palsy with 378 randomly selected control infants. The children who had spastic cerebral palsy were more likely to have been exposed to a maternal temperature that exceeded 38°C in labor (odds ratio, 9.3) as well as a clinical diagnosis of chorioamnionitis (odds ratio, 9.3). One or more indicators of maternal infection were found in 22% of the children who had cerebral palsy, but in only 3% of the controls. Grether and Nelson estimated that maternal infection might account for 12% of all cases of spastic cerebral palsy, 19% of cases of unexplained cerebral palsy, and 35% of cases of unexplained spastic quadriplegia. Most of the infants who developed cerebral palsy following maternal infection had signs that were consistent with birth asphyxia; these infants had a significant increase in the need for medication to maintain blood pressure, intubation in the delivery room, neonatal seizures (without meningitis), and a diagnosis of hypoxic-ischemic encephalopathy. Ninety percent of the children who had cerebral palsy following maternal infection had one or more of these findings, and 88% had a 5-minute Apgar score of 5 or less. These data are consistent with the authors' belief that the most likely mechanism for maternal infection to cause cerebral palsy in the term infant is by causing placental dysfunction and birth asphyxia.

Numerous mechanisms have been proposed to explain the occurrence of birth asphyxia in infants who are born after IAI. Chorioamnionitis results in increased cytokine and prostaglandin production. With prolonged chorioamnionitis the concentrations of toxins and cytokines increase, myometrial function is impaired, and labor abnormalities develop. Maternal hemorrhage, an increased need for oxytocin and cesarean delivery, uterine atony, and an increased incidence of first- and second-stage labor abnormalities are all more frequent in women who have IAIs [33,88–90]. In a large, prospective, multicentered trial, uterine atony, 5-minute Apgar score of 3 or less, and neonatal mechanical ventilation within 24 hours of birth were associated significantly with increased duration of IAI [91].

Several mechanisms have been proposed to explain the occurrence of birth asphyxia following IAI. These include placental dysfunction that is due to villous edema [92], placental abruption [90,91], an increase in oxygen consumption that is due to maternal hyperthermia [33], and a primary endotoxic effect upon the fetus [33]. In a study of pregnant sheep, maternal hyperthermia with subsequent hyperventilation and respiratory alkalosis led to a 53% reduction in uterine blood flow, a 30% reduction in umbilical blood flow, and the onset of fetal acidosis [93].

Combined exposure to infection and intrapartum asphyxia may exert a synergistic harmful effect upon the fetal brain [94]. Neonates who are exposed to infection in utero who also had potentially asphyxiating obstetric complications are at a much higher risk for cerebral palsy than are those with only one or no other risk factor [95,96]. Nelson and Grether [97] found that combined exposure to infection and intrapartum hypoxia dramatically increased the risk for spastic cerebral palsy (odds ratio, 78) compared with hypoxia alone. The mechanism for this synergistic effect has not been determined.

Intra-amniotic infection and cytokine-induced brain damage in the term newborn

Shalak and colleagues [98] determined cord blood cytokine levels in 61 term infants who were exposed to chorioamnionitis and admitted to a neonatal ICU and compared the values with those of 50 healthy term infants. Cord cytokine (IL-6, IL 8, and RANTES) levels were higher in infants who were born with chorioamnionitis. Infants who were born following chorioamnionitis and who had hypoxic-ischemic encephalopathy had significantly higher cytokine levels than did those who were exposed to chorioamnionitis but not hypoxic-ischemic encephalopathy. Long-term follow-up was not provided; however, if the pro-inflammatory cytokines are harmful to the term neonatal brain, then it would be expected that those who had the highest cytokine levels (ie, those who had chorioamnionitis and hypoxic-ischemic encephalopathy) would be at the greatest risk for brain injury.

Nelson and colleagues [99] examined the stored blood from 31 neonates (25 of whom were term) who had spastic cerebral palsy and from 65 controls. The infants who had cerebral palsy had statistically increased levels of IL-1, IL-8, IL-9, tumor necrosis factor-α, and RANTES. The infants who had elevated cytokine levels and spastic cerebral palsy also had lower Apgar scores, and proinflammatory cytokines are known to increase following hypoxia-ischemia [100,101]; infants with the most severe stages of asphyxia have the highest levels of IL-6 in the cerebrospinal fluid [102]. It remains possible that many of the infants in Nelson and colleagues' [99] study were asphyxiated at birth, and the birth asphyxia caused the cerebral palsy; the elevated cytokine levels were only a marker of the IAI, the birth asphyxia, or both. Further studies of term infants without evidence of birth asphyxia but with elevated cytokine levels should help to clarify this. Insufficient evidence exists to conclude that direct cytokine-induced brain injury occurs in the term and near-term neonate.

Neonatal infections

A variety of neonatal viral, bacterial, protozoan, and fungal infections is known to cause cerebral palsy. The damage may occur because of a direct effect of the infection (eg, meningitis or persistent pulmonary hypertension [PPHN]) or as a result of a systemic inflammatory response that causes shock and multi-system failure.

Early-onset bacterial infections

Pneumonia
PPHN with severe hypoxemia is a common complication of neonatal pneumonia. This tends to be one of the more severe forms of PPHN because of the release of vasoactive substance. In infants who have PPHN that is due to pneumonia, initially there is severe arterial spasm without changes in the morphometry of the pulmonary vasculature [103–105]; changes probably are mediated by the prostaglandin thromboxane A_2 [106,107]. This is followed by increased capillary permeability with increased lung fluid content. The increased capillary permeability is believed to be due to bacterial endotoxins that sequester white

blood cells in the lungs where they release vasoactive agents, such as tumor necrosis factor [105,108]. Treatment of PPHN that is associated with sepsis is extremely difficult because of the hypotension and coagulation disturbances that are associated with overwhelming sepsis [109]; 30% to 40% of the survivors have permanent brain injury, most notably cerebral palsy [109]. Because of the low incidence of GBS pneumonia today, pneumonia with PPHN is an uncommon cause of cerebral palsy.

Meningitis

Meningitis complicates 5% to 20% of the cases of early-onset neonatal sepsis [110]. CNS damage follows as a result of intense inflammatory vasculitis that results in small or large vessel obstruction and infarctions. Following the infarctions bacteria invade the brain and produce necrotizing lesions, which is followed by liquefaction and cavitation [111]. Additionally, an adhesive arachnoiditis leads to a rapidly progressive hydrocephalus in approximately one third of the cases [112]. The associated cardiorespiratory instability of the coincident sepsis and shock can cause additional brain injury. Ultimately, severe encephalopathic damage occurs that results in diffuse cerebral atrophy [111].

Older data suggested that infants who had GBS infection had better outcomes than did those who were infected with gram-negative meningitis [113,114]; however, more recent data demonstrate that the outcome of early-onset GBS meningitis is comparable to the outcome of gram-negative meningitis [115]. Infants who have early-onset GBS meningitis have worse outcomes than do infants who have late-onset GBS meningitis [116]. Other factors that are associated with worse outcomes include the presence of septic shock, coma, neutropenia, seizures, a very high cerebral spinal fluid protein content, and parenchymal injury on CT or MRI [10,115].

CNS damage, including cerebral palsy, is present in 20% to 50% of the survivors of neonatal meningitis [117,118]. In 1977, Haslam and associates [119] reported major neurologic sequelae in 2 of 15 survivors of GBS meningitis. In a prospective assessment of 20 survivors of GBS meningitis from 1974 to 1982, major handicaps were found in 15%, mild cognitive impairments were present in 15%, and 70% were functioning normally [120]. A third study from the 1970s found that following neonatal meningitis, 29% of 6-year-old children had severe sequelae, 21% had mild to moderate sequelae, and 50% were functioning normally [121]. Wald and colleagues [122] reported on 74 patients who had early- or late-onset GBS meningitis; 12% had major neurologic sequelae. As with pneumonia, this is an uncommon cause of cerebral today.

Infected preterm newborns

Infected preterm newborns are at a higher risk for cerebral palsy than are preterm newborns who escape infection. Wheater and Rennie [123] studied 508 very low–birth weight newborns. Of 389 who did not experience neonatal sepsis, 31 (8%) developed cerebral palsy. Of 119 who experienced neonatal sepsis, 38 (32%) developed cerebral palsy (odds ratio, 4.0). Murphy and colleagues [124] also found that neonatal sepsis increased the risk for cerebral palsy in infants who were born at less than 32 weeks' gestation (odds ratio, 3.6).

Systemic inflammatory response syndrome, sepsis, septic shock, and multiple organ dysfunction syndrome

Infections progress along a continuum of inflammatory reactions from the SIRS to sepsis, severe sepsis, septic shock, MODS, and death [125]. The signs of SIRS can be subtle and consist of only vital sign instability and white blood cell changes. The advanced signs of inflammation—MODS—include metabolic acidosis, shock, renal failure, cardiac dysfunction, adult respiratory distress syndrome (ARDS), disseminated intravascular coagulopathy (DIC), and CNS disturbances.

The progression of sepsis [126] starts with a release of the proinflammatory cytokines. The body then regulates the inflammation with a release of anti-inflammatory cytokines and cytokine inhibitors. The progression of disease and clinical symptoms is dependant upon an intricate, and only partially understood, balance between the proinflammatory and anti-inflammatory factors. The cytokines and their secondary mediators, including nitric oxide, thromboxanes, leukotrienes, platelet-activating factor, prostaglandins, and complement, cause activation of the coagulation cascade, the complement cascade, and the production of prostaglandins and leukotrienes. Clots lodge in the blood vessels and lower perfusion of the organs. In time the activation of the coagulation cascade depletes the patient's ability to clot, which results in DIC and ARDS. The cumulative effect of this cascade is an unbalanced state with inflammation dominant over anti-inflammation, and coagulation dominant over fibrinolysis. Microvascular thrombosis, hypoperfusion, ischemia, and tissue injury result. Severe sepsis, shock, and multiple organ dysfunction and failure follow, which often lead to death. The survivors are at a increased risk for cerebral palsy that is due to cerebral ischemia.

SIRS and MODS are nonspecific inflammatory reactions and are not confined to patients who have infections. Although asphyxia, trauma, hemorrhagic shock, burns, pancreatitis, malignancies, and autoimmune disorders each can cause a release of the proinflammatory cytokines and result in SIRS and MODS, infections and asphyxia are by far the most common causes in neonates.

With MODS as the common end point of inflammatory symptoms, the MODS of asphyxia can be difficult to distinguish from the MODS of sepsis. Both conditions may follow fetal distress, be associated with low Apgar scores and metabolic acidosis, and demonstrate hypo- or hyperglycemia, thrombocytopenia, DIC, elevated nucleated red blood cells [127], neutrophilia, bandemia, renal dysfunction or failure, cardiac dysfunction or failure, respiratory dysfunction or failure, and CNS dysfunction. Therefore, it often becomes a challenge for clinicians to differentiate SIRS and MODS of asphyxia from SIRS and MODS of sepsis. Certain clues may help differentiate the initiating processes:

The "gold standard" for differentiating infectious SIRS and MODS from noninfections causes is a positive culture; however, cultures may produce false-negative results if the mother or infant received antibiotics before collection of the cultures. Slow-growing or fastidious bacteria and virus may be difficult to isolate by culture. Bacterial autolysis [128] and inadequate sample size also can result in false-negative blood cultures.

Maternal risks factors that are associated with neonatal sepsis include untreated GBS, prolonged rupture of the fetal membranes, IAI, urinary tract infection, and fever; however chorioamnionitis can cause placenta dysfunction that results in asphyxia and asphyxial MODS. Therefore, the presence of maternal risk factors does not necessarily indicate that neonatal MODS was only of an infectious cause.

Neonatal leukopenia and neutropenia are more likely to be the result of an infection. Leukocytosis, neutrophilia, and bandemia are seen with infectious and noninfectious SIRS and MODS.

Spinal fluid pleocytosis indicates infection.

A sentinel event, such as a cord prolapse or ruptured uterus, is indicative of asphyxia.

Infants who are born severely depressed from infectious MODS are difficult to resuscitate and stabilize. Their mortality within hours of birth is high. Infants who are born with asphyxial MODS are more likely to be resuscitated and stabilized, albeit in a critical condition. They are more likely to survive, although they have a substantial risk for brain damage.

Recent investigations reported that sophisticated heart rate pattern analysis may differentiate infectious SIRS from noninfectious SIRS [129–131].

Several laboratory markers of inflammation, including many of the cytokines, have been studied to differentiate infectious from noninfections SIRS and MODS. Of these, procalcitonin and C-reactive protein levels seem to hold the most promise in diagnosing infection [132–134].

Summary

Although there are many mechanism by which maternal, intrauterine, fetal, or neonatal infections can result in cerebral palsy, the mechanisms with the strongest evidence and greatest frequency are the transplacental (TORCH) infections, maternal infections that cause preterm birth (IAI, histologic chorioamnionitis, bacterial vaginosis, and periodontal disease), and birth asphyxia following IAI and placental dysfunction (Table 1). IAI can result in the release of pro-inflammatory cytokines that cause white matter injury in the preterm infant, but scant evidence exists for such a process in term newborns. Infectious MODS can be difficult to differentiate from asphyxia MODS, and it is common for the two

Table 1
Infectious mechanisms in the etiology of cerebral palsy

Mechanism	Strength of evidence	Relative incidence
TORCH infections cause brain damage	++++	++++
IAI causes prematurity	++++	++
Histologic chorioamnionitis causes prematurity	++	+++
Preterm infants born after IAI or histologic chorioamnionitis have worse outcomes than those not exposed to infection	+++	++
Bacterial vaginosis causes prematurity	+++	++++
Maternal nongenital infections (eg, pneumonia) cause prematurity	++	+
Maternal periodontal infections cause prematurity	++	+++
IAI causes cytokine-induced brain damage in preterm neonates	+++	++
Maternal GBS colonization causes neonatal sepsis	++++	+
IAI causes placental insufficiency and birth asphyxia	+++	++
Synergistic brain damage occurs with IAI and asphyxia	++	++
IAI causes cytokine-induced brain damage in term neonates	+	+
Neonatal pneumonia with PPHN causes hypoxic brain damage	++++	+
Neonatal meningitis causes brain damage	++++	+
Fetal inflammation causes MODS and brain injury independent of asphyxia	++	+

processes to coexist. Infants who are born after exposure to infection and asphyxia have worse outcomes than do infants who are born after only one or other of the two processes.

References

[1] Stanley F, Blair E, Alberman E. Causal pathways initiated preconceptionally or in early pregnancy. In: Cerebral palsies: epidemiology and causal pathways. London: MacKeith Press; 2000. p. 48–59.

[2] Remington JS, Klein JO. Infectious diseases of the fetus and newborn infant. 5th edition. Philadelphia: W.B. Saunders Co.; 2001.

[3] Guerina NG, Hsu H-W, Ceissner C, et al. Neonatal screening and early treatment for congenital *Toxoplasma gondii* infection. N Engl J Med 1994;330:1858–63.

[4] Roizen N, Swisher C, Stein M, et al. Neurologic and developmental outcome in treated congenital toxoplasmosis. An Pediatr (Barc) 1995;95:11–20.

[5] Demmler GJ. Summary of a workshop on surveillance for congenital cytomegalovirus disease. Rev Infect Dis 1991;13:315–29.

[6] Fowler KB, Stagno S, Pass RF, et al. The outcome of congenital cytomegalovirus infection in relation to maternal antibody status. N Engl J Med 1992;326(10):663–7.

[7] Newell ML, and the European Collaborative Study. Mother to child transmission of cytomegalovirus. Br J Obstet Gynaecol 1994;101:122–34.

[8] Conboy T, Pass RF, Stagno S, et al. Early clinical manifestations and intellectual outcome in children with symptomatic congenital cytomegalovirus infection. J Pediatr 1987;111:343–8.

[9] Pass RF, Fowler KB, Boppana S. Progress in cytomegalovirus research. In: Landini MP, editor. Proceedings of the Third International Cytomegalovirus Workshop. London: Excerpta Medica; 1991. p. 3–10.

[10] Bale Jr JF, Bell WE. Prenatal and perinatal infectious causes of cerebral palsy. In: Miller G, Clark GD, editors. The cerebral palsies. Boston: Butterworth-Heinemann; 1998. p. 209–44.

[11] Stone KM, Brooks CA, Guinan ME, et al. National surveillance for neonatal herpes simplex virus infections. Sex Transm Dis 1989;16:152–6.

[12] Whitley R, Arvin A, Prober C, et al. A controlled trial comparing vidarabine with acyclovir in neonatal herpes simplex virus infection. N Engl J Med 1991;324:444–9.

[13] Whitley RJ, Nahmias J, Soong SJ, et al. Vidarabine therapy of neonatal herpes simplex virus infection. Pediatrics 1980;66(4):495–501.

[14] McCormick MC. The contribution of low birth weight to infant mortality and childhood morbidity. N Engl J Med 1985;312:82–90.

[15] Goncalves LF, Chaiworapongsa T, Romero R. Intrauterine infection and prematurity. Ment Retard Dev Disabil Res Rev 2002;8:3–13.

[16] Watts DH, Krohn MA, Hillier LI, et al. The association of occult amniotic fluid infection with gestational age and neonatal outcome among women in preterm labor. Obstet Gynecol 1992;79(3):351–7.

[17] Gibbs RS, Duff P. Progress in pathogenesis and management of clinical IAI. Am J Obstet Gynecol 1991;164:1317–26.

[18] Newton ER. Chorioamnionitis IAI. Clin Obstet Gynecol 1993;36(4):795–808.

[19] Smulian JC, Schen-Schwarz S, Vintzileos AM, et al. Clinical chorioamnionitis and histologic placental inflammation. Obstet Gynecol 1999;94:1000–5.

[20] Knox Jr IC, Hoerner JK. The role of infection in premature rupture of the membranes. Am J Obstet Gynecol 1950;59:190–4.

[21] Goldenberg RL, Hauth JC, Andrews WW. Intrauterine infection and preterm delivery. N Engl J Med 2000;342:1500–7.

[22] Goldenberg RL, Culhane JF, Johnson DC. Maternal infection and adverse fetal and neonatal outcomes. Clin Perinatol 2005;32:523–59.

[23] Dammann O, Leviton A. Maternal intrauterine infection, cytokines, and brain damage in the preterm newborn. Pediatr Res 1996;42:1–8.

[24] Dammann O, Leviton A. The role of perinatal brain damage in developmental disabilities: an epidemiologic perspective. Ment Retard Dev Disabil Res Rev 1997;3:13–21.

[25] Zupan V, Gonzalez P, Lacaze-Masmonteil T, et al. Periventricular leukomalacia: risk factors revisited. Dev Med Child Neurol 1996;38:1061–7.

[26] Perlman JM, Risser R, Broyles RS. Bilateral cystic periventricular leukomalacia in the premature infant: associated risk factors. Pediatrics 1996;97:822–7.

[27] Alexander JM, Gilstrap LC, Cox SM, et al. Clinical chorioamnionitis and the prognosis for very low birth weight infants. Obstet Gynecol 1998;91(5):725–9.

[28] Wu YW, Colford Jr JM. Chorioamnionitis as a risk factor for cerebral palsy: a meta-analysis. JAMA 2000;284:1417–24.

[29] Dong Y, St. Clair PJ, Ramzy I, et al. A microbiologic and clinical study of placental inflammation at term. Obstet Gynecol 1987;70(2):175–82.

[30] Aquino TI, Zhan J, Kraus FT, et al. Sub-chorionic fibrin cultures for bacteriologic study of the placenta. Am J Clin Pathol 1984;81:482–6.

[31] Chellam VG, Rushton DI. Chorioamnionitis and funiculitis in the placentas of 200 births weighing less than 2.5 kg. Br J Obstet Gynaecol 1985;92(8):808–14.

[32] Romero R, Gonzalez R, Sepulveda W, et al. Infection and labor: VIII. Microbial invasion of the amniotic cavity in patients with suspected cervical incompetence: prevalence and clinical significance. Am J Obstet Gynecol 1992;167:839–51.

[33] Newton ER. Preterm labor, preterm premature rupture of membranes, and chorioamnionitis. Clin Perinatol 2005;32:571–600.

[34] Guzick DS, Winn K. The association of chorioamnionitis with preterm delivery. Obstet Gynecol 1985;65:11–6.

[35] Hillier SL, Martius J, Krohn M, et al. A case-control study of chorioamnionic infection and histologic chorioamnionitis in prematurity. N Engl J Med 1988;319(15):972–8.

[36] Grafe MR. The correlation of prenatal brain damage with placental pathology. J Neuropathol Exp Neurol 1994;53:407–15.

[37] Salafia CM, Minior VK, Rosenkrantz TS, et al. Maternal, placental, and neonatal associations with early germinal matrix/intraventricular hemorrhage in infants born before 23 weeks' gestation. Am J Perinatol 1995;12:429–36.

[38] DeFelice C, Toti P, Laurini RN, et al. Early neonatal brain injury in histologic chorioamnionitis. J Pediatr 2001;138:101–4.

[39] Kraus FT. Cerebral palsy and thrombi in placental vessels of the fetus: insights from litigation. Hum Pathol 1997;28:246–8.

[40] Arias F, Tomich P. Etiology and outcome of low birth weight and preterm infants. Obstet Gynecol 1982;60(3):277–81.

[41] Romero R, Chaiworapongsa T. Preterm labor, intrauterine infection, and the fetal inflammatory response syndrome. NeoReviews 2002;3(5):e73–84.

[42] Romero R, Mazor M. Infection and preterm labor. Clin Obstet Gynecol 1988;31:553–84.

[43] Hay PE, Lamont RF, Taylor-Robinson D, et al. Abnormal bacterial colonization of the lower genital tract as a marker for subsequent preterm delivery and late miscarriage. BMJ 1994; 308:295–8.

[44] Meis PJ, Goldenberg RL, Mercer B, et al. The preterm prediction study: significance of vaginal infections. National Institute of Child Health and Human Development Maternal-Fetal Medicine Units Network. Am J Obstet Gynecol 1995;173(4):1231–5.

[45] Hillier SL, Nugent RP, Eschenbach DA, et al for the Vaginal Infections and Prematurity Study Group. Association between bacterial vaginosis and preterm delivery of a low-birth-weight infant. N Engl J Med 1995;333:1737–42.

[46] Martius J, Krohn MA, Hillier SL, et al. Relationships of vaginal lactobacillus species, cervical Chlamydia trachomatis, and bacterial vaginosis to preterm birth. Obstet Gynecol 1988;72: 89–95.

[47] McGregor JA, French JI, Richter R, et al. Antenatal microbiologic and maternal risk factors associated with prematurity. Am J Obstet Gynecol 2002;187(1):157–63.

[48] Gravett MG, Hummel D, Eschenbach DA, et al. Preterm labor associated with subclinical amniotic fluid infection and with subclinical bacterial vaginosis. Obstet Gynecol 1986;67: 229–37.

[49] Silver HM, Sperling RS, St. Clair PJ, et al. Evidence relating bacterial vaginosis to intra-amniotic infection. Am J Obstet Gynecol 1989;161:808–12.

[50] Hillier SL, Krohn MA, Cassen E, et al. The role of bacterial vaginosis and vaginal bacteria in amniotic fluid infection in women in preterm labor with intact fetal membranes. Clin Infect Dis 1993;20(Suppl 2):S276–8.

[51] McDonald H, Brocklehurst P, Parsons J. Antibiotics for treating bacterial vaginosis in pregnancy. Cochrane Database Sys Rev 2005;1:CD000262.

[52] Leitich H, Bodner-Adler B, Brunbauer M, et al. Bacterial vaginosis as a risk factor for preterm delivery: a meta-analysis. Am J Obstet Gynecol 2003;189(1):139–47.

[53] Romero R, Ovarzun E, Mazor M, et al. Meta-analysis of the relationship between asymptomatic bacteriuria and preterm delivery low birthweight. Obstet Gynecol 1989;73:576–82.

[54] Jeffcoat MK, Geurs NC, Reddy MS, et al. Periodontal infection and preterm birth: results of a prospective study. J Am Dent Assoc 2001;132:875–80.

[55] Offenbacher S, Katz V, Fertik G, et al. Periodontal infection as a possible risk factor for preterm low birthweight. J Periodontol 1996;67(Suppl 10):1103–13.

[56] Mitchell-Lewis D, Engebretson SP, Chen J, et al. Periodontal infections and pre-term birth: early findings from a cohort of young minority women in New York. Eur J Oral Sci 2001; 109(1):34–9.

[57] Lopez NJ, Smith PC, Gutierrez J. Periodontal therapy may reduce the risk of preterm low birthweight in women with periodontal disease: a randomized controlled trial. J Periodontol 2002;73(8):911–24.

[58] Jeffcoat MK, Hauth JC, Geurs NC, et al. Periodontal disease and preterm birth: results of a pilot intervention study. J Periodontol 2003;74(8):1214–8.

[59] Leviton A. Preterm birth and cerebral palsy: is tumor necrosis factor the missing link? Dev Med Child Neurol 1993;35:553–8.

[60] Dammann O, Leviton A. Maternal intrauterine infection, cytokines, and brain damage in the preterm newborn. Pediatr Res 1997;42:1–8.

[61] Adinolfi M. Infectious diseases in pregnancy, cytokines and neurological impairment: an hypothesis. Dev Med Child Neuro 1993;35:549–58.

[62] Dammann O, Leviton A. Brain damage in preterm newborns: biological response modification as a strategy to reduce disabilities. J Pediatr 2000;136:433–8.

[63] Dammann O, Leviton A. Brain damage in preterm newborns: might enhancement of developmentally regulated endogenous protection open a door for prevention. Pediatrics 1999; 204(3 Pt 1):541–50.

[64] Chao CC, Hu S, Ehrlich L, et al. Interleukin 1 and TNF α synergistically mediate neurotoxicity: involvement of nitric oxide and of NMDA receptors. Brain Behav Immun 1995;9: 355–67.

[65] Okusawa S, Gelfand JA, Ikejima T, et al. Interleukin-1 induces a shock like state in rabbits. Synergism with tumor necrosis factor and the effect of cyclooxygenase inhibition. J Clin Invest 1988;81:1162–72.

[66] Yoon BH, Jun JK, Romero R, et al. Amniotic fluid inflammatory cytokines (interleukin-6, interleukin-1β, and tumor necrosis factor-α), neonatal brain white matter lesions, and cerebral palsy. Am J Obstet Gynecol 1997;177:19–26.

[67] Yoon BH, Park JS, Romero R, et al. Interleukin-6 concentrations in umbilical cord plasma are elevated in neonates with white matter lesions associated with periventricular leukomalacia. Am J Obstet Gynecol 1996;174:1433–40.

[68] Yoon BH, Romero R, Kim CJ, et al. High expression of tumor necrosis factor-α and interleukin-6 in periventricular leukomalacia. Am J Obstet Gynecol 1997;177:406–11.

[69] Gomez R, Romero R, Ghezzi F, et al. The fetal inflammatory response syndrome. Am J Obstet Gynecol 1998;197:194–202.

[70] Yoon BH, Romero R, Park JS, et al. Fetal exposure to an intra-amniotic inflammation and the development of cerebral palsy at the age of three years. Am J Obstet Gynecol 2000; 182:675–81.

[71] Okumura A, Hayakawa F, Kato T, et al. Hypocarbia in preterm infants with periventricular leukomalacia: the relation between hypocarbia and mechanical ventilation. Pediatrics 2001; 107(3):469–75.

[72] Martens SE, Rijken M, Stoelhorst GM, et al. Is hypotension a major risk factor for neurological morbidity at term age in very preterm infants? Early Hum Dev 2003;75(1–2):79–80.

[73] Grether JK, Nelson KB. Maternal infection and cerebral palsy in infants of normal birth weight. JAMA 1997;278:207–11.

[74] Neufeld MD, Frigon C, Graham AS, et al. Maternal infection and risk of cerebral palsy in term and preterm infants. J Perinat 2005;25:108–13.

[75] Wu YW, Escobar GJ, Grether JK, et al. Chorioamnionitis and cerebral palsy in term and near-term infants. JAMA 2003;290:2677–84.

[76] Edwards MS, Baker CJ. Group B streptococcal infection. In: Remington J, Klein JO, editors. Infectious diseases of the fetus and newborn infant. Philadelphia: Saunders; 2001. p. 1091–156.

[77] Dillon HC, Khare S, Gray BM. Group B streptococcal carriage and disease: a 6-year prospective study. J Pediatr 1987;110(1):31–6.

[78] Anderson DC, Hughes BJ, Edwards MS, et al. Impaired chemotaxigenesis by type III group B streptococci in neonatal sera: relationship to diminished concentration of specific anticapsular antibody and abnormalities of serum complement. Ped Res 1983;17:496–502.

[79] Baker CJ, Kasper DL. Correlation of maternal antibody deficiency with susceptibility to neonatal group B streptococcal infection. N Engl J Med 1976;294:753–6.

[80] Zangwill KM, Schuchat A, Wenger JD. Group B streptococcal disease in the United States, 1990: report from a multistate active surveillance system. MMWR CDC Surveill Summ 1992; 41(6):25–32.

[81] Schrag S, Gorwitz R, Fultz-Butts K, et al. Prevention of perinatal group B streptococcal disease: Revised guidelines from CDC. MMWR Recomm Rep 2002;51(RR-11):1–22.

[82] Schrag SJ, Zywicki S, Farley MM, et al. Group B streptococcal disease in the era of intrapartum antibiotic prophylaxis. N Engl J Med 2000;342:15–20.

[83] Lukacs S, Schoendorf K, Schuchat A. Trends in sepsis-related mortality in the United States, 1985–98. Pediatr Inf Dis J 2004;23:599–603.

[84] Alexander JM, McIntire DM, Leveno KJ. Chorioamnionitis and the prognosis for term infants. Obstet Gynecol 1999;94:274–8.

[85] Badawi N, Kurinczuk JJ, Keogh JM, et al. Intrapartum risk factors for newborn encephalopathy: the Western Australian case-control study. BMJ 1998;317:1554–8.

[86] Inflammation, infection, coagulation abnormalities, and autoimmune disorders. Neonatal Encephalopathy Committee Opinion-2003. Neonatal Encephalopathy and Cerebral Palsy. Washington, DC: American College of Obstetricians and Gynecologists and The American Academy of Pediatrics; 2003.

[87] Maberry MC, Ramin SM, Gilstrap III LC, et al. Intrapartum asphyxia in pregnancies complicated by intra-amniotic infection. Obstet Gynecol 1990;76(3 Pt 1):351–4.

[88] Rouse DJ, Landon M, Leveno KJ, et al. The Maternal-Fetal Medicine Unit's cesarean registry: chorioamnionitis at term and its duration-relationship to outcomes. Am J Obstet Gynecol 2004; 191:211–6.

[89] Satin AJ, Maberry MC, Leveno KJ, et al. Chorioamnionitis: a harbinger of dystocia. Obstet Gynecol 1992;79:913–5.

[90] Mark SP, Croughan-Minihane MS, Kilpatrick SJ. Chorioamnionitis and uterine function. Obstet Gynecol 2000;95:909–12.

[91] Rouse DJ, Landon M, Leveno KJ, et al. The Maternal-Fetal Medicine Unit's cesarean registry: chorioamnionitis at term and its duration-relationship to outcomes. Am J Obstet Gynecol 2004; 191:211–6.

[92] Ilagan NB, Elias EG, Liang KC, et al. Perinatal and neonatal significance of bacteria-related placental villous edema. Acta Obstet Gynecol Scan 1990;69:287–90.

[93] Oakes GK, Walker AM, Ehrenkranz RA, et al. Uteroplacental blood flow during hyperthermia with and without respiratory alkalosis. J Appl Physiol 1976;41(2):197–201.

[94] Peebles DM, Wyatt JS. Synergy between antenatal exposure to infection and intrapartum events in causation of perinatal brain injury at term. BJOG 2002;109:737–9.

[95] Nelson KB, Willoughby RE. Infection, inflammation and the risk of cerebral palsy. Curr Opin Neurol 2000;13:133–9.

[96] Nelson KB, Grether JK. Causes of cerebral palsy. Curr Opin Pediatr 1999;11:487–91.

[97] Nelson KB, Grether JK. Potentially asphyxiating conditions and spastic cerebral palsy in infants of normal birth weight. Am J Obstet Gynecol 1998;179(1 Pt 1):507–13.

[98] Shalak LF, Laptook AR, Jafri HS, et al. Clinical chorioamnionitis, elevated cytokines, and brain injury in term infants. Pediatrics 2002;110(4):673–80.

[99] Nelson KB, Dambrosia JM, Grether JK, et al. Neonatal cytokines and coagulation factors in children with cerebral palsy. Ann Neurol 1998;44(4):665–75.

[100] Bona E, Andersson A, Blomgren K, et al. Chemokine and inflammatory cell response to hypoxia-ischemia in immature rats. Pediatr Res 1999;45:500–9.

[101] Hagberg H, Gilliaud E, Bona E, et al. Enhanced expression of IL-1 and IL-6 m-RNA and bioactive protein after hypoxia ischemia in neonatal rats. Pediatr Res 1999;40:603–9.

[102] Tekgul H, Yalaz M, Kutukculer N, et al. Value of biochemical markers for outcome in term infants with asphyxia. Pediatr Neurol 2004;31(5):326–32.

[103] Philips III JB, Lyrene RK, Godoy G, et al. Hemodynamic responses of chronically instrumented piglets to bolus injections of group B streptococcus. Ped Res 1988;23:81–5.

[104] Rojas J, Larsson LE, Hellerqvist CG, et al. Pulmonary hemodynamic and ultrastructural changes associated with group B streptococcal toxemia in adult sheep and newborn lambs. Ped Res 1983;70:1002–8.

[105] Sandberg K, Engelhardt B, Hellerqvist C, et al. Pulmonary response to group B streptococcal toxin in your lambs. J Appl Physiol 1987;63:2024–30.

[106] Gibson RL, Truog WE, Redding GJ. Thromboxane-associated pulmonary hypertension during three types of Gram positive bacteremia in piglets. Ped Res 1988;23:553–6.

[107] Hammerman C, Lass N, Strates E, et al. Prostanoids in neonates with persistent pulmonary hypertension. J Pediatr 1987;110:470–2.

[108] Rojas J, Stahlman M. The effects of group B streptococcus and other organism on the pulmonary vasculature. Clinics Perinal 1984;11:591–9.

[109] Greenough A, Roberton NRC. Acute respiratory disease in the newborn. In: Rennie J, Roberton NRC, editors. Textbook of neonatology. 3rd edition. Edinburgh (Scotland): Churchill Livingston; 2000. p. 481–607.

[110] Isaacs D, Barfield CP, Grimwood K, et al. Systemic bacterial and fungal infections in infants in Australian neonatal units. Australian Study Group for Neonatal Infections. Med J Aust 1995;162:198–201.

[111] Berman PH, Banker BQ. Neonatal meningitis: a clinical and pathological study of 29 cases. Pediatrics 1966;38:6–24.

[112] Hristeva L, Booy R, Bowler I, et al. Prospective surveillance of neonatal meningitis. Arch Dis Child 1993;69:514–7.

[113] Chin KC, Fitzhardinge PM. Sequelae of early onset group B hemolytic streptococcal neonatal meningitis. J Pediatr 1985;106:819–22.

[114] Haslam RH, Allen JR, Dorsen MM, et al. The sequelae of group B beta-hemolytic streptococcal meningitis in early infancy. Am J Dis Child 1977;131:845–9.

[115] Edwards MS, Rench MA, Haffar AAM, et al. Long-term sequelae of group B streptococcal meningitis in infants. J Pediatr 1985;106:717–22.

[116] Franco SM, Cornelius VE, Andrews BF. Long-term outcome of neonatal meningitis. Am J Dis Child 1992;146:567–71.

[117] McCracken GH. Management of bacterial meningitis; current status and future prospects. Am J Med 1984;76:215–23.

[118] Franco SM, Cornelius VF, Andrews BF. Long-term outcome of neonatal meningitis. Am J Dis Child 1992;146:567–71.

[119] Haslam RHA, Allen JR, Dorsen MM, et al. The sequelae of group B β-hemolytic streptococcal meningitis in early infancy. Am J Dis Child 1977;121:845–9.

[120] Chin KC, Fitzhardinge PM. Sequelae of early-onset group B streptococcal neonatal meningitis. J Pediatr 1985;106:819–22.

[121] Edwards MS, Rench MA, Haffar AAM, et al. Long-term sequelae of group B streptococcal meningitis in infants. J Pediatr 1985;105:717–22.

[122] Wald ER, Bergman I, Taylor HG, et al. Long-term outcome of group B streptococcal meningitis. Pediatrics 1986;77:217–21.

[123] Wheater M, Rennie JM. Perinatal infection is an important risk factor for cerebral palsy in very-low-birthweight infants. Devel Med Child Neuro 2000;42:364–7.

[124] Murphy DJ, Hope PL, Johnson AM. Neonatal risk factors for cerebral palsy in very preterm babies: case-control study. BMJ 1997;314:404–8.

[125] American College of Chest Physicians. Society of Critical Care Medicine Consensus Conference. Definitions for sepsis and organ failure and guidelines for the use of innovative therapies in sepsis. Crit Care Med 1992;20:864–75.

[126] Chamberlain NR. From systemic inflammatory response syndrome (SIRS) to bacterial sepsis with shock. Available at: http://www.kcom.edu/faculty/chamberlain/Website/lectures/lecture/sepsis.htm. Accessed April 22, 2006.

[127] Hermansen MC. Nucleated red blood cells in the fetus and newborn. Arch Dis Child Fetal Neonatal Ed 2001;84(3):F211–5.

[128] Fischer GW, Smith LP, Hemming VG, et al. Avoidance of false-negative blood culture results by rapid detection of pneumococcal antigen. JAMA 1984;252(13):1742–3.

[129] Griffin PM, Lake D, Moorman JR. Heart rate characteristics and laboratory tests in neonatal sepsis. Pediatrics 2005;115(4):937–41.

[130] Goldstein B. Heart rate characteristics in neonatal sepsis: a promising test that is still premature. Pediatrics 2005;115(4):1070–2.

[131] Kovatchev BP, Farhy LS, Cao H, et al. Sample asymmetry analysis of heart rate characteristics

with application to neonatal sepsis and systemic inflammatory response syndrome. Pediatr Res 2003;54:892 – 8.

[132] Marik PE. Definition of sepsis: not quite time to dump SIRS? Crit Care Med 2002;30(3): 706 – 8.

[133] Joram N, Boscher C, Denizot S, et al. Umbilical cord blood procalcitonin and C reactive protein concentrations as markers for early diagnosis of very early onset neonatal infection. Arch Dis Child Fetal Neonatal Ed 2006;91(1):F65 – 6.

[134] Meisner M. Biomarkers of sepsis: clinically useful? Curr Opin Crit Care 2005;11(5):473 – 80.

CLINICS IN
PERINATOLOGY

Clin Perinatol 33 (2006) 335–353

Intrapartum Asphyxia and Cerebral Palsy: Is There a Link?

Jeffrey M. Perlman, MB ChB

Department of Pediatrics, Weill Cornell Medical Center, 525 East 68th Street, N-506, New York, NY 10021, USA

Brain injury that occurs during the perinatal period remains one of the most commonly recognized causes of severe long-term neurologic deficits in infants and children, which often is termed "cerebral palsy" (CP) [1]. The injury is invariably secondary to interruption of placental blood flow—a state that often is referred to as "asphyxia." A much-debated question relates to the extent of contribution of asphyxia to CP [2]. This is a complex issue; in this article the author frames a template that attempts to link events during labor with subsequent CP, which is based on pathophysiologic principles, rather than empiric definitions. This article includes definitions of CP and asphyxia; describes the fetal adaptive mechanisms to preserve cerebral perfusion and oxygen delivery following interruption of placental blood flow; and highlights the major brain lesions that evolve as a consequence of hypoxia-ischemia, the accompanying neonatal neurologic syndrome, and finally, the associated systemic organ involvement. The minimal inclusion and exclusion criteria that are necessary to link intrapartum asphyxia and subsequent CP are presented.

Definition of cerebral palsy

The definition of CP is highly variable. One recent description defined CP "as a non-progressive motor disorder of the development of movement and posture, causing activity limitation that is attributed to non-progressive disturbances that occurred in the developing fetal or infant brain. The motor disorders of CP are often accompanied by disturbances of sensation, cognition, communication, per-

E-mail address: jmp2007@med.cornell.edu

ception or behavior or seizure disorder" [2]. As a second definition, a Task Force on Neonatal Encephalopathy and Cerebral Palsy convened by the American College of Obstetricians and Gynecologists (ACOG) defined CP "as a chronic disability of central nervous system origin characterized by aberrant control of movement and posture appearing early in life and not as a result of progressive neurologic disease." The statement goes on to state, "spastic quadriplegia, especially with an associated movement disorder is the only type of CP associated with acute interruption of placental blood flow. Purely dyskinetic or ataxic CP especially when there is an associated learning difficulty commonly has a genetic origin and is not caused by intrapartum or peripartum asphyxia. Similarly absent CP, neither epilepsy, nor mental retardation nor attention-deficit hyperactivity disorder is caused by birth asphyxia" [3].

How does one reconcile these two definitions? The first is more global and reflects an onset of injury that includes the fetal and perinatal periods, whereas the second definition is targeted to the intrapartum period. This is more appropriate when trying to link events during labor (asphyxia) and subsequent CP. Thus, the origin of the brain injury that results in CP may occur during the antepartum, intrapartum, or postpartum period. Accumulating evidence suggests that the brain injury occurs during the antepartum period in approximately 70% to 80% of cases of CP [4–6]. The proportion of CP that may be attributed to perinatal events (eg, birth asphyxia) is small and is estimated to be approximately 20%. Given that CP affects approximately 2 to 3 per 1000 school-aged children, the contribution of intrapartum events or asphyxia is small and is less than 1 per 1000 term deliveries [3–6]; however, this is the most relevant and important group of infants who has CP, because therapeutic strategies to reduce or prevent cerebral injury are possible and are being investigated [7,8].

Definition of asphyxia

The definition of birth asphyxia is imprecise. The process occurs during the first and second stages of labor secondary to interruption of placental blood flow; a fairly consistent description is that of a condition of impaired gas exchange which leads, if persistent, to hypoxemia and hypercapnia. The process is identified by fetal acidosis (as measured in umbilical arterial blood), which reflects the degree of anaerobic metabolism that is required during periods of hypoxia or increased oxygen demand [9]. The umbilical arterial pH that best defines asphyxia remains unclear. Traditionally, asphyxia was defined as a cord umbilical arterial pH of less than 7.20. With this definition the rate of "asphyxia" ranges from 5% to 20% [10]. If a pH of less than 7.10 is used, the rate ranges from 2% to 8% [11]. Evidence suggests that an umbilical arterial pH of less than 7.00 reflects a degree of acidosis that often is referred to as pathologic or severe fetal acidemia, whereby the risk of adverse neurologic sequelae is increased [12,13]. A cord pH of less than 7.0 complicates approximately 0.3% of all deliveries [12]; however, even with this degree of acidemia, the likelihood of subsequent brain injury is low. Thus, most infants (>60%) exhibit no difficulties in the deliveryroom, are triaged to the regular newborn nursery, and are discharged home following an uncomplicated neonatal course in almost all cases [14]. Even when infants who have severe fetal acidemia are admitted to intensive care (usually because of respiratory difficulties) about 80% to 90% exhibit a benign neurologic course [15–17]; only a small percentage progresses to the degree of encephalopathy that is associated with severe brain injury. (Fig. 1).

In one study, 8 of 47 infants (12%) who had severe fetal acidemia that required neonatal intensive care developed hypoxic-ischemic encephalopathy, including seizures [17]. Infants with seizures were 234 times more likely to require cardiopulmonary resuscitation (CPR) in the delivery room as compared with infants who had severe fetal acidemia without seizures (see Fig. 1) [17]. Clearly, the presence of severe fetal acidemia, although a distinct marker of stress, does not provide insight into the fetal adaptive ability to maintain cerebral perfusion (see later discussion). The coupling of bradycardia with severe fetal acidosis that necessitates intensive delivery room resuscitation for correction provides initial objective evidence of a severe intrapartum insult of sufficient duration to compromise cerebral perfusion and oxygen delivery. This resistance of the brain to asphyxia, even when profound, is extraordinary, and is based, in part, on the ability of the fetus to adapt to interruption of placental blood flow to preserve cerebral perfusion and oxygen delivery (see later discussion).

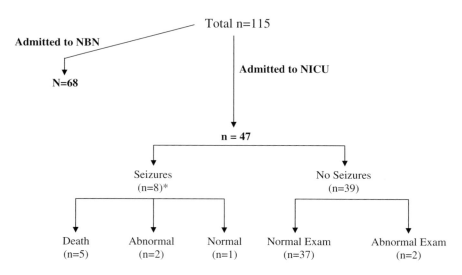

Fig. 1. Severe fetal acidemia (cord umbilical arterial pH <7.00) and short-term neurologic outcome in term infants who were admitted to the neonatal ICU at Parkland Hospital in Dallas, Texas. *Six of the eight infants received CPR in the delivery room. The odds ratio estimate for developing seizures following CPR is 234. (*Data from* Perlman JM, Risser R. Severe fetal acidemia: neonatal neurological features and short term outcome. Pediatr Neurol 1993;9:277–82.)

Fetal adaptive mechanisms

The fetal adaptive mechanisms to preserve neuronal integrity with interruption of placental blood flow include circulatory and noncirculatory responses. Each is discussed briefly.

Circulatory responses

The important circulatory manifestations of asphyxia have been well categorized in experimental studies. These include (1) a redistribution of cardiac output to preserve blood flow to the more vital organs (ie, brain, myocardium, adrenal gland), at the expense of flow to less vital organs, i.e., kidney, intestine, and muscle; (2) loss of cerebral vascular autoregulation resulting in a pressure passive circulation, and (3) eventual diminution in cardiac output with resultant hypotension, and ultimately, a decrease in cerebral blood flow (CBF) (Fig. 2) [18–23]. With regard to the latter, in the experimental model with initial arterial hypoxemia, fetal vascular resistance can decrease by at least 50% to maintain CBF with a minimal decrease in oxygen delivery [24–26]. Critical to this state is a normal or elevated mean arterial blood pressure; however, with persistent hypoxemia, and eventual hypotension, cerebral vascular resistance cannot decrease further, which results in a marked reduction in CBF [27]. The critical ischemic threshold for neuronal necrosis in developing brain remains unclear. Postnatal observations indicate that this likely is a complex issue. In adults, CBF "thresholds" have been identified; below a critical threshold functional disturbances (electroencephalographic slowing) occur [28], and below an even lower CBF threshold ion pump failure occurs [29,30]. Yet values in preterm and term infants that are less than those associated with pump failure in adults have been associated with normal neurologic development [31].

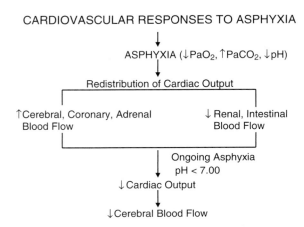

Fig. 2. The circulatory responses to interruption of placental blood flow. Note the increased blood flow to brain, heart, and adrenal glands at the expense of blood flow to the less vital organs.

Noncirculatory factors that contribute to neuronal preservation

In addition to the circulatory responses that were described above, factors that are considered to be potentially important in preserving neuronal integrity with asphyxia include biologic alterations that accompany maturation. Some examples include an increasing rate of brain metabolism during early development with resultant slower depletion of high-energy compounds during hypoxia-ischemia in the fetus as compared with the term or adult [32,33], the use of alternate energy substrate, the neonatal brain having the capacity to use lactate and ketone bodies for energy production [34,35], the relative resistance of the fetal and neonatal myocardium to hypoxia-ischemia [36,37], the potential protective role of fetal hemoglobin [38], and the potential for ischemic preconditioning [39].

Specific placental conditions increase risk for brain injury

The primary mechanism that contributes to interruption of placental blood flow seems to be a critical determinant of neurologic outcome Thus, the systemic and cerebral impact of an acute event (eg,, placental abruption) differs from that of a more chronic process (eg, repetitive decelerations). For example, prolonged partial asphyxia damages cerebral cortex and white matter in parasagittal regions, whereas brief total asphyxia damages subcortical nuclei in the thalamus and brainstem—and if preceded by subthreshold partial asphyxia—includes basal ganglia [40,41]. Moreover, specific placental abnormalities may increase the likelihood of brain injury and subsequent CP. For example, decelerations may be related to cord compression, underlying occult placental inflammation, or placental vascular changes. Thus, there is an unexplained increased association between clinical or histologic chorioamnionitis and CP [42]. The mechanisms that link these two conditions remain obscure and may include interruption of placental blood flow, fever, or cytokine release [43]. A recent report described an association between placental vasculopathies and subsequent CP [44].

Clinical measures of asphyxia

Several markers that are suggestive of stress and may be a proxy for "asphyxia" have been used during and following delivery in an attempt to identify the infant who is at highest risk for brain injury.

Assessment during labor

Readily identified markers of fetal stress/distress during labor include fetal heart rate abnormalities and meconium staining of the amniotic fluid.

Fetal heart rate monitoring

Fetal heart rate monitoring was designed to detect changes in heart rate response, which might identify asphyxia in utero. The introduction of fetal heart monitoring in the 1970s raised expectations of identifying the infant who is at greatest risk for developing hypoxic-ischemic cerebral injury. It was postulated that fetal heart rate monitoring would reduce the incidence of deficits that were attributed to perinatal events by 50% [45]. Despite a near 3-decade experience with intensive fetal heart rate monitoring, the impact on subsequent neurologic outcome has been minimal. Although the incidence of seizures may be reduced by fetal heart rate monitoring [46], long-term neurologic and cognitive outcome is unaffected [47]. Even fetal bradycardia—considered to be a sign of severe or prolonged hypoxia-ischemia—is associated rarely with CP, and only when the subsequent Apgar score is low [48]. This is a postpartum association.

Meconium-stained amniotic fluid

Meconium-stained amniotic fluid (MSAF) is a common observation during labor and occurs in approximately 10% to 20% of infants [49]. Meconium, particularly when thick, is considered to reflect in utero stress by some investigators [50,51], whereas others have reported no association with fetal hypoxia, acidosis, or asphyxia [52,53]. Thus, it should not be a surprise that despite its common presence, most infants with MSAF do not develop CP.

The above observations should not be unanticipated because neither marker in isolation provides insight with regard to an asphyxial process, the duration of such an event, or the fetal adaptive mechanism to maintain cerebral perfusion and metabolism.

Delivery room markers

Apgar scores

In many studies, the Apgar score has been used as a major criterion for the diagnosis of birth asphyxia; however, it is inappropriate to define birth asphyxia when used in isolation [54]. Thus, the presence of a low Apgar score is not indicative of intrapartum asphyxia; several studies demonstrated false positive (low Apgar score, normal pH) and false negative (normal Apgar score, low pH) results [54]. A persistent low Apgar score at 5, 10, or 20 minutes, despite intensive resuscitation, is associated with increasing mortality and morbidity [55–57]. Moreover, a low 5-minute Apgar score in combination with other markers—notably pathologic fetal acidemia and the need for intubation with or without intensive resuscitation—is indicative of a significant intrapartum insult and greatly increases the risk for injury to the brain. Thus, such infants are 340-fold more likely to progress to moderate to severe encephalopathy than are infants without these markers [58].

Cardiopulmonary resuscitation

The need for CPR (ie, chest compressions with or without medications) in the delivery room significantly increases the risk for abnormal neurologic outcome, particularly when associated with severe fetal acidemia [59]. This should be

Table 1
Death or moderate to severe encephalopathy in term infants administered cardiopulmonary resuscitation in the presence or absence of severe fetal acidemia Delivered at Parkland Memorial Hospital, Dallas, Texas, 1992–2002

Event	Abnormal outcome	Normal outcome
CPR, cord pH <7.00	25	3
CPR, cord pH >7.00	4	37

Sensitivity 86%; specificity 92%; positive predictive value 89%; odds ratio 77; 95% confidence interval, 15–374.

obvious from Fig. 2, because it implies failure of the adaptive mechanisms and cerebral hypoperfusion as a consequence of cardiac or pump failure. When CPR is related to postdelivery events (eg, consequence of ineffective initial ventilatory support—infants with normal cord pH), the short-term neurologic outcome is favorable in more than 95% of infants [58]. Extending these initial observations, over a 10-year experience (1992–2002), 25 of 28 term infants who were delivered at Parkland Memorial Hospital in Dallas, Texas with severe fetal acidemia and who were administered CPR developed an abnormal neurologic outcome as compared with 4 of 41 infants with a pH of more than 7.00 who received CPR (Table 1).

Combination of perinatal markers

The cumulative data clearly indicate that a single marker of in utero stress provides little useful information regarding the "asphyxial process" or the fetal adaptive responses, and thus, the relationship to neonatal brain injury or subsequent CP. Rather a constellation of markers is of far greater value in identifying infants who are at greatest risk for evolving neonatal brain injury, and as a consequence, is more valuable in linking "asphyxia" and CP. For example, in the evaluation of 96 "high-risk" term infants who were derived from 14,000 deliveries, which were admitted to neonatal intensive care, 5 infants developed moderate to severe encephalopathy, including seizures. They could be identified within the first hour of life by a combination of 5-minute Apgar score of 5 or less, the need for delivery room intubation or CPR, and a cord umbilical arterial pH of less than 7.00. The presence of these markers increased the risk for seizures by 340-fold with an 80% positive predictive value, a sensitivity of 80%, and a specificity of 98.8%. When used in isolation, the same markers were far less predictive of seizures [59]. Infants who have moderate to severe encephalopathy are more likely to progress to CP [1].

Neuropathology attributed to intrapartum hypoxia-ischemia

Failure to adapt to the asphyxial process results in a critical reduction in cerebral perfusion and oxygen delivery and subsequent hypoxic-ischemic injury. The topography of the major lesions that are seen with intrapartum asphyxia in the term infant commonly has a vascular distribution. The lesions include parasagittal cerebral injury; selective neuronal necrosis (SNN), including basal ganglia injury; periventricular leukomalacia; and focal/multifocal ischemic injury [1].

Parasagittal cerebral injury

Parasagittal cerebral injury refers to bilateral cortical and adjacent subcortical white matter necrosis that involves the superior medial, and particularly, the posterior aspects of the cerebral convexities. The necrosis occurs within border zones, also referred to as "watershed areas," between the end branches of the major cerebral vessels; these regions are extremely vulnerable to decreases in cerebral perfusion pressure [1,60]. Injury to this region involves the motor cortex that subserves proximal extremity function; the upper extremities are affected more severely than are the lower extremities [1]. Spastic quadriplegia is the most frequent long-term consequence of injury to this region.

Selective neuronal necrosis

SNN is the most common variety of injury that is observed in hypoxic-ischemic encephalopathy [1]. Specific vulnerable neurons include the CA1 region and subiculum of the hippocampus; the lateral geniculate body and thalamus of the diencephalon; caudate nucleus, putamen, and globus pallidus of the basal ganglia; the fifth and seventh cranial motor nuclei nerves within the pons; and the dorsal vagal nuclei. The basal ganglia seem to be particularly vulnerable to hypoxia [40,41] (see later discussion). The pathogenesis of SNN includes hypoperfusion followed by reperfusion and a prominent role for glutamate-induced injury [1]. The neonatal consequences of SNN include seizures and sucking and swallowing difficulties; the long-term sequelae include mental retardation and seizures [1].

Basal ganglia injury

Basal ganglia injury is characterized by neuronal injury within the basal ganglia (ie, thalamus, caudate nucleus, globus pallidus, putamen) [1]. Following the near-routine evaluation of the brain by MRI, this injury has been recognized with increasing frequency, and is identified in approximately two thirds of "asphyxiated" infants [1,41,61].

Periventricular leukomalacia

Periventricular leukomalacia is the primary ischemic lesion of the preterm infant. It involves bilateral white matter necrosis adjacent to the external angles of the lateral ventricles that includes the centrum semiovale, optic and acoustic radiations—a region that resides within border zones between the penetrating branches of the major cerebral vessels [1]. These border zones, which correspond to the parasagittal areas of the term infant, also are exquisitely sensitive to decreases in cerebral perfusion [62]. Descending fibers from the motor cortex traverse this region of cerebral white matter. The long-term manifestations include spastic diplegia and spastic quadriplegia, with visual and cognitive deficits with more severe injury [63,64].

Focal/multifocal ischemic injury

Focal/multifocal ischemic cerebral necrosis is characterized by injury to all cellular elements, and is caused by an infarction within a vascular distribution. Experimental data in monkeys support the importance of ischemia in the genesis of this lesion [65]. The long-term neurologic manifestations reflect the location and extent of the primary lesion, and include spastic hemiplegia, spastic quadriplegia, or seizures [1]. In isolation, this lesion is associated rarely with perinatal markers of asphyxia, and often presents in apparently healthy infants with seizures or apnea on the first or second postnatal day [66,67].

Neonatal encephalopathy

Neonatal encephalopathy is defined clinically on the basis of a constellation of findings that include abnormal consciousness, tone and reflexes, feeding, or respiration and seizures; it can result from a myriad of conditions [1]. Neonatal encephalopathy may or may not result in permanent neurologic impairment. It can be stated with certainty, however, that the pathway from an intrapartum hypoxic-ischemic injury to subsequent CP must progress through neonatal encephalopathy. Thus, there will be abnormalities in the neurologic examination that are noted shortly after delivery and become prominent within 12 to 24 hours after birth. The examination is characterized by abnormalities in cortical function (ie, hyperalertness, lethargy, stupor, coma plus seizures; brainstem function (ie, pupillary and cranial nerve abnormalities); tone (ie, hypotonia, hypertonia); and reflexes (ie, notably absent, hyporeflexia, hyperflexia). These findings vary depending on the time of examination and the severity of the underlying brain injury [1]. The Sarnat staging method is used most commonly to grade the degree of encephalopathy. Outcome is related to the maximum grade of severity [68]. Thus, outcome is invariably favorable for infants who have mild encephalopathy (Sarnat stage 1), whereas an abnormal outcome is observed in approximately 20% to 25% of cases of moderate encephalopathy (Sarnat stage 2); severe encephalopathy (Sarnat stage 3) is associated with a poor outcome in all cases [1]. When faced with an encephalopathic neonate, it is critical to exclude other potential causes (ie, meningitis, inborn errors of metabolism, focal cerebral infarction, traumatic brain injury) [67,69].

Multiorgan injury

It should be apparent from the preceding sections that interruption of umbilical blood flow with resultant redistribution of cardiac output may be followed by systemic organ injury of varying severity, which is determined, in part, by the duration and the severity of the insult (Fig. 3). For example, studies in fetal lambs demonstrated that partial occlusion of the umbilical cord caused a prompt reduction in urinary output and in glomerular filtration rate [70]. A lack of uniformity in the renal response to experimental hypoxia seems to be due to varying levels of CO_2. Thus, studies in hypoxic fetal lambs showed that superimposed hypercapnia, as opposed to hypocapnia on an asphyxial process, caused a sharp reduction in renal blood flow [71]. This may explain, in part, why certain infants who have sustained a perinatal insult with brain injury do not

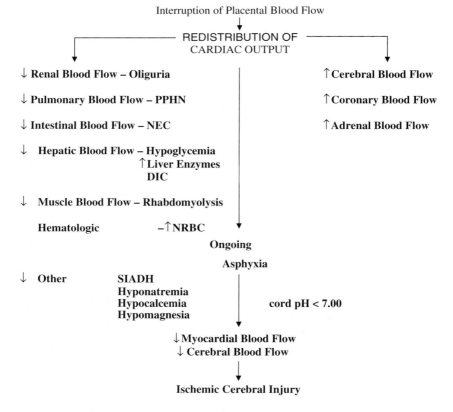

Fig. 3. Potential systemic organ involvement following interruption of placental blood flow. DIC, disseminated intravascular coagulation; NEC, necrotizing enterocolitis; NRBC, nucleated red blood cells; PPHN, persistent pulmonary hypertension of the newborn; SIADH, syndrome of inappropriate antidiuretic hormone release.

exhibit overt renal dysfunction. Clinical studies indicate that the proximal tubule (PT) is exquisitely vulnerable to a reduction in renal blood flow. Elevated urinary B_2 microglobulin levels (a sensitive marker of proximal tubule function) was noted in otherwise healthy term infants with normal urine output and who delivered with MSAF, when compared with infants with clear amniotic fluid [72]. If the decrease in renal perfusion is marked, necrosis of the tubular epithelium may occur, which results in the clinical syndrome of acute tubular necrosis with oliguria and azotemia [73]. Other organs/systems that may be adversely affected by the reduction in blood flow include: 1. the gastrointestinal tract with an increased potential for necrotizing enterocolitis; 2. pulmonary circulation with an increased risk for pulmonary hypertension; 3. liver with an increased risk for hepatocellular injury potentially resulting in abnormal liver enzymes, hypoglycemia, and disseminated intravascular coagulopathy; 4. muscle, with an increased risk for cellular injury and rhabdomyolysis; 5. hematologic—release of nucleated red blood cells [74,75]; 6. fluid and electrolytes—a reduction in blood flow may be associated with release of antidiuretic hormone, which when coupled with acute tubular necrosis, increases the potential for fluid retention and hyponatremia; and 7. endocrine—suppression of parathyroid hormonal release with the potential for hypocalcemia and hypomagnesemia.

Relationship between systemic organ injury and central nervous system injury

In one prospective study, approximately 60% of "asphyxiated" term newborn infants exhibited single or multiple organ injury [76]. In a second prospective study, 80% of infants exhibited single or multiple organ involvement. Notably, severe CNS injury always occurred with involvement of other organs [77]; however, moderate CNS involvement only was noted in 20% of cases. Renal injury is the best systemic marker of potential brain injury. Thus, the presence of altered renal function—and specifically oliguria—when associated with an abnormal neurologic examination is related to a poor long-term neurologic outcome [78]. Specifically, the odds ratio estimates of poor neurologic outcome in infants who had transient oliguria (urine output <1mL/kg/h for <24 hours) was 2.8 (95% CI, 0.96–8); with persistent oliguria the odds ratio was 5.1 (95% CI, 1.95–13.3) [78]. Most "asphyxiated" babies who have transient oliguria do not exhibit neurologic injury. Finally, up to 10% of "asphyxiated" infants who have normal urine output may exhibit moderate to severe encephalopathy (Table 2). This observation is consistent with the findings of a subsequent study [79].

Neonatal brain imaging

MRI provides the best opportunity to define the extent of CNS injury as well as to determine the potential timing of the insult [1,80–85]. Diffusion-weighted

Table 2
Short- and long-term outcome in term infants with and without oliguria

Population	Persistent oliguria: 36 hours (n=6)	Transient oliguria: 24 hours (n=8)	Normal urine output (n=22)	Total (n=36)
Short-term outcome				
HIE	6	2	2	10
Death	1	0	1	2
Long-term outcome				
Abnormal CNS Examination	4	1	2	7
Normal	1[a]	7	16	24

Abbreviation: HIE, hypoxic-ischemic encephalopathy.
  [a] Significant speech delay.
Adapted from Perlman JM, Tack EC. Renal injury in the asphyxiated newborn infant: relationship to neurological outcome. J Pediatr 1998;113:875–9.

imaging with increased signal intensity secondary to reduced water diffusivity in tissue may be observed within the first 24 to 48 hours following an insult. The distribution of MRI signal abnormalities can be subdivided according to the severity of the insult, and is consistent with the experimental changes [40]. Thus, mild to moderate hypoperfusion is characterized by parasagittal-perirolandic changes, whereas basal ganglia–thalamic changes are observed alone or with cerebral cortical changes with more profound insults [1]. The postnatal evolution of changes over time (ie, hemorrhage or focal cerebral infarction in the context of markers of perinatal stress) strongly supports a relationship with "intrapartum asphyxia." Macroscopic abnormalities (eg, cystic periventricular leukomalacia) on any neuroimaging modality in the immediate neonatal period are indicative of an antepartum insult of long-standing duration [1,86].

Findings necessary to link events during labor with subsequent cerebral palsy

Inclusion criteria

1. A sentinel event that occurs during labor. The healthy fetus has many special physiologic mechanisms to protect the brain from recurrent transient mild hypoxic episodes during labor. For a neurologically intact fetus, who is not compromised by chronic hypoxia, to sustain a neurologically damaging acute insult, a serious pathologic event has to occur [87]. Examples include a fetus with absent fetal heart rate variability with persistent late or variable decelerations, or bradycardia [88], ruptured uterus, placental abruption, cord prolapse, or massive fetal maternal hemorrhage.
2. Evidence of metabolic acidosis in umbilical arterial cord or early neonatal blood, notably a pH of less than 7.00 and a base deficit of greater than 12 mmol/mL [12–17].

3. An Apgar score of less than 3 at 10 minutes or longer is indicative of some form of active resuscitation in the delivery room (eg, intubation with or without CPR) [1,58,89].
4. Early onset of moderate or severe neonatal encephalopathy in infants who are born at greater than 36 weeks' gestation in the absence of other causes of encephalopathy. The pathway from an intrapartum hypoxic-ischemic injury to CP must progress through neonatal encephalopathy [1,3]. In a recent retrospective study, more than 90% of term infants who had neonatal encephalopathy, seizures, or both, and who did not have specific syndromes or major congenital anomalies, had evidence of perinatal-acquired insults [90].
5. Early evidence of multi-system organ involvement [76,77].
6. Neuroimaging that is consistent with acute cerebral injury [1,80–85].

Three points are worthy of further amplification. First, as opposed to the ACOG Task Force criteria [3], the author considers a sentinel event to be the critical and essential first step in linking an intrapartum event to neonatal encephalopathy, and as a potential consequence, CP. Most term infants who are delivered in the presence of severe fetal acidemia are not recognized by intrapartum events and are triaged to the regular nursery and have an uneventful course [14]. Entry criteria for postnatal neuroprotective studies have as one entry criteria, a sentinel event to treat infants who are likely to have had a period of cerebral hypoperfusion shortly before delivery [7,8]. Approximately 50% of infants who present with hypoxic-ischemic encephalopathy do not have evidence of severe fetal acidemia [58] (see later discussion). Second, except for a history of a sentinel event, all of the criteria

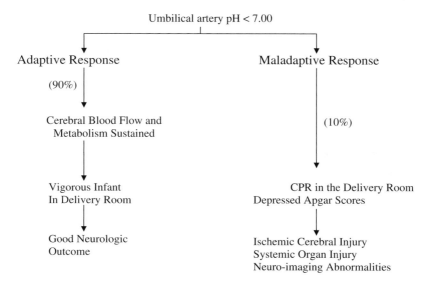

Fig. 4. The response of the fetus to interruption of blood flow with severe fetal acidemia. Note that the overwhelming majority adapt adequately.

are postdelivery assessments. Thus "asphyxia" is a postdelivery diagnosis, and in hindsight is indicative of a maladaptive fetal response to stress (Fig. 4). Finally, a question that is always asked is whether all six criteria are essential to establish the link between intrapartum events and subsequent CP. In the cumulative experience of this author, all criteria are present in greater than 90% of cases.

Exclusion criteria

It is necessary to exclude the following criteria before linking intrapartum asphyxia to hypoxic-ischemic cerebral injury: the absence of previous antenatal injury, no major or multiple congenital or metabolic abnormalities, systemic or central nervous system infection, congenital coagulation disorders, focal cerebral infarction, and no traumatic brain injury [44,68,91–94].

Neonatal encephalopathy occurring in the absence of markers of asphyxia secondary to presumed interruption of placental blood flow

There is a group of term infants that is triaged initially to the regular nursery without any markers of stress; these infants develop a syndrome of neonatal encephalopathy with seizures in the first 12 to 24 hours, exhibit systemic organ dysfunction, and have acute neuroimaging changes in the distribution that are consistent with chronic intermittent interruption of placental blood flow (Figs. 5 and 6). It is the author's experience that this subset of infants accounts for approximately 50% of the cases of neonatal encephalopathy [68]; this is consistent with observations that were made by other investigators [94]. It was

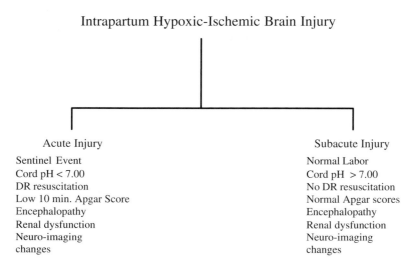

Intrapartum Hypoxic-Ischemic Brain Injury

Acute Injury

Sentinel Event
Cord pH < 7.00
DR resuscitation
Low 10 min. Apgar Score
Encephalopathy
Renal dysfunction
Neuro-imaging
changes

Subacute Injury

Normal Labor
Cord pH > 7.00
No DR resuscitation
Normal Apgar scores
Encephalopathy
Renal dysfunction
Neuro-imaging
changes

Fig. 5. Acute and subacute hypoxic-ischemic brain injury. (DR, delivery room.)

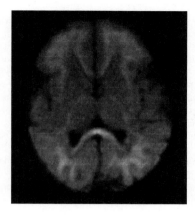

Fig. 6. Diffusion-weighted MRI obtained at 72 hours of age from a term infant who presented with a history of decreased fetal movements 24 hours before a vaginal delivery. Cord arterial pH was normal; the infant required brief bag mask ventilation, had a 5-minute Apgar score of 8, a neurologic examination that was pertinent for marked proximal hypotonia but no seizures, a normal EEG, and transient oliguria. Note the restricted bilateral diffusion within subcortical white matter as well as the posterior limb of the internal capsule.

postulated that these infants suffer a cerebral insult before labor and have a sufficient recovery to exhibit an uncomplicated labor, and then develop a post-natal encephalopathy [94].

Summary

Perinatal hypoxic-ischemic cerebral injury, secondary to intrapartum asphyxia, that results in CP is a rare event in most delivery rooms and neonatal ICUs. The ability to link an intrapartum event to subsequent CP should include a history of a sentinel event during labor, which is followed by the delivery of a depressed acidemic infant, and the subsequent evolution of neonatal encephalopathy, systemic organ injury, and acute neuroimaging abnormalities.

References

[1] Volpe JJ. Neurology of the newborn. 4th edition. Philadelphia: WB Saunders Company; 2001.
[2] Paneth N, Damiano D, Rosenbaum P, et al. The classification of cerebral palsy. Dev Med Child Neuro 2005;46:571–6.
[3] American College of Obstetricians and Gynecologists. Task Force on Neonatal Encephalopathy and Cerebral. Neonatal encephalopathy and cerebral palsy. Washington, DC: American College of Obstetricians and Gynecologists; 2003.
[4] Nelson KB. The epidemiology of cerebral palsy in term infants. Ment Retard Dev Disabil Res Rev 2002;8:146–50.
[5] Blair E, Stanley FJ. Intrapartum asphyxia—a rare cause of cerebral palsy. J Pediatr 1988;112: 515–9.

[6] Torfs CP, Van der berg BJ, Oeschali FW. Prenatal and perinatal factors in the etiology of cere-
     bral palsy. J Pediatr 1990;116:615–9.
[7] Gluckman PD, Wyatt JS, Azzopardi D, et al. Selective head cooling with mild systemic hypo-
     thermia after neonatal encephalopathy: multicentre randomized trial. Lancet 2005;365:663–70.
[8] Shankaran S, Laptook AR, Ehrenkrantz RA, et al. Whole body hypothermia for neonates with
     hypoxic-ischemic encephalopathy. N Engl J Med 2005;353:1574–84.
[9] Low JA, Panagiotopoulos C, Derrick EJ. Newborn complications after intrapartum asphyxia
     with metabolic acidosis in the preterm fetus. Am J Obstet Gynecol 1995;172:805–9.
[10] Freeman JM, Nelson KB. Intrapartum asphyxia and cerebral palsy. Pediatrics 1988;82:240–9.
[11] Towell ME. The rationale for biochemical monitoring of the fetus. J Perinat Med 1988;
     16(Suppl 1):55–70.
[12] Goldaber KG, Gilstrap LC, Leveno KJ, et al. Pathologic fetal acidemia. Obstet Gynecol 1991;
     78:1103–7.
[13] Sehdev HM, Stamilio DM, Macones GA, et al. Predictive factors for neonatal morbidity in
     neonates with an umbilical arterial cord pH less than 7.00. Am J Obstet Gynecol 1997;177:
     1030–4.
[14] King T, Jackson G, Burks M, et al. Unanticipated severe umbilical artery acidemia in term
     infants admitted to a newborn nursery: is it benign? J Pediatr 1998;132:624–9.
[15] Fee SC, Malee K, Deddish R, et al. Severe acidosis and subsequent neurologic status. Am J
     Obstet Gynecol 1990;162:802–6.
[16] Goodwin TM, Belai I, Hernandez P, et al. Asphyxial complications in the term newborn with
     severe umbilical acidemia. Am J Obstet Gynecol 1992;162:1506–12.
[17] Perlman JM, Risser R. Severe fetal acidemia: neonatal neurological features and short term
     outcome. Pediatr Neurol 1992;9:277–82.
[18] Lassen NA, Christensen MS. Physiology of cerebral blood flow. Br J Anaesth 1976;48:719–34.
[19] Behrman RE, Lees MH, Petersen EN, et al. Distribution of circulation in the normal and
     asphyxiated fetal primate. Am J Obstet Gynecol 1970;108:956–69.
[20] Cohn EH, Sacks EJ, Heyman MA, et al. Cardiovascular responses to hypoxemia and acidemia in
     fetal lambs. Am J Obstet Gynecol 1974;120:817–24.
[21] Peeters L, Sheldon R, Jones M, et al. Blood flow to fetal organs as a function of arterial oxygen
     content. Am J Obstet Gynecol 1979;135:637–46.
[22] Vannucci RC, Duffy TE. Cerebral metabolism in newborn dogs during reversible asphyxia. Am
     Neurol 1977;1:528–34.
[23] Dawes G. Foetal and neonatal physiology. Chicago: Year Book Medical Publishers, Inc.; 1968.
[24] Jones Jr MD, Sheldon RE, Peeters LL, et al. Regulation of cerebral blood flow in the ovine
     fetus. Am J Physiol 1978;235:H162–6.
[25] Koehler RC, Jones Jr MD, Traystman RJ. Cerebral circulation response to carbon monoxide and
     hypoxic hypoxia in the lamb. Am J Physiol 1982;243:H27–32.
[26] Ashwal S, Dale PS, Longo ID. Regional cerebral blood flow: studies in the fetal lamb during
     hypoxia, hypercapnia, acidosis and hypotension. Pediatr Res 1984;18:1309–16.
[27] Johnson EW, Palahniwk RJ, Tween WA, et al. Regional cerebral blood flow changes during
     severe fetal asphyxia produced by slow partial umbilical cord compression. Am J Obstet
     Gynecol 1979;135:48–52.
[28] Powers WJ, Grubb Jr RL, Darriet D, et al. Cerebral blood flow and cerebral metabolic rates of
     oxygen requirements for cerebral function and viability in humans. J Cereb Blood Flow Metab
     1985;5:600–8.
[29] Heiss WD, Rosner G. Functional recovery of cortical neurons as related to the degree and
     duration of ischemia. Ann Neurol 1983;14:294–301.
[30] Astrup J, Symon L, Branston NM, et al. Cortical evoked potential and extracellular K^+ and H^+
     at critical levels of brain ischemia. Stroke 1977;8:51–7.
[31] Altman DI, Powers WI, Perlman JM, et al. Cerebral blood flow requirement for brain viability
     in newborn infants is lower than in adults. Ann Neurol 1988;24:218–26.
[32] Duffy TE, Kohle SJ, Vannucci RC. Carbohydrate and energy metabolism in perinatal rat brain:
     relation to survival in anoxia. J Neurochem 1975;24:271–6.

[33] Holowach-Thurston J, McDougal Jr DB. Effects of ischemia on metabolism of the brain of the newborn mouse. Am J Physiol 1964;216:348–52.

[34] Yager J, Heitjan DF, Towfighi J, et al. Effect of insulin-induced and fasting hypoglycemia on perinatal hypoxic ischemic brain damage. Pediatr Res 1992;31:138–42.

[35] Cremer JE. Substrate utilization and brain development. J Cereb Blood Flow Metab 1982;2: 394–407.

[36] Dawes GS, Mott JC, Shelley HJ. The importance of cardiac glycogen for the maintenance of life in foetal lambs and newborn animals during anoxia. J Physiol 1959;146:519–38.

[37] Wells RJ, Friedman WF, Sobel BE. Increased oxidative metabolism in the fetal and neonatal lamb heart. Am J Physiol 1972;222:1488–93.

[38] Wimberley PD. A review of oxygen and delivery in the neonate. Scand J Clin Lab Invest 1982; 160(Suppl):114–8.

[39] Ferreiro DM. Protecting neurons. Epilepsia 2005;46(Suppl 7):45–51.

[40] Myers RE. Four patterns of perinatal brain damage and their conditions of occurrence in the primate. Adv Neurology 1975;10:223–34.

[41] Pasternak JF, Gorey MT. The syndrome of near total asphyxia in the term infant. Pediatr Neurol 1998;18:391–8.

[42] Wu YW, Colford JM. Chorioamnionitis as a risk factor for cerebral palsy. JAMA 2000;284: 1417–24.

[43] Shalak L, Laptook A, Ramilo O, et al. Clinical chorioamnionitis, elevated cytokines and brain injury in term infants. Pediatrics 2002;110:673–80.

[44] Kraus FT, Acheen VI. Fetal thrombotic vasculopathy in the placenta: cerebral thrombi and infarcts, coagulopathies and cerebral palsy. Hum Pathol 1999;30:759–69.

[45] Quilligan EJ, Paul RH. Fetal monitoring: is it worth it. Obstet Gynecol 1975;45:96–110.

[46] Grant A, O'Brien N, Marie-Theriese J, et al. Cerebral palsy among children born during the Dublin randomized trial of intrapartum monitoring. Lancet 1989;111:1233–6.

[47] Painter MJ, Scott M, Hirsch RP, et al. Fetal heart rate patterns during labor: neurologic and cognitive development at six to nine years of age. Am J Obstet Gynecol 1988;159:854–8.

[48] Nelson KB, Ellenberg JH. Obstetric complications as risk factors for cerebral palsy or seizure disorders. JAMA 1984;251:1843–8.

[49] Gregory GA, Gooding CA, Phibbs RH, et al. Meconium aspiration in infants—a prospective study. J Pediatr 1974;85:848–52.

[50] Miller FC, Sacks DA. Significance of meconium during labor. Am J Obstet Gynecol 1975;122: 573–80.

[51] Meis PJ, Hall III M, Marshall JR, et al. Meconium passage. A new classification for risk assessment during labor. Am J Obstet Gynecol 1978;131:509–13.

[52] Abramovici H, Brandes JM, Fuchs K, et al. Meconium during delivery: a sign of compensated fetal distress. Am J Obstet Gynecol 1974;118:251–4.

[53] Yeomans ER, Gilstrap LC, Leveno KJ, et al. Meconium in the amniotic fluid and fetal acid-base status. Obstet Gynecol 1989;73:175–8.

[54] American Academy of Pediatrics. American College of Obstetrics and Gynecologists. Use and abuse of the Apgar score. ACOG Committee Opinion 174. Elk Grove Village (IL): AAP; 1996.

[55] Nelson KB, Ellenberg JH. Apgar score as predictors of chronic neurologic disability. Pediatrics 1981;68:36–44.

[56] Casey BM, McIntire DD, Leveno KJ. The continuing value of the Apgar score for the assessment of newborn infants. N Engl J Med 2001;344:467–71.

[57] Moster D, Lie RT, Irgens LM, et al. The association of Apgar score with subsequent death and cerebral palsy in term infants. J Pediatr 2001;138:798–803.

[58] Perlman JM, Risser R. Cardiopulmonary resuscitation in the delivery room: associated clinical events. Arch Pediatr Adolesc Med 1995;149:20–5.

[59] Perlman JM, Risser R. Can infants with neonatal seizures secondary to perinatal asphyxia be rapidly identified by current high risk markers. Pediatrics 1996;97:456.

[60] DeReuck J. The human periventricular arterial blood supply and the anatomy of cerebral infarctions. Eur Neurol 1973;5:321–34.

[61] Roland EH, Hill A, Rodriguez E, et al. Perinatal hypoxia-ischemic thalamic injury: clinical features and neuroimaging. Ann Neurol 1998;44:161–6.

[62] Takashima S, Tanaka K. Development of cerebrovascular architecture and its relationship to periventricular leukomalacia. Arch Neurol 1978;35:11–6.

[63] Perlman JM, Risser R, Broyles RS. Bilateral cystic periventricular leukomalacia in the premature infant: associated risk factors. Pediatrics 1996;97:822–6.

[64] Rogers B, Msall M, Owens T, et al. Cystic periventricular leukomalacia and type of cerebral palsy in preterm infants. J Pediatr 1994;125:S1–8.

[65] Myers RE. Cerebral ischemia in the developing primate fetus. Biomed Biochim Acta 1989; 48:S137–42.

[66] Perlman JM, Rollins NK, Evans D. Neonatal stroke: clinical characteristics and cerebral blood flow velocity measurements. Pediatr Neurol 1994;11:281–4.

[67] Perlman JM. Brain injury in the term infant. Semin Perinatol 2004;28:415–24.

[68] Sarnat HB, Sarnat MS. Neonatal encephalopathy following fetal distress. A clinical and electro-encephalographic study. Arch Neurol 1976;33:696–705.

[69] Nelson KB, Levinton A. How much of neonatal encephalopathy is due to birth asphyxia? Am J Dis Child 1991;315:81–6.

[70] Dauber IM, Krauss AN, Symchych PS, et al. Renal failure following perinatal anoxia. J Pediatr 1976;88:851–5.

[71] Begwin F, Dunnihood DB, Quilligan EJ. Effect of carbon dioxide elevation on renal blood flow in the fetal lamb in utero. Am J Obstet Gynecol 1974;199:630–5.

[72] Cole JJW, Portman RJ, Lim Y, et al. Urinary B_2 microglobulin in full term infants: evidence for proximal tubular dysfunction in term infants with meconium stained amniotic fluid. Pediatrics 1985;76:958–63.

[73] Stork H, Geiger R. Renal tubular dysfunction following vascular accidents of the kidneys in the newborn period. J Pediatr 1973;83:933–7.

[74] Korst LM, Phelan JP, Ahn MO, et al. Nucleated red blood cells: an update on the marker for fetal asphyxia. Am J Obstet Gynecol 1996;175:843–6.

[75] Phelan JP, Korst LM, Ahn MO, et al. Neonatal nucleated red blood cell and lymphocyte counts in fetal brain injury. Obstet Gynecol 1998;91:485–9.

[76] Perlman JM, Tack EC, Martin T, et al. Acute systemic organ injury in term infants after asphyxia. Am J Dis Child 1989;143:617–20.

[77] Martinancel A, Garcia-Alix A, Gaya F, et al. Multiple organ involvement in perinatal asphyxia. J Pediatr 1995;127:786–93.

[78] Perlman JM, Tack EC. Renal injury in the asphyxiated newborn infant: relationship to neuro-logical outcome. J Pediatr 1998;113:875–9.

[79] Phelan JP, Nelson KB, Ellenberg JH, et al. Intrapartum fetal asphyxial brain injury with absent multiorgan system dysfunction. J Matern Fetal Med 1998;7:19–22.

[80] Barkovich AJ. The encephalopathic neonate: choosing the proper imaging technique. AJNR Am J Neuroradiol 1997;18:1816–20.

[81] Barkovich AJ, Westmark K, Partridge C, et al. Perinatal asphyxia: MR-findings in the first 10 days. AJNR Am J Neuroradiol 1995;16:427–38.

[82] Mercuri E, Guzzetta A, Haataja L, et al. Neonatal neurological examination in infants with hyp-oxic ischemic encephalopathy: correlation with MRI findings. Neuropediatrics 1999;30:83–9.

[83] Robertson R, Ben Sira L, Barnes P, et al. MR line-scan diffusion-weighted imaging of term neonates with perinatal brain ischemia AJNR. AJNR Am J Neuroradiol 1999;20:1658–70.

[84] Saul JS, Robertson RL, Tzika AA, et al. Time course of changes in diffusion-weighted magnetic resonance imaging in a case of neonatal encephalopathy with defined onset and duration of hypoxic-ischemic insult. Pediatrics 2001;35(2):148–51.

[85] Rutherford M, Counsell S, Allsop J, et al. Diffusion-weighted magnetic resonance imaging in term perinatal brain injury. A comparison with site of lesion and time from birth. Pediatrics 2004; 144:1004–14.

[86] Perlman JM. Intrapartum hypoxic-ischemic cerebral injury and subsequent cerebral palsy: medicolegal issues. Pediatrics 1997;99:851–9.

[87] Badawi N, Watson L, Petterson B, et al. What constitutes cerebral palsy? Dev Med Child Neurol 1998;40:520–7.

[88] National Institute of Child Health and Human Development Research Planning Workshop. Electronic fetal heart rate monitoring: research guidelines for interpretation. Am J Obstet Gynecol 1997;177:1385–90.

[89] Nelson KB, Ellenberg JH. Apgar scores as predictors of chronic neurologic disability. Pediatrics 1981;68:36–44.

[90] Cowan F, Rutherford M, Groenendaal F, et al. Origin and timing of brain lesions in term infants with neonatal encephalopathy. Lancet 2003;361:736–42.

[91] Nelson KB, Ellenberg JH. Antecedents of cerebral palsy multivariate analysis of risk. N Engl J Med 1986;315:81–6.

[92] Nelson KB, Grether JK. Potentially asphyxiating conditions and spastic cerebral palsy in infants of normal birth weight. Am J Obstet Gynecol 1998;179:507–13.

[93] Nelson KB, Dambrosia JM, Grether JK, et al. Neonatal cytokines and coagulation factors in children with cerebral palsy. Ann Neurol 1998;44:665–75.

[94] Hull J, Dodd K. What is birth asphyxia? Br J Obstet Gynaecol 1991;98:953–5.

ELSEVIER
SAUNDERS

CLINICS IN
PERINATOLOGY

Clin Perinatol 33 (2006) 355–366

Perinatal Trauma and Cerebral Palsy

Michael J. Noetzel, MD

*Department of Neurology, St. Louis Children's Hospital, Room 12E25, One Children's Place,
St. Louis, MO 63110, USA*

At the outset it must be acknowledged that the term "perinatal trauma" has been used by a variety of investigators to describe a myriad of situations and, thus, if it is to be understood in any meaningful context, a limited definition must be applied. In this article "perinatal trauma" is restricted to injuries that are sustained by the infant during the labor and delivery primarily as a result of mechanical factors [1], with the understanding that even under optimal circumstances, the process of birth is traumatic. Mechanical insults to the perinatal brain may result in primarily a hypoxic or ischemic injury to the cerebral tissues; those conditions are not discussed in this article. Although there are multiple types of perinatal trauma, this article is restricted mainly to those types that impact upon the subsequent development of cerebral palsy, although when applicable, other adverse developmental outcomes are mentioned.

The actual incidence of perinatal trauma that causes injury to central nervous system tissues is difficult to ascertain, even using the restricted definition that was supplied above. It has been estimated that significant birth-related injuries of a physical-traumatic nature—that typically involve the head—account for roughly 2% of all neonatal deaths [2]. Although "traumatic" injuries to the central nervous system can be seen in normal spontaneous births [3], the incidence increases sharply in cases of instrumented delivery or abnormal presentation of the fetus. Over the last 20 years there has been a significant reduction in the occurrence of perinatal trauma to central nervous system structures [1]. Not surprisingly during this same time course, there has been a marked decline in the frequency of forceps- and vacuum-assisted delivery. The latest birth figures for the year 2003 indicate that the combined rate of forceps and vacuum extraction is 5.6%, which represents a 41% decrease compared with the high of 9.5% in 1994

E-mail address: noetzelm@neuro.wustl.edu

[4]. Nonetheless, even in 2003, nearly 230,000 infants were delivered with the assistance of forceps or vacuum extraction.

Perinatal intracranial injuries

Subdural hemorrhage

The prevalence of subdural hemorrhage reported in the literature varies considerably, in part depending upon the route and manner of delivery at the reporting institution. In two large studies the prevalence of subdural or cerebral hemorrhage in spontaneous vaginal deliveries ranged between 1.0 and 2.9 per 10,000 infants (Table 1) [5,6]. In infants who were delivered with the use of vacuum extraction or forceps the prevalence increased considerably to 7 to 9.8 per 10,000 infants; if vacuum and forceps were applied the prevalence increased to 21.3 per 10,000 infants. The combined results of these studies do not indicate any statistically significant increase in intraventricular hemorrhage or subarachnoid bleeding with forceps use. Vacuum extraction, however, was associated with an increased incidence of subarachnoid blood, but no real alteration in the incidence of intraventricular hemorrhage. In one interesting prospective study, MRI scans were obtained on a cohort of normal term asymptomatic babies who were born in the Central Sheffield University Hospitals [3]. Subdural hematomas were identified in 3 of the 49 children who had undergone a spontaneous vaginal delivery, which confirms the concept that apparently "traumatic injuries" to the central nervous system can be seen in normal spontaneous birth.

Table 1
Prevalence of major neonatal intracranial complications associated with methods of delivery

Intracranial condition	Reference	Spontaneous vaginal	Vacuum	Forceps	Both	CS no labor[a]	CS during labor[b]
ICH: all forms	[5]	5.3	11.7	15.7	35.7	4.9	10.5
	[6]	3.0	12	10	n.d.	n.d.	n.d.
	[9]	9	19	11	21	n.d.	n.d.
Subdural/cerebral	[5]	2.9	8.0	9.8	21.3	4.1	6.8
	[6]	1	7	7	n.d.	n.d.	n.d.
Subarachnoid	[5]	1.3	2.2	3.3	10.7	0	1.1
	[6]	1	6	1	n.d.	n.d.	n.d.
IVH	[5]	1.1	1.5	2.6	3.7	0.8	2.6
	[6]	1	1	1	n.d.	n.d.	n.d.

The prevalence is expressed as the number of cases per 10,000 infants.
Abbreviations: ICH, intracranial hemorrhage; IVH, intraventricular hemorrhage; n.d., not determined.
   [a] CS no labor indicates a cesarean delivery before the onset of labor.
   [b] CS during labor refers to a cesarean delivery after the onset of labor, but with no attempt at operative vaginal delivery.

Pathology

Newborn subdural hemorrhage is related most commonly to laceration or injury to the sinuses and veins of the brain. There are three predominant locations for subdural hemorrhage. The first is within the subdural space over the cerebral convexity. Typically, this injury is caused by rupture to the superficial draining veins that cross between the cerebrum and the dura, frequently as a result of rotational movement of the brain within the skull. A newborn brain is particularly at risk for this type of injury because of the large head size combined with the weaker neck musculature that permits greater rotational movement with angular acceleration. These subdural hemorrhages typically are unilateral, but bilateral locations have been described [7]. Concomitant subarachnoid hemorrhages often are diagnosed on CT scan or by way of examination of cerebrospinal fluid. Convexity and other supratentorial hemorrhages also are caused by superior extension of primary posterior fossa hemorrhages (see later discussion).

Posterior fossa hemorrhages, typically located behind the cerebellum, is the second form of traumatic subdural hemorrhages that is seen in infants (Fig. 1). These subdural hemorrhages usually result from tentorial laceration or injury to the transverse or straight sinuses or the vein of Galen. Less commonly, tearing of the cerebellar bridging veins may cause an infratentorial hemorrhage. In rare cases, traumatic breech deliveries can result in posterior fossa subdural hemorrhage and cerebellar lacerations because of mechanical disruption of the squamous and occipital bones with damage to the occipital sinuses. About 50% of the time, tentorial lacerations cause bleeding that spreads superiorly and anteriorly to result in supratentorial hematomas [8]. Parenchymal hemorrhagic injury to the cerebrum or the cerebellum is much less common, and occurs in roughly 10% to 20% of the cases; however, the location and extent of this type of injury may be one of the most important factors in determining long-term outlook.

The third and least consequential form of subdural hemorrhage occurs when there is an injury to the inferior sagittal sinus, typically from a laceration of the

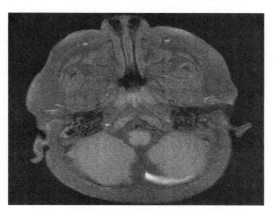

Fig. 1. MRI scan (subtraction views) of a 3-day-old infant who was delivered after vacuum extraction. Image reveals subdural hemorrhage along the left side of the cerebellum in the posterior fossa.

falx. This produces an intrahemispheric bleed along the longitudinal cerebral fissure. As an isolated phenomenon, this type of injury is uncommon compared with the above described entities; however, it often is found in conjunction with, and as an extension of, a posterior fossa hemorrhage.

Pathogenesis

Difficult delivery that mandates vacuum extraction, forceps use, or both is noted frequently in instances of newborn subdural hemorrhage [5,6,9]. The mechanism by which vacuum extraction causes subdural hemorrhage secondary to tentorial laceration or hemorrhage is well delineated [10]. The forces that are generated on the newborn head by a vacuum extractor can result in oblique elongation of the cranium and, in some instances, tentorial laceration or venous stretching and rupture of vessels. In contrast, cerebral convexity subdural hemorrhages are believed to relate to extreme vertical molding with resultant tearing of the bridging cortical vessels [11]. In addition to instrumented delivery, however, a variety of considerations and factors impact upon or predispose to the manner of delivery, as well as the duration and progression of labor. For example, an instrumented assisted delivery is much more frequent in infants with higher birth weights and greater gestational ages. In addition, forceps delivery, in particular, tends to occur more frequently in pregnancies that are complicated by dystocia, pregnancy-induced hypertension, abruptio placentae, or amniotic fluid infection, and in mothers who have delivered babies by previous cesarean section [6]. Older mothers, who also are more likely to have instrumented deliveries, may have more rigid pelvic structures and often experience labor that is unusually brief (not allowing enough time for dilation of the pelvic structures) or unusually long (subjecting the head to prolonged molding and compression). There are some data to suggest that intracranial hemorrhage in neonates (as well as other forms of newborn injury) may be due to dysfunctional labor, rather than the resultant operative intervention [5]. In a study using a large California database, researchers demonstrated that the rate of intracranial hemorrhage associated with cesarean section before the onset of labor did not differ significantly from that seen in uncomplicated spontaneous vaginal delivery (see Table 1). In contrast, the frequency of subdural or cerebral hemorrhage in neonates who were born by cesarean delivery during labor with no attempted vacuum extraction or forceps use did not differ significantly from the rates that were observed in newborns who were delivered by operative vaginal delivery. Thus, the investigators suggested that the method of delivery may not be the primary factor associated with traumatic newborn intracranial hemorrhage [5]. A more recent smaller study failed to duplicate these findings. Using Washington state birth certificate data, the investigators noted that the incidence of intracranial hemorrhage in infants who were exposed to vacuum extraction and forceps did not decrease, even when adjustment was made for labor augmentation, dysfunctional labor, and other pregnancy complications, such as chronic hypertension, preeclampsia, and diabetes [9].

Trauma in isolation is not the only consideration in the pathogenesis of newborn intracranial hemorrhage. Subdural hemorrhage, and, in fact, all serious intracranial hemorrhages have been reported to occur in utero, sometimes in the context of fetal–maternal trauma [7]. In more recent reports the association of fetal and newborn hemorrhage has been documented in cases of disorders that affect the coagulation pathways and delayed-onset vitamin K deficiency, including infants whose delivery was by way of instrumentation [12,13].

Diagnosis, clinical features, and outcome

The advent of imaging technology (especially CT and MRI) has enhanced greatly our ability to diagnosis neonatal subdural hemorrhage [14]. Brain imaging also provides detailed information regarding the size and extent of the bleed. Not surprisingly, we also are recognizing that radiologically apparent subdural hemorrhage need not produce any clinical or neurologic signs or can be manifest by minimal and nonspecific difficulties. Improvement in brain imaging also has provided greater prognostic information.

Cerebral convexity subdural hemorrhages. Depending upon their size and location, these subdural hemorrhages may not produce any disturbance in newborn neurologic function or abnormalities on examination. In larger lesions, focal signs of hemiparesis or impaired extraocular motions are seen typically, and often are associated with seizures. In these patients, detailed imaging studies may reveal intracerebral hemorrhagic contusions. The outcome for convexity subdural hemorrhages mirrors the clinical and radiologic presentation. Death is uncommon and when it occurs it typically relates to other factors, such as an underlying coagulation disorder [12]. Infants who have no or minimal neurologic abnormalities can expect uniformly normal developmental outcomes. In patients who have signs of focal or cortical disturbance (and hence, most of those who have intracerebral hemorrhage underlying the subdural) the outlook is still good with roughly 60% to 80% of the infants being normal (although in these studies the length of follow-up often is only 1–2 years) [12,15]. Those children who are affected long-term often have alterations in tone (hypotonia and hypertonia) along with psychomotor delay, and less frequently, findings that are consistent with cerebral palsy [16].

Posterior fossa subdural hematomas. Infants who have these hemorrhages have a higher incidence of morbidity and mortality, related mainly to the degree of subdural bleeding and the presence of major lacerations of the tentorium. In cases of massive infratentorial bleeding, infants typically demonstrate signs of brainstem dysfunction shortly after delivery with rapid progression to bradycardia and coma, as the clot further compresses the brainstem. In the absence of neurosurgical intervention, death ensues within 1 or 2 days. This rapidly lethal syndrome typifies roughly 5% of cases of all posterior fossa subdural hemorrhage, whereas previously as many as 40% to 50% of infants left unoperated expired. The neurologic outcome for children who survive this injury is judged to be quite good. Approximately 80% of surgically treated infants and 88% of infants who do not require evacuation of their hematoma are believed to be normal or to have minor neurologic deficits on follow-up [11], although some of these infants do develop communicating hydrocephalus that necessitates placement of a shunt system. Increased intracranial pressure (ICP) has been recognized as a strong predictor of poor outcome. In one report of 6 infants with an ICP of less than 300 mm H_2O, all were judged to be neurologically normal at follow-up ranging between 6 months and 3 years [15]. In contrast, only 4 of 7 infants with an ICP of more than 300 mm H_2O were normal. Volpe's [11] review of the literature, combined with his personal cases, indicated that major neurologic sequelae were found in 7% of the unoperated patients; 13% of those infants required surgical evacuation of subdural hemorrhages. Included in this group are cases of spastic and hypotonic cerebral palsy [10]. In another series from Toronto, 15 neonates who had posterior fossa subdural hemorrhage were managed between 1986 and 1995; 7 children were neurologically normal and 3 had only mild neurologic findings [17]. Length of follow-up ranged from 2 to 10 years, with a mean of 4.5 years. In contrast, 3 survivors had a profound neurologic disorder, including 2 patients who had hemiplegic cerebral palsy. There was no consistent relationship between the location of subdural hematoma and the pattern of neurologic deficits; however, on follow-up scans the 3 severely affected children had CT evidence of supratentorial parenchymal injury in conjunction with the posterior fossa subdural hemorrhages, including cerebral atrophy, porencephaly, and cortical calcification [17].

Epidural hemorrhage

Epidural hemorrhage or hematoma occurs rarely in a newborn (Fig. 2). Review articles suggest that less than 50 cases have been reported in the literature

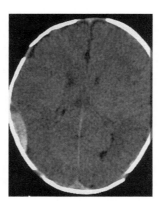

Fig. 2. CT scan on a newborn who was delivered with forceps use. An elliptical-shaped hyperdense extra-axial fluid collection in the right parietal region is diagnostic of an epidural hematoma. There is some mass effect on the underlying brain. A linear skull fracture was noted on other images.

[18,19]. Autopsy information indicates that epidural hemorrhage constitutes roughly 2% of all cases of intracranial hemorrhage in newborns [20]. The rarity of this condition often has been ascribed to one of two factors. First, at this stage of development the middle meningeal artery has not developed fully. Second, in infants the dura mostly is contiguous with the inner periosteum and cannot be detached easily from the overlying skull.

Pathology

In most newborns, epidural hematomas are believed to result from bleeding into this space as a result of laceration or tearing of major veins, the venous sinuses, or branches of the middle meningeal artery.

Pathogenesis

Most cases described in the literature suggest that neonatal epidural hematoma results from instrumented deliveries or other complications during labor and delivery [18,19]. Excessive molding or forces that are generated during delivery produce local stress that causes the dura mater to detach from the skull. This results in a severing of the vessels that connect the inner periosteum and the skull. Data combined from three large series that were published over the last several years indicate that trauma does play a major role in the generation of epidural hematomas, but may not explain each case examined in isolation (Table 2) [12,18,19]. In one study roughly half of the patients were delivered by forceps or with vacuum extraction [18]. In a second report, instrumentation was used in 9 of the 15 infants; 3 of these infants ultimately were delivered by cesarean section because the attempted instrumented delivery was unsuccessful. In the three reports, skull fractures were diagnosed in 21 of the 36 infants (58%) and cephalohematomas were found in 19 (53%). Abnormal position during labor, including breech and occipito-sacral presentation, were noted in 5 infants. Only 8 of the 36 had a spontaneous vaginal delivery (22%; including one infant whose injury occurred after being dropped on the labor room floor). This combination of data strongly suggests that epidural hematomas in neonates is a trauma-related phenomenon, primarily through the use of forceps or vacuum extraction.

Table 2
Modes of delivery and clinical features associated with neonatal epidural hemorrhage

Reference	Abnormal position[a]	Instrumented	Spontaneous vaginal	C-section	Skull fracture	Cephalohematoma	Seizures
[12]	1/3	2/3	0	0	2/3	3/3	1/3
[18]	4/18	8/18	5/18	1/18	9/18	11/18	n.r.
[19]	n.r.	9/15	3/15	6/15[b]	10/15	5/15	8/15

Abbreviation: n.r., not recorded.
  [a] Includes breech in four cases and an occipitosacral presentation in one infant.
  [b] Includes three infants who failed attempts at instrumented (forceps or vacuum) vaginal delivery.

Diagnosis, clinical features, and outcome

A typical presentation in an infant who has an epidural hematoma is progressive scalp swelling (secondary to the commonly associated cephalohematoma), followed by signs of raised intracranial pressure (typically within the first day of life), including a bulging anterior fontanel and hypotonia, and subsequently, stupor and coma. Seizures have been reported in approximately 50% of the cases (Table 2) [12,18,19]. Diagnosis is confirmed by CT or MRI. Ultrasound is not reliable in diagnosing extradural hematomas in neonates [19]. After the hematoma has been identified, surgical evacuation of a clot can be performed, if indicated. Alternatively, successful treatment has been rendered through needle aspiration of the hematoma itself or of the overlying cephalohematoma if there is communication with the epidural space through a fracture site [18,19,21].

The outcome of newborn epidural hematoma as described in the literature is polar. In Akiyama and colleagues' [18] survey article on 18 patients who had birth trauma–related epidural hematomas, 5 patients died, including 3 infants whose injuries were complicated by subdural and intraventricular hemorrhage. Of the 13 survivors, however, 12 were judged to have a good outcome and only a single child had psychomotor delay. In a large study from France that spanned 24 years (1979–2002), Heyman and colleagues [19] reported on 15 newborns who had epidural hematomas (including the one whose epidural hematoma occurred after being dropped on the labor room floor). There were no deaths among these infants. Of the 12 patients who were available for testing, 8 children had normal neurologic and psychomotor examination at follow-up (range, 6 months to 6 years). Three children had moderate neurologic deficits or psychomotor delay and a single child had severe neurologic disability that included cerebral palsy.

Intraparenchymal hemorrhage

Intracerebral hemorrhage in a neonate rarely is an isolated phenomenon, if the injury stems primarily from mechanical factors. More commonly it is associated with depressed skull fractures and subarachnoid hemorrhage [12], as well as epidural hematomas (Fig. 3). In one study, 20% of newborns who had epidural hematomas had evidence of a cortical contusion, some of which evolved into porencephalic cavities [19]. Additionally, ischemic cortical involvement can be related to direct trauma or a stretch injury of an intracranial vessel [22,23]. Isolated trauma-induced cerebellar hemorrhage also is uncommon. More typically, traumatic tentorial laceration and injury to the sinuses or the vein of Galen produce a posterior fossa hematoma that is associated with a cerebellar parenchymal hemorrhage in about 16% of the cases [8].

Subarachnoid hemorrhage

Trauma seems to play some role in the genesis of primary subarachnoid hemorrhage (SAH) in neonates, given the increased frequency with which it is docu-

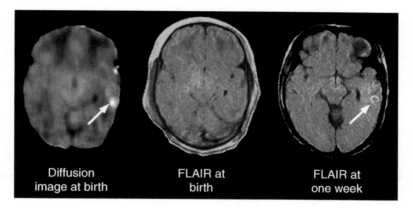

Fig. 3. MRIs of a term infant who has a temporal lobe injury that was sustained at birth in relation to a forceps delivery and skull fracture. The leftmost two images were obtained within 24 hours of birth. The diffusion image shows the lesion as a bright area of low water apparent diffusion coefficient (*arrow*). The fluid-attenuation inversion recovery (FLAIR) image does not show the injury at this time. At 1 week, the injury is confirmed on the FLAIR image (*arrow*). At one week, the injury was not detectable on the diffusion image (image not shown). This reflects the usual progression of MRI findings following trauma. (Courtesy of J.J. Neil, MD, PhD, St. Louis, MO).

mented in instrumented deliveries, especially those in which forceps and vacuum are used [5,6]. In addition, SAH often is associated with skull fractures [12]. The prognosis for neonates who have SAH is dependent mainly on the presence, size, and extent of other traumatic central nervous system injuries. Thus, the overwhelming majority do well, especially the patients who have isolated SAH. The small subset of infants that demonstrates a catastrophic deterioration, followed shortly thereafter by death, typically sustained overwhelming perinatal asphyxia in addition to any traumatic events [11].

Perinatal extracranial injuries

Skull fractures

Typically, skull fractures that are diagnosed in newborns are linear or depressed. Linear fractures have been observed anywhere on the cranium, but usually occur in the parietal region. Linear fractures may result from pressure of the skull against the maternal bony pelvis before delivery or as a result of instrumentation, in particular, the use of forceps. Skull fractures may reflect other intracranial complications, but most commonly are an isolated phenomenon. In an otherwise neurologically normal newborn there are no data to indicate that further imaging studies of the brain are warranted; however, follow-up skull radiographs should be obtained after several months to document that there has not been interval development of a leptomeningeal cyst. Depressed or ping-pong skull fractures also are believed to be closely related to instrumented delivery. In one study, 87.5% of the infants who had a depressed skull fracture were delivered with the use of forceps [24]. In contrast to linear fractures, infants who have depressed skull fractures require close neurologic assessment, as well as a CT scan of the brain to assess for the possibility of extradural and subdural hemorrhage or other intraparenchymal injury. In the absence of these, normal development is expected.

Cephalohematomas

Cephalohematomas occur in approximately 2% of all live births. The incidence increases in individuals who were delivered with the use of vacuum extraction or forceps [6]. The blood is localized below the periosteum, and thus, is confined by the anatomy of cranial sutures. Although the size of a cephalohematoma often increases after birth, it rarely grows large enough to cause neurologic issues. Cephalohematomas may be accompanied by more significant intracranial pathology. By themselves, however, they have no clinical impact and do not affect neurodevelopmental outcome.

Subgaleal hemorrhage

In contrast to cephalohematomas, subgaleal hemorrhage occurs beneath the aponeurosis covering the scalp. The overall prevalence was reported to range between 4 and 60 per 10,000 live births [25]. Subgaleal hemorrhage occurs more commonly in deliveries that are performed by vacuum extraction; in those instances it is believed to be secondary to external compression and dragging forces. Infants who have abnormalities in the coagulation system also have been described [13]. In general, neonatal subgaleal hematomas are benign and the long-term outlook is good, even in cases that are associated with other head trauma and the clinical features of neonatal encephalopathy [26]. There are rare instances, however, in which a large hematoma results in consumption of intravascular clotting factors with continued rebleeding, ultimately causing massive hemorrhage into the subgaleal space. Hypovolemia and exsanguination have been reported, although uncommonly. Additionally, there is a report of two newborn infants whose subgaleal hematomas became so large that there was subsequent vascular compromise of the head and neck that caused diffuse cerebral edema [25]. Although one patient made a good recovery, the other infant died.

Summary

Intracranial injuries from perinatal trauma are associated strongly with vacuum extraction and use of forceps during delivery. There is, however, some evidence to suggest that intracranial hemorrhage in newborns may be due to dysfunctional labor rather than to the resultant operative intervention. In general, the outcome for recovery from the traumatic injuries is good. Death occurs infrequently and then usually as a consequence of overwhelming hemorrhage into the posterior fossa or as a result of a disorder in coagulation. Most infants who have perinatal intracranial trauma develop in a normal fashion, but approximately 10% to 15% demonstrate severe neurologic sequelae, including spastic and hypotonic forms of cerebral palsy.

Acknowledgments

The author wishes to thank Dr. Jeffrey J. Neil for his kind assistance in providing Fig. 3, along with its detailed interpretation.

References

[1] Volpe JJ. Injuries of extracranial, cranial, intracranial, spinal cord and peripheral nervous system structures. In: Neurology of the newborn. 4th edition. Philadelphia: W.B. Saunders; 2001. p. 813–38.

[2] Leestma JE. Forensic neuropathology. In: Duckett S, editor. Pediatric neuropathology. Baltimore: Williams and Wilkins; 1995. p. 243–83.

[3] Whitby EH, Griffiths PD, Rutter S, et al. Frequency and natural history of subdural heamorrhages in babies and relation to obstetric factors. Lancet 2003;362:846–51.

[4] Martin JA, Hamilton BE, Sutton PD, et al. Births: final data for 2003. Natl Vital Stat Rep 2005;54(2):1–116.

[5] Towner D, Castro MA, Eby-Wilkens E, et al. Effect of mode of delivery in nulliparous women on neonatal intracranial injury. N Engl J Med 1999;314:1709–14.

[6] Wen SW, Liu S, Kramer MS, et al. Comparison of maternal and infant outcomes between vacuum extraction and forceps deliveries. Am J Epidemiol 2001;153:103–7.

[7] Stephens RP, Richardson AC, Lewin JS. Bilateral subdural hematomas in a newborn infant. Pediatrics 1997;99(4):619–21.

[8] Welch K, Strand R. Traumatic and parturitional intracranial hemorrhage. Dev Med Child Neurol 1986;28:156–64.

[9] Gardella C, Taylor M, Benedetti T, et al. The effect of sequential use of vacuum and forceps for assisted vaginal delivery on neonatal and maternal outcomes. Am J Obstet Gynecol 2001; 185:896–902.

[10] Hanigan WC, Morgan AM, Stahlberg LK, et al. Tentorial hemorrhage associated with vacuum extraction. Pediatrics 1990;85(4):534–9.

[11] Volpe JJ. Intracranial hemorrhage: subdural, primary subarachnoid, intracerebellar, intraventricular (term infant), and miscellaneous. In: Neurology of the newborn. 4th edition. Philadelphia: W.B. Saunders; 2001. p. 397–427.

[12] Vinchon M, Pierrat V, Tchofo PJ, et al. Traumatic intracranial hemorrhage in newborns. Childs Nerv Syst 2005;21:1042–8.

[13] Guilcher GMT, Scully M-F, Harvey M, et al. Treatment of intracranial and extracranial haemorrhages in a neonate with severe haemophilia B with recombinant factor IX infusion. Haemophilia 2005;11:411–4.

[14] McKinstry RC, Miller JH, Snyder AZ, et al. A prospective, longitudinal diffusion tensor imaging study of brain injury in newborns. Neurology 2002;59:824–33.

[15] Hayashi T, Hashimoto T, Fukuda S, et al. Neonatal subdural hematoma secondary to birth injury. Clinical analysis of 48 survivors. Childs Nerv Syst 1987;3(1):23–9.

[16] Hanigan WC, Powell FC, Miller TC, et al. Symptomatic intracranial hemorrhage in full term infants. Childs Nerv Syst 1995;11(12):698–707.

[17] Perrin RG, Rutka JT, Drake JM, et al. Management and outcomes of posterior fossa subdural hematomas in neonates. Neurosurg 1997;40(6):1190–200.

[18] Akiyama Y, Moritake K, Maruyama N, et al. Acute epidural hematoma related to cesarean section in a neonate with Chiari II malformation. Childs Nerv Syst 2001;17:290–3.

[19] Heyman R, Heckly A, Magagi J, et al. Intracranial epidural hematoma in newborn infants: clinical study of 15 cases. Neurosurg 2005;57:924–9.

[20] Takagi T, Nagai R, Wakabayashi S, et al. Extradural hemorrhage in the newborn as a results of birth trauma. Childs Brain 1978;4:306–18.

[21] Vachharajani A, Mathur A. Ultrasound-guided needle aspiration of cranial epidural hematoma in a neonate: treating a rare complication of vacuum extraction. Am J Perinatol 2002;19(8):401–4.

[22] Govaert P, Vanhaesebrouck P, de Praeter C. Traumatic neonatal intracranial bleeding and stroke. Arch Dis Child 1992;67(7 Spec):339–40.

[23] Kumar M, Avdic S, Paes B. Contralateral cerebral infarction following vacuum extraction. Am J Perinatol 2004;21(1):15–7.

[24] Harwood-Nash DC, Hendrick EB, Hudson AR. The significance of skull fracture in childhood: a study of 1,187 patients. Radiology 1971;101:151–6.

[25] Amar AP, Aryan HE, Meltzer HS, et al. Neonatal subgaleal hematoma causing brain compression: report of two cases and review of the literature. Neurosurg 2003;52:1470–4.

[26] Chadwick LM, Pemberton PJ, Kurinczuk JJ. Neonatal subgaleal haematoma: associated risk factors, complications and outcome. J Paediatr Child Health 1996;32(3):228–32.

ELSEVIER
SAUNDERS

CLINICS IN
PERINATOLOGY

Clin Perinatol 33 (2006) 367–386

Cerebral Palsy Secondary to Perinatal Ischemic Stroke

Adam Kirton, MD, MSc, FRCPC, Gabrielle deVeber, MD, MHSc, FRCPC*

Children's Stroke Program, Division of Neurology, The Hospital for Sick Children, 555 University Avenue, Toronto, Ontario M5G1X8, Canada

Arterial ischemic stroke (AIS) in the neonate is a clinicoradiographic diagnosis of cerebral infarction within an arterial distribution and accounts for more than two thirds of ischemic neonatal strokes [1]. The incidence of pediatric AIS is highest in the perinatal period, when symptomatic diagnosis occurs in about 1 in 4000 live births [2–4], although some studies suggest a higher incidence [5–7]. For the discussion in this article, perinatal arterial ischemic stroke (PAS) is defined as occurring between birth and 28 days postnatal age in term or near-term infants, with subsequent distinctions for premature infants and presumed pre- or perinatal AIS to be made.

Approximately half of PAS presents acutely, usually as seizures [3,8,9], which are more likely to be focal clonic convulsions beginning after the first 12 hours of life and without other signs of encephalopathy [10]. Focal neurologic signs such as hemiparesis are present in less than 25% of cases [1,11,12]. Large cortically based infarcts are the most common pattern, the vast majority occurring in the middle cerebral artery (MCA) territory, and, for unknown reasons, there is preferential involvement of the left side (Fig. 1) [5,13–18]. AIS recurrence rates are low in neonates (approximately 3% to 5%) [1,19] and typically affect only children with chronic risk factors such as congenital heart disease or prothrombotic disorders [19]. Case fatality rates may be up to tenfold higher when compared with those for older children [20].

AIS in the preterm neonate and presumed pre- or peri-natal AIS are two additional forms of AIS that deserve consideration. Less is known about AIS

---

* Corresponding author.
E-mail address: gabrielle.deveber@sickkids.ca (G. deVeber).

doi:10.1016/j.clp.2006.03.008

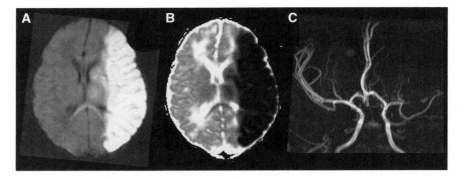

Fig. 1. Neonatal AIS. A day 3 term neonate presented with focal right-sided seizures at 9 hours of life. (*A*) Bright signal on diffusion-weighted MRI coupled with (*B*) decreased signal on the apparent diffusion coefficient map were consistent with ischemic infarction in the left MCA territory. (*C*) Time-of-flight MR angiography demonstrates loss of flow distal to the left MCA bifurcation.

in the preterm infant, although evidence supports its occurrence [18,21,22]. In one study of selected neonatal intensive care unit patients screened with cranial ultrasound, MCA infarcts were detected at comparable frequencies in infants born before and after 34 weeks' gestation [18]. Lenticulostriate branches and multifocal lesions may be more common in premature neonates, whereas main MCA branch occlusions dominate at term [18,23]. The development of cerebral palsy after preterm AIS is not well described and is complicated by other more common mechanisms of vascular preterm brain injury, such as periventricular leukomalacia and germinal matrix hemorrhage, which may co-occur [18].

Presumed pre- or perinatal AIS refers to a group of children who are neurologically normal in the neonatal period but are subsequently recognized retrospectively to have had a stroke at or around the time of birth. Most of these patients present with signs of hemiparesis in the first year of life, usually between 4 and 8 months, although seizures and other neurologic deficits are often present

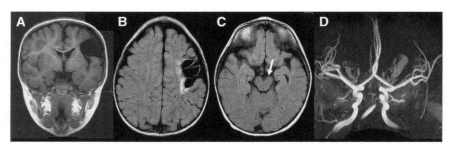

Fig. 2. Presumed perinatal stroke. A 2-year-old boy presented with chronic right spastic hemiparesis. (*A*) Coronal T1 and (*B*) axial FLAIR MRI demonstrated a well-demarcated, focal area of cystic encephalomalacia with surrounding gliosis consistent with an old branch MCA infarct. (*C*) There was atrophy of the left cerebral peduncle (*arrow*) secondary to Wallerian degeneration of the descending corticospinal tracts. (*D*) MR angiogram demonstrates patency of major vessels with mild decreased arborization in the left hemisphere.

[14,16,24]. Structural neuroimaging reveals remote AIS, with most events occurring in the MCA territory, although large and small vessel patterns are observed (Fig. 2).

Perinatal cerebral sinovenous thrombosis

Cerebral sinovenous thrombosis (CSVT) refers to thrombosis within the cerebral venous system. The incidence is highest in the neonatal period, when it accounts for about 30% of perinatal ischemic strokes and may be underrecognized [25]. Neonatal CSVT can present with seizures or, infrequently, neurologic deficits [25,26]. Between 40% and 50% of patients sustain a venous infarction, with hemorrhagic transformation of the infarct and intraventricular hemorrhage being common additional complications [25–27].

Diagnosis

Because of the lack of sensitive or specific clinical markers, accurate diagnosis of perinatal strokes relies on neuroimaging, advances in which have greatly improved recognition in the last decade. Cranial ultrasound can diagnose perinatal stroke [18] but is insensitive [5,28]. CT is helpful in confirming the diagnosis of AIS and CSVT, and CT venography is particularly useful in the diagnosis of neonatal CSVT (Fig. 3) [29]. CT can usually be performed rapidly without sedation and is effective in excluding hemorrhage. Limitations include a lack of sensitivity in the acute time frame, insensitivity to small or infratentorial lesions, and the risk of radiation to the neonatal brain.

MRI is the investigation of choice for most neonatal cerebrovascular disorders including AIS and preterm cerebral lesions. Diffusion-weighted imaging (DWI) is the gold standard for the diagnosis of cerebral infarction in the acute time frame in the neonate [3], although the time window for capturing DWI signal after stroke may be narrower than in adults [30]. Demonstration of restricted diffusion within a vascular territory (see Fig. 1) is highly suggestive of infarction and limits the time of occurrence to approximately within the preceding week. Structural MR recognizes specific chronic changes that occur after stroke (well-circumscribed cystic encephalomalacia, gliosis, focal ventricular dilatation) and allows the diagnosis of presumed perinatal infarction to be made retrospectively (Fig. 2) [16,31,32]. For retrospective and, in particular, acute diagnosis of all neonatal strokes, the dramatic improvements in diagnostic sensitivity and specificity in the last 10 to 20 years should not be underestimated. It is likely that the insensitivity of previous methods often missed the diagnoses, which may explain, in part, why the relative importance of perinatal stroke in cerebral palsy pathogenesis has only recently been appreciated.

MR angiography further increases diagnostic accuracy by confirming arterial occlusion in some infants with perinatal AIS (see Fig. 1) [3,5,33,34]. MR venog-

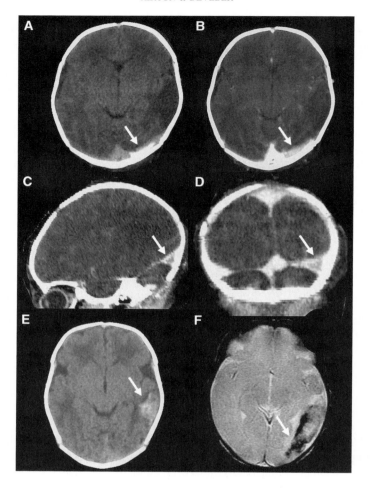

Fig. 3. Neonatal CSVT. A day 3 term neonate presented with focal clonic seizures. (*A*) Unenhanced CT demonstrates hyperdense thrombus in the left transverse sinus (LTS) (*arrow*) and venous infarction of the left temporal lobe. (*B*) Contrast-enhanced CT venography demonstrates a corresponding filling defect (*arrows*) in the LTS that is best appreciated on (*C*) sagittal and (*D*) coronal reformats. MRI performed 4 days later demonstrated hemorrhagic transformation of the infarct (*arrows*) on contiguous T1 (*E*) and gradient echo (*F*) sequences.

raphy can provide supporting evidence of CSVT in the neonate, although the diagnosis can be difficult [25,29]. Contrast-enhanced, rather than time-of-flight, MR angiography and MR venography may increase the accuracy of cerebrovascular imaging in stroke but have not been applied routinely to the neonatal population. Advanced MR neuroimaging is rapidly expanding in neonatal stroke research. Diffusion tensor imaging (DTI) can image functional white matter tracts in the brain, may offer valuable prognostic information in adult stroke [35], and appears feasible in neonates [36]. Functional MRI (fMRI) studies are providing valuable understanding of reorganization patterns after neonatal stroke [37,38]. In addition to neuroimaging, extensive investigations are required to screen for the multitude of potential risk factors for neonatal strokes. Electroencephalography (EEG) is an important investigational tool in perinatal stroke in which seizures are often subclinical and may worsen secondary brain injury [4,10].

Stroke mimics and other patterns of neonatal ischemic brain injury

Global hypoxic-ischemic insults, a common mechanism of ischemic brain injury in the term neonate [39], are not always easily distinguishable from stroke, and the two may occur together [40]. The previously held belief that much of cerebral palsy was related to global injuries and birth "asphyxia" in the term infant has gradually faded, supporting the importance of other contributors such as stroke [39,41]. Different patterns of global hypoxic-ischemic brain injury are well described elsewhere [39]. Watershed infarction occurs when global cerebral hypoperfusion generates ischemic lesions in terminal vascular beds between different vascular territories. Such lesions can mimic AIS, particularly when they are asymmetrical or other patterns of hypoxic-ischemic encephalopathy are absent. Watershed infarction may also occur in the brainstem, where it has been suggested as a cause of several congenital neurologic syndromes [42]. Abnormal arteriography or venography, combined with the absence of recognized global patterns of injury such as basal ganglia lesions or elevated lactate on MR spectroscopy, favors the diagnosis of ischemic stroke. When asymmetrical, they can also resemble ischemic stroke. Another example is the recent suggestion that hemiparetic cerebral palsy secondary to in utero unilateral periventricular venous infarction may occur with similar but distinctly different neuroimaging features from neonatal AIS [43].

Pathophysiology: shared risk factors for perinatal stroke and cerebral palsy

A unique aspect of stroke-induced cerebral palsy is the relatively clear pathophysiologic event that underlies it. Blockage of a cerebral artery or vein leads to regional ischemia, hypoxia, and infarction that produce a focal circumscribed lesion usually isolated to a single well-defined region of the developing brain with sparing of remaining parenchyma. A long list of risk factors and associations have been described for AIS and CSVT in the neonate and can be defined in about two thirds of cases [3,16,25]. These associations also overlap with known risk factors for cerebral palsy, and possible connections between the two are proposed. Because of the small volume and relatively recent onset of active research into the causes of perinatal stroke, the strength of many proposed associations is weak, and the evidence required to establish a true causative role of

Table 1
Summary of investigational approaches in neonatal stroke

Investigations	Comments
Neuroimaging	Brain parenchyma: In all cases, MRI with diffusion is ideal; use CT as needed.
	Arterial: Consider MR angiography of the head and neck if concern for vasculopathy (eg, infection, dissection, trauma); need for cerebral angiography is rare.
	Venous: Obtain MR or CT venogram if unable to rule out CSVT/venous infarction.
History	Prenatal history: Document infertility, recurrent early pregnancy loss, fetal growth and movements, infections, bleeding, diabetes, hypertension, drug abuse (cocaine), smoking.
	Perinatal history: Document maternal fever, placental abnormality, cord abnormality, fetal status (heart rate, decelerations, gases), mode of delivery, prolonged rupture of membranes (>24 h), prolonged second stage of labor (>2 h), Apgar score, cord gas, resuscitation.
	Past medical history: Document cardiac disease, systemic thrombosis, feeding and growth, hydration, infection, interventions.
	Family history: Document maternal or family history of thrombosis (DVT, recurrent early pregnancy loss, young myocardial infarction, or stroke).
Physical	Document vital signs, growth parameters, fluid status.
	Look at fontanelle (bulging, pulsatile), dilated head and neck veins (CSVT), papilledema, asymmetric movements or primitive reflexes, seizure activity, focal neurologic deficits (uncommon).
Laboratory	
Cardiac	Obtain echocardiogram and perform ECG with or without cardiac monitoring for rhythm disturbance.
	Consider venous ultrasound if potential R$\rightarrow$L shunting.
Infectious/ inflammatory	Obtain CBC, CRP, blood cultures; perform TORCH screen as indicated. Check CSF for cells, protein, glucose, cultures.
Hematology	Obtain CBC to rule out anemia/polycythemia/thrombocytosis.
Prothrombotic	Initial screen[a]: Perform assay for protein C, protein S, APCR, fibrinogen, antithrombin, lipoprotein (a), ACLA, LAC, PTT, INR.
	Follow-up (3–6 months): Perform assay for factor V Leiden, prothrombin gene mutation, MTHFR, lipoprotein (a), homocysteine, factors VIII/IX/XI.
	Consider evaluating mother or parents if positive maternal or family history.
EEG	Obtain EEG for any suspected seizures.
Systemic	Consider liver enzymes, renal function, cardiac enzymes/troponin, as well as MR spectroscopy to assess for diffuse hypoxic or ischemic injury.
Placenta	Perform pathologic examination if available.

Once a diagnosis is made from neuroimaging, a systematic evaluation for potential risk factors should be completed. A causal relationship for many risk factors remains unproven (see text). Reasonable routine investigations are listed, although some would be considered experimental. Additional historical, physical, or investigational approaches may be indicated.

Abbreviations: ACLA, anticardiolipin antibodies; APCR, activated protein C resistance; CBC, complete blood count; CRP, C-reactive protein; CSF, cerebrospinal fluid; DVT, deep vein thrombosis; INR, international normalized ratio; LAC, lupus anticoagulant; MTHFR, methylene tetrahydrofolate reductase; PTT, partial thromboplastin time.

[a] Initial prothrombotic screen should precede administration of heparin if possible.

most factors is lacking. In addition, the presence of multiple risk factors is common in neonatal AIS and CSVT [3,8,25,26,44], and their interaction is most likely important in disease pathogenesis, an argument commonly made in cerebral palsy studies as well [7,45]. An overview of the appropriate diagnostic evaluation is provided in Table 1.

Infection and inflammation

Inflammatory markers, often but not exclusively related to infection, are commonly associated with neonatal stroke and cerebral palsy. Bacterial meningitis is a risk factor for AIS and CSVT, with evidence of vascular ischemic injury occurring in as many as 75% of neonatal and young infant cases and predicting a poor neurologic outcome [46,47]. Some recognizable congenital infections may predispose to AIS, and other less diagnosable infections also may have a role [3,48,49]. Although accurate case definitions are problematic, chorioamnionitis has been independently associated with perinatal stroke and cerebral palsy [8,49–51]. Intrauterine exposure to non-TORCH infections (toxoplasmosis, others; rubella; cytomegalovirus; and herpes simplex) without evidence of neonatal sepsis or meningitis seems to be increased in cases of otherwise idiopathic cerebral palsy and is suggested to account for over 10% of such cases [50]. Term infants with evidence of in utero infection exposure are also at risk for early depression and neonatal encephalopathy, and the mechanisms linking such infections to cerebral palsy are poorly understood [52]. Whether findings of elevated interferons in children with cerebral palsy relate to infection or other noninfectious inflammation has not been determined, although this association seems to be specific to children with bilateral cerebral palsy and not hemiplegia, perhaps downplaying a connection to perinatal stroke [53].

Maternal/prenatal

Multiple gestational and obstetric variables have been associated with stroke in the newborn. A recent population-based, multivariate analysis of maternal factors associated with perinatal AIS identified infertility, chorioamnionitis, prolonged rupture of membranes, and pre-eclampsia as factors [8]. Another study selecting only children with motor impairment identified pre-eclampsia and intrauterine growth retardation as risks [54]. Other common maternal factors, such as hypertension or diabetes, are seen in less than 20% of cases of neonatal CSVT [25,26]. Presumed perinatal stroke may be associated with maternal factors, including pre-eclampsia, bleeding, and diabetes, although studies have been small [16]. The risk for cerebral palsy in multiple gestation pregnancy is highest with death of a co-twin but does not appear to be related to delivery parameters, the order of birth, or genetics [55,56]. Cases of neonatal stroke in a surviving twin [57,58] have been reported but not explored in detail.

Placental

A variety of pathologic lesions of the placenta have been described in association with cerebral palsy and adverse neurologic outcomes. Thrombi have been the most common of multiple placental pathologies reported in series of placentas reviewed for cerebral palsy litigation [59,60]. Many of these studies failed to distinguish the pattern of cerebral palsy, although they suggest that hemiplegia is less common than bilateral involvement [59]. Postmortem studies suggest that systemic fetal thromboemboli, including strokes, are common in fetal thrombotic vasculopathy and associated with prothrombotic states in the mother [61]. Other studies have associated placental abnormalities with perinatal stroke and suggested a thromboembolic mechanism [62,63]. Abnormal thrombosis of the placenta strongly suggests the stroke mechanism, whereas coexistent inflammatory changes may be associated with a poorer neurologic outcome [64]. The confirmation of a substantial etiologic role for such mechanisms has been difficult, in part owing to the difficulty in performing pathologic examination of placental tissue. Despite enormous research efforts into the thrombotic complications of pregnancy, none have seriously explored the risks or potential benefits of maternal treatment on the neurologic outcome of the fetus [7].

Prothrombotic/hematologic

Congenital and acquired prothrombotic states have been associated with more than 50% of neonatal AIS [16,65–69]. Consistent abnormalities include protein C deficiency, factor V Leiden, and elevated lipoprotein (a) [68,70]. Cardiogenic and artery-to-artery thromboemboli are suspected to contribute to some perinatal AIS but are probably less common [3]. Pregnancy, particularly the peripartum period, is a generally prothrombotic state, which is likely important in some cases of perinatal AIS [71]. A hypercoagulable risk may also be conferred on the fetus by inheriting a genetic prothrombotic disorder or via transfer of antiphospholipid antibodies [3]. Stroke may also complicate acquired coagulopathic states in the neonate, particularly disseminated intravascular coagulation and sepsis [23]. Coagulation abnormalities may also be found in later testing of more than half of presumed perinatal strokes [16]. Although the risk of venous thrombosis is generally considered even higher in prothrombotic states, most studies have suggested an incidence around 20% in neonatal CSVT [25,72]. Evidence also supports immune-mediated alterations in the coagulation systems of neonates in whom cerebral palsy develops [73]. Anemia, usually related to iron deficiency, is clearly a risk factor for CSVT in children but has not been well studied in neonates [74,75]. Polycythemia may also increase the risk for perinatal stroke [68,70]. A complete hematologic and prothrombotic evaluation is required in most cases, although certain studies will be altered in the acute setting and may need to be repeated. Screening of the parents may be indicated, particularly if there is a positive family history of thrombosis.

Cardiac

Although the relative risk is better established in older children, cardiac disease also predisposes neonates to strokes, and cardiac evaluation is indicated [3,76–78]. Structural and flow abnormalities can generate thromboemboli while diagnostic or surgical procedures further increase the probability of stroke [3,79]. Congenital heart disease accounts for most cases. The risk is greatest in the periprocedural period when AIS may complicate as many as 1 in 150 to 400 procedures [80,81], with the risk associated with the Fontan procedure being 3% to 19% [82]. Strokes also occur preoperatively, when they are usually clinically silent [76]. Cardiac causes other than structural congenital heart disease, such as cardiomyopathy, valve disease, and arrhythmia, are less common but should be considered [1,83]. Any potential right-to-left shunt carries a risk of paradoxical neonatal AIS secondary to venous thrombosis, with patent foramen ovale being the most common [77]. Cardiac investigations of children diagnosed at an older age with presumed perinatal stroke are usually normal, most likely owing to the fact that most patent foramen ovale's close after the newborn period [16]. The relationship between congenital heart disease and neonatal CSVT is less clear. A large population-based study identified no abnormalities in 69 neonates [25], whereas a tertiary care study found congenital heart disease in 23% of 30 cases [26]. This later study also identified extracorporeal membrane oxygenation as a risk factor for CSVT.

Congenital/genetic

Male gender seems to increase the risk for AIS and CSVT in the neonate [84]. Congenital vascular malformations may accompany recognizable syndromes, such as posterior fossa malformations, hemangiomas, arterial abnormalities, co-arctation of the aorta, eye abnormalities, sternal pit (PHACES) syndrome, [85] or occur spontaneously and predispose to AIS [86]. Although certain polymorphisms may confer an increased risk of cerebral palsy in certain at-risk populations [87], such studies have not been applied to the perinatal stroke population. An increased incidence of congenital malformations in children with cerebral palsy supports early prenatal etiologies [88], although any relationship to cerebrovascular disease has not been established.

Systemic disease

Acute systemic disease was the most common risk factor identified in the largest cohort of neonatal CSVT [25]. Dehydration is a major risk factor and occurs commonly in neonates who have difficulty establishing early feeding [25]. Acute neonatal conditions such as sepsis, meconium aspiration, and disseminated intravascular coagulation seem to be associated with CSVT in the neonate [26]. Chronic systemic diseases including hematologic disorders are not commonly seen in neonatal CSVT [25]. Drug or toxin exposure can be associated with perinatal stroke, which occurred in 17% of infants born to mothers abusing cocaine [89].

Trauma and delivery

A relatively increased proportion of neonates with AIS are delivered by cesarean section; however, this observation may represent an increased incidence of fetal distress requiring urgent delivery related to placental or other peripartum events [3,54]. Arterial dissection, a common cause of AIS in older children, has rarely been diagnosed in the neonate [90]. Strokes can also be seen with nonaccidental trauma and the shaken baby syndrome [91]. Other potential trauma in the perinatal period, including the use of forceps, vacuum delivery, or prolonged labor, has not been clearly related to perinatal stroke [8,54].

Neonatal encephalopathy

The coexistence of neonatal "asphyxia" or encephalopathy (suggested by low Apgar scores, fetal heart rate anomalies, low cord pH, and other factors) and stroke may be less common than previously suggested [4], although, when present in combination, may portend a worse neurologic prognosis [40]. A recent population-based study of children with motor impairment and PAS suggested an association with delivery complications including the need for resuscitation, low Apgar scores, and emergency cesarean section [54]. Perinatal complications are identified in more than half of neonates with CSVT, the most common of which is evidence of hypoxia [25,26]. Although neonatal encephalopathy remains the best predictor of cerebral palsy in term neonates [7], less than 25% of cases may have such a history [92]. A search for other associated risks must occur, because simple birth asphyxia is not supported clinically in most cases, and its use as a "default" etiology is no longer considered acceptable [7].

Cerebral palsy: motor outcome from perinatal stroke

It has further been determined that a large number of cases of infantile cerebral palsy is caused by the same factors that bring about the majority of cases of cerebral paralysis of adults: by tearing, embolism, and thrombosis of cerebral vessels.

—Sigmund Freud, 1895 [93]

The known causes of cerebral palsy account for only a minority of the total cases.

—Karin B. Nelson, 2003 [41]

The previous statements seem suspiciously paradoxical in their degree of certainty, being inversely related to the chronologic advancement of neuroscience over more than a century, yet they are both accurate. Congenital hemiplegia is the most common form of cerebral palsy in children born at term [94]. Despite the lack of good epidemiologic studies, experts suggest that perinatal stroke is the most common cause of hemiparetic cerebral palsy while also contributing to some cases of bilateral motor impairment [3,41]. Even though approximately half of children with cerebral palsy are born at term, research efforts and the understanding of pathogenesis are inferior to that in the preterm population [7,41]. The fact that the incidence of cerebral palsy has failed to decrease despite fetal monitoring and other research efforts over the past decades underscores the need to look more broadly at the root causes, which include neonatal stroke [41].

Neurologic deficits or epilepsy occur in 50% to 75% of survivors of perinatal strokes, and sensorimotor deficits are most common [17,34,95,96]. Estimates of the frequency of cerebral palsy after perinatal stroke are similar [16,97,98]. A recent population-based study of neonatal AIS [97] demonstrated good agreement with previous outcome studies, documenting cerebral palsy in 32% of infants with AIS diagnosed acutely in the neonatal period and in 82% of those with "presumed perinatal" AIS. By nature of the mode of presentation leading to diagnosis, it is not surprising that the vast majority of cases of presumed perinatal AIS also have hemiparesis [14,16], and that a delay to diagnosis is associated with an increased risk of cerebral palsy [97]. Outcomes from CSVT are similarly unfavorable, with only half of children being neurologically normal, with motor impairment being the most common adverse outcome, occurring in as many as 80% of impaired survivors [25]. Walking ability and milestones are impaired in a small minority of patients who have perinatal AIS and CSVT and usually only in those with bilateral infarcts [99], a finding possibly related to selective involvement of the MCA and relative sparing of lower extremity motor function.

Contemporary definitions of cerebral palsy include "a group of disorders of the development of movement and posture causing activity limitation that are attributable to non-progressive disturbances that occurred in the developing fetal or infant brain" [100]. Although such reclassifications of cerebral palsy terminology avoid limiting descriptions to simple anatomic or functional localizations, consideration of lesion-specific outcomes may be relevant in cases of cerebral palsy related to perinatal stroke, given the focal nature of the injury. Recent suggestions also support the retention of concepts such as dyskinetic or ataxic cerebral palsy [100]. Dyskinetic, choreoathetoid, or dystonic cerebral palsy has historically been associated with selective injuries to the basal ganglia, such as kernicterus or certain patterns of neonatal encephalopathy. Although strokes causing focal injury to unilateral basal ganglia structures occur more frequently in older children [101], these structures can be affected in AIS and CSVT of term and preterm neonates [18,25]. Despite this observation, hyperkinetic movement disorders are not a common adverse motor outcome of perinatal strokes [16,101]. Ataxic cerebral palsy might be expected after perinatal stroke affecting the brainstem or cerebellum, although the posterior circulation is not commonly affected in perinatal AIS [16,17], and the deep venous thrombosis that might cause infratentorial injury is also uncommon in neonatal CSVT [25].

Also consistent with contemporary definitions of cerebral palsy [100] is the common co-occurrence of other neurologic deficits in children with neonatal or presumed perinatal stroke. Disorders of language, vision, and cognition, as well as epilepsy, are common, each occurring in 20% to 60% of cases [14,16,17, 34,83]. The life-long morbidity of stroke in a child lasts decades, amplifying the huge economic burden demonstrated in adult stroke [102] and the impact on quality of life for the child and their family.

Prediction of neurologic outcome

Overt focal neurologic deficits or other clinical means of assessing acute stroke severity are usually absent in the neonate; therefore, potential predictors of outcome tend to focus on neuroimaging features. Not surprisingly, motor and other neurologic outcomes have been correlated with MRI findings of very large areas of infarction [96–98,103]. Lesion topography and combined involvement of structures including the motor cortex, basal ganglia, or internal capsule on MRI may help predict motor outcome in perinatal AIS [96–98,101,104]. Adding EEG information to MRI findings may slightly increase motor outcome prediction [98]. Certain clinical features, such as the severity of early seizures or neurologic examination abnormalities at discharge, may help predict disability [34]. The presence of seizures or venous infarction predicts a worse outcome from neonatal CSVT [25]. Certain prothrombotic states may also portend a worse outcome in perinatal stroke, including elevated factor VIII, D-dimer, or factor V Leiden [105,106].

Recent evidence suggests that restricted diffusion signal within the cerebral peduncle may represent pre–Wallerian degeneration and correlate with poor motor outcome [107]. Previous studies have shown that the degree of Wallerian degeneration in the descending corticospinal tracts on follow-up imaging correlates with the severity of motor outcome after perinatal stroke [108]. The authors recently discovered that computer-assisted measurement of the extent of acute restricted DWI signal within the descending corticospinal tracts remote from the area of infarction appears to be an accurate predictor of motor outcome (A. Kirton et al, 2006, unpublished data). An example is shown in Fig. 4.

The outcomes from perinatal stroke are often assumed to be better than that for older children, which are, in turn, better than that for adults [3], a finding often attributed to the increased "plasticity" of the immature brain. Nevertheless, such trends have not always been seen [109,110], and the mechanisms of plasticity remain poorly understood. Neonatal stroke provides an ideal model for studying the response of the developing brain to injury with focal, well-defined lesions that can be contrasted with homotopic healthy brain regions in the contralateral hemisphere. Applying functional neuroimaging modalities such as fMRI, DTI, and transcranial magnetic stimulation has the potential to describe and quantify

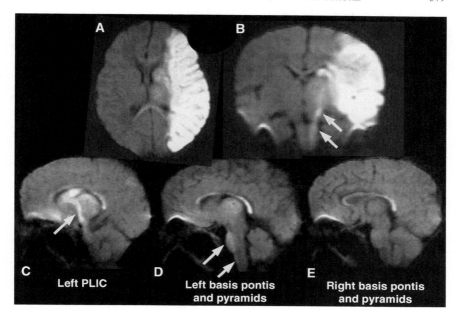

Fig. 4. (*A*) Large left MCA infarction in a term neonate. (*B*) Coronal and (*C,D,E*) sagittal images demonstrate restricted diffusion of ipsilateral descending corticospinal tracts remote from the area of infarct (*arrows*). This finding may represent pre–Wallerian degeneration, and its extent is predictive of motor outcome. (PLIC, posterior limb of internal capsule.)

mechanisms of recovery, provide measurable evidence of brain plasticity, and improve therapeutic interventions.

Therapeutic strategies for stroke-induced cerebral palsy

An important difference between cerebral palsy secondary to stroke versus that due to other causes is the often unilateral and focal nature of the brain injury. As a result, intact adjacent areas of the ipsilesional hemisphere, as well as the entire contralesional hemisphere, have the potential to contribute to motor outcome in ways that a more globally injured brain does not. Recent progress in the understanding of motor reorganization and recovery in adult stroke [111] has yet to be paralleled in pediatric stroke despite potentially greater insights gained from studying plasticity in the developing brain. A discussion of brain plasticity mechanisms after stroke is beyond the scope of this review. This is an active area of research, and an improved understanding of such mechanisms will facilitate therapeutic strategies for children with cerebral palsy secondary to perinatal stroke. No studies of stroke prevention have been undertaken in perinatal AIS or attention paid to preventing fetal or perinatal strokes in mothers with known risk factors such as a prothrombotic disorder [3]. The importance of education and family support must not be forgotten [112]. Assessment of the psychosocial impact and development of complementary educational and supportive resources need to parallel other advances in perinatal stroke research.

Acute care and neuroprotection

Acute pharmacologic and supportive care has the potential to minimize secondary brain injury after PAS and improve motor outcome. Although not as well studied as other forms of neonatal encephalopathy, there is reason to suspect that many of the unique pathophysiologic mechanisms of other ischemic brain injuries in the neonate [123] also apply to the focal ischemic injury of stroke. For PAS, published consensus guidelines support the use of anticoagulant therapy with unfractionated heparin or low molecular weight heparin for 3 months in neonates with a cardioembolic source only while no pharmacologic intervention is recommended for other etiologies [113]. The evidence base for this recommendation is weak with no randomized trails to date. For neonatal CSVT, a similar degree of evidence and opinion support the safety and use of anticoagulation therapy [113,114]. Supportive care is essential in the acute management of all children with stroke to prevent extension of the acute infarct and secondary brain injury [115]. Based primarily on animal models [116,117] and evidence from adult stroke [118], this care should include attention toward the normalization of blood sugar, temperature, ventilation/oxygenation, blood volume, and blood pressure, although ideal parameters have not been established. Sources of infection should be sought and aggressively treated, and seizures should be treated promptly with anticonvulsants, because hyperthermia and seizures are likely to worsen ischemic brain injury in the neonate [119,120]. Recent evidence for neuroprotection with hypothermia in neonatal encephalopathy [121] is untested in focal ischemic injury. The development of anti-excitotoxic or other neuroprotective therapies faces unique challenges in perinatal AIS, in which the mechanisms of brain injury likely differ from those in older children and adults, and special approaches and cautions are required [39].

Rehabilitation

As is true in most cases of cerebral palsy, rehabilitation is the therapeutic mainstay for children with motor sequelae from perinatal stroke; however, unique issues arise related to the focal unilateral nature of the brain injury. In general, early and aggressive therapy including physical, occupational, and speech modalities is essential in pediatric stroke patients of all ages [112,113]. Most rehabilitation research has focused on motor function, most likely because this is the most common neurologic deficit after stroke in childhood as well as the most amenable to clinical evaluation. Numerous interventions have been suggested but generally lack supporting evidence. An exception is a randomized controlled trial demonstrating the effectiveness of constraint-induced therapy in children with congenital hemiplegia [122]. Other strategies include inhibitive casting, Lycra splinting, treadmill training, and functional electrical stimulation. Recently published guidelines [112] suggest the following strategies should be considered: muscle strengthening to improve function and minimize contractures, Botox injections for spasticity, and ankle-foot orthoses for gait and contracture prevention. Limited studies have been performed regarding the rehabilitation of other associated consequences of pediatric stroke, such as vision impairment, somatosensory deficits, and language or cognitive and behavioral disorders. The optimal frequency, duration, and intensity of different therapies have not been well studied and are most likely dependent on the child's age, injury, and duration of recovery, as well as parental factors, family dynamics, school environments, and community resources.

Formal evaluation of different rehabilitation strategies is unavoidably complex in the developing brain, particularly in pediatric stroke, which is less common and underrecognized. The use of standardized measures such as the Pediatric Stroke Outcome Measure [95] facilitates the study of pediatric stroke outcomes and rehabilitative strategies. Advanced neuroimaging techniques, such as fMRI, DTI, and transcranial magnetic stimulation, have enormous potential to improve understanding of brain reorganization strategies and plasticity mechanisms, quantify brain recovery, and function as powerful tools for the evaluation of different rehabilitation strategies. Such approaches are currently underway in pediatric stroke research and offer new avenues of hope for improving outcomes from stroke in the neonate, older children, and adults.

Summary

Perinatal stroke is a unique and important contributor to the pathogenesis of cerebral palsy. The significant overlap between the risk factors for the cerebral vaso-occlusion underlying perinatal stroke and other forms of cerebral palsy is not coincidental, and a closer look at their interrelation promises to yield insight to both. Treatment approaches focused on antithrombotics and neuroprotective strategies are evolving. The adverse outcomes from perinatal stroke have motivated a rapid expansion of research efforts, including the development of large research networks. These efforts, coupled with rapid advances in available technologic tools, offer real potential for improved understanding and a decrease in the substantial burdens of stroke-induced cerebral palsy.

References

[1] deVeber G, Roach ES, Riela AR, et al. Stroke in children: recognition, treatment, and future directions. Semin Pediatr Neurol 2000;7:309–17.

[2] Lynch JK, Nelson KB. Epidemiology of perinatal stroke. Curr Opin Pediatr 2001;13(6): 499–505.

[3] Nelson KB, Lynch JK. Stroke in newborn infants. Lancet Neurol 2004;3(3):150–8.

[4] Estan J, Hope P. Unilateral neonatal cerebral infarction in full term infants. Arch Dis Child Fetal Neonatal Ed 1997;76(2):F88–93.

[5] Schulzke S, Weber P, Luetschg J, et al. Incidence and diagnosis of unilateral arterial cerebral infarction in newborn infants. J Perinat Med 2005;33(2):170–5.

[6] Andrew ME, Monagle P, deVeber G, et al. Thromboembolic disease and antithrombotic therapy in newborns. Hematology (Am Soc Hematol Educ Program) 2001:358–74.

[7] Nelson KB. The epidemiology of cerebral palsy in term infants. Ment Retard Dev Disabil Res Rev 2002;8(3):146–50.

[8] Lee J, Croen LA, Backstrand KH, et al. Maternal and infant characteristics associated with perinatal arterial stroke in the infant. JAMA 2005;293(6):723–9.

[9] deVeber G, Adams M, Andrew M, on behalf of the Canadian Pediatric Ischemic Stroke Study Group. Cerebral thromboembolism in neonates: clinical and radiographic features. Thromb Haemostas 1997;Suppl:725.

[10] Rafay MF, Tan-Dy C, Al-Futaisi A, et al. Predictive value of seizure and EEG features in the diagnosis of neonatal stroke and hypoxic ischemic encephalopathy. Ann Neurol 2005;58:S104.

[11] Miller V. Neonatal cerebral infarction. Semin Pediatr Neurol 2000;7(4):278–88.

[12] Mercuri E, Cowan F. Cerebral infarction in the newborn infant: review of the literature and personal experience. Eur J Paediatr Neurol 1999;3(6):255–63.

[13] Levy SR, Abroms IF, Marshall PC, et al. Seizures and cerebral infarction in the full-term newborn. Ann Neurol 1985;17(4):366–70.

[14] Trauner DA, Chase C, Walker P, et al. Neurologic profiles of infants and children after perinatal stroke. Pediatr Neurol 1993;9:383–6.

[15] Sran S, Baumann R. Outcome of neonatal stroke. Am J Dis Child 1988;142:1086–7.

[16] Golomb MR, MacGregor DL, Domi T, et al. Presumed pre- or perinatal arterial ischemic stroke: risk factors and outcomes. Ann Neurol 2001;50(2):163–8.

[17] deVeber G, MacGregor D, Curtis R, et al. Neurological outcome in survivors of neonatal arterial ischemic stroke. Pediatr Res 2003;53(4):537A.

[18] de Vries LS, Groenendaal F, Eken P, et al. Infarcts in the vascular distribution of the middle cerebral artery in preterm and full term infants. Neuropediatrics 1997;28(2):88–96.

[19] Kurnik K, Kosch A, Strater R, et al. Recurrent thromboembolism in infants and children suffering from symptomatic neonatal arterial stroke: a prospective follow-up study. Stroke 2003;34(12):2887–92.

[20] Murphy SL. Deaths: final data for 1998. Natl Vital Stat Rep 2000;48(11):1–105.

[21] de Vries LS, Regev R, Connell JA, et al. Localized cerebral infarction in the premature infant: an ultrasound diagnosis correlated with computed tomography and magnetic resonance imaging. Pediatrics 1988;81(1):36–40.

[22] Amato M, Huppi P, Herschkowitz N, et al. Prenatal stroke suggested by intrauterine ultrasound and confirmed by magnetic resonance imaging. Neuropediatrics 1991;22(2):100–2.

[23] Barmada MA, Moossy J, Shuman RM. Cerebral infarcts with arterial occlusion in neonates. Ann Neurol 1979;6(6):495–502.

[24] Uvebrant P. Hemiplegic cerebral palsy: aetiology and outcome. Acta Paediatr Scand Suppl 1988;345:1–100.

[25] deVeber G, Andrew M, Canadian Pediatric Ischemic Stroke Study Group. Cerebral sinovenous thrombosis in children. N Engl J Med 2001;345(6):417–23.

[26] Wu YW, Miller SP, Chin K, et al. Multiple risk factors in neonatal sinovenous thrombosis. Neurology 2002;59(3):438–40.

[27] Wu YW, Hamrick SE, Miller SP, et al. Intraventricular hemorrhage in term neonates caused by sinovenous thrombosis. Ann Neurol 2003;54(1):123–6.

[28] Golomb MR, Dick PT, MacGregor DL, et al. Cranial ultrasonography has a low sensitivity for detecting arterial ischemic stroke in term neonates. J Child Neurol 2003;18(2):98–103.

[29] Shroff M, deVeber G. Sinovenous thrombosis in children. Neuroimaging Clin North Am 2003; 13(1):115–38.

[30] Mader I, Schoning M, Klose U, et al. Neonatal cerebral infarction diagnosed by diffusion-weighted MRI: pseudonormalization occurs early. Stroke 2002;33(4):1142–5.

[31] Okumura A, Hayakawa F, Kato T, et al. MRI findings in patients with spastic cerebral palsy. I. Correlation with gestational age at birth. Dev Med Child Neurol 1997;39(6):363–8.

[32] Okumura A, Kato T, Kuno K, et al. MRI findings in patients with spastic cerebral palsy. II. Correlation with type of cerebral palsy. Dev Med Child Neurol 1997;39(6):369–72.

[33] Lynch JK, Hirtz DG, deVeber G, et al. Report of the National Institute of Neurological Disorders and Stroke workshop on perinatal and childhood stroke. Pediatrics 2002;109(1): 116–23.

[34] Sreenan C, Bhargava R, Robertson CM. Cerebral infarction in the term newborn: clinical presentation and long-term outcome. J Pediatr 2000;137(3):351–5.

[35] Sotak CH. The role of diffusion tensor imaging in the evaluation of ischemic brain injury: a review. NMR Biomed 2002;15(7–8):561–9.

[36] Seghier ML, Lazeyras F, Zimine S, et al. Combination of event-related fMRI and diffusion tensor imaging in an infant with perinatal stroke. Neuroimage 2004;21(1):463–72.

[37] Heller SL, Heier LA, Watts R, et al. Evidence of cerebral reorganization following perinatal stroke demonstrated with fMRI and DTI tractography. Clin Imaging 2005;29(4):283–7.

[38] Staudt M, Grodd W, Gerloff C, et al. Two types of ipsilateral reorganization in congenital hemiparesis: a TMS and fMRI study. Brain 2002;125(Pt 10):2222–37.

[39] Ferriero DM. Neonatal brain injury. N Engl J Med 2004;351(19):1985–95.

[40] Ramaswamy V, Miller SP, Barkovich AJ, et al. Perinatal stroke in term infants with neonatal encephalopathy. Neurology 2004;62(11):2088–91.

[41] Nelson KB. Can we prevent cerebral palsy? N Engl J Med 2003;349(18):1765–9.

[42] Sarnat HB. Watershed infarcts in the fetal and neonatal brainstem: an aetiology of central hypoventilation, dysphagia, Moibius syndrome and micrognathia. Eur J Paediatr Neurol 2004; 8(2):71–87.

[43] Takanashi J, Barkovich AJ, Ferriero DM, et al. Widening spectrum of congenital hemiplegia: periventricular venous infarction in term neonates. Neurology 2003;61(4):531–3.

[44] Heller C, Heinecke A, Junker R, et al. Cerebral venous thrombosis in children: a multifactorial origin. Circulation 2003;108(11):1362–7.

[45] Nelson KB, Grether JK. Potentially asphyxiating conditions and spastic cerebral palsy in infants of normal birth weight. Am J Obstet Gynecol 1998;179(2):507–13.

[46] Chang CJ, Chang WN, Huang LT, et al. Cerebral infarction in perinatal and childhood bacterial meningitis. Q J Med 2003;96(10):755–62.

[47] Takeoka M, Takahashi T. Infectious and inflammatory disorders of the circulatory system and stroke in childhood. Curr Opin Neurol 2002;15(2):159–64.

[48] Ment LR, Ehrenkranz RA, Duncan CC. Bacterial meningitis as an etiology of perinatal cerebral infarction. Pediatr Neurol 1986;2(5):276–9.

[49] Walstab J, Bell R, Reddihough D, et al. Antenatal and intrapartum antecedents of cerebral palsy: a case-control study. Aust N Z J Obstet Gynaecol 2002;42(2):138–46.

[50] Grether JK, Nelson KB. Maternal infection and cerebral palsy in infants of normal birth weight. JAMA 1997;278(3):207–11.

[51] Wu YW, Escobar GJ, Grether JK, et al. Chorioamnionitis and cerebral palsy in term and near-term infants. JAMA 2003;290(20):2677–84.

[52] Nelson KB, Willoughby RE. Infection, inflammation and the risk of cerebral palsy. Curr Opin Neurol 2000;13(2):133–9.

[53] Grether JK, Nelson KB, Dambrosia JM, et al. Interferons and cerebral palsy. J Pediatr 1999; 134(3):324–32.

[54] Wu YW, March WM, Croen LA, et al. Perinatal stroke in children with motor impairment: a population-based study. Pediatrics 2004;114(3):612–9.

[55] Scher AI, Petterson B, Blair E, et al. The risk of mortality or cerebral palsy in twins: a collaborative population-based study. Pediatr Res 2002;52(5):671–81.

[56] Pharoah PO. Twins and cerebral palsy. Acta Paediatr Suppl 2001;90(436):6–10.

[57] Cole-Beuglet C, Aufrichtig D, Cohen A, et al. Ultrasound case of the day: twin pregnancy, intrauterine death of one twin with disseminated intravascular coagulation resulting in the development of a cerebral infarct in the surviving twin. Radiographics 1987;7(2):389–94.

[58] de Laveaucoupet J, Ciorascu R, Lacaze T, et al. Hepatic and cerebral infarction in the survivor after the in utero death of a co-twin: sonographic pattern. Pediatr Radiol 1995;25(3):211–3.

[59] Redline RW. Severe fetal placental vascular lesions in term infants with neurologic impairment. Am J Obstet Gynecol 2005;192(2):452–7.

[60] Kraus FT. Cerebral palsy and thrombi in placental vessels of the fetus: insights from litigation. Hum Pathol 1997;28(2):246–8.

[61] Kraus FT, Acheen VI. Fetal thrombotic vasculopathy in the placenta: cerebral thrombi and infarcts, coagulopathies, and cerebral palsy. Hum Pathol 1999;30(7):759–69.

[62] Burke CJ, Tannenberg AE, Payton DJ. Ischaemic cerebral injury, intrauterine growth retardation, and placental infarction. Dev Med Child Neurol 1997;39(11):726–30.

[63] Burke CJ, Tannenberg AE. Prenatal brain damage and placental infarction: an autopsy study. Dev Med Child Neurol 1995;37(6):555–62.

[64] Redline RW, Pappin A. Fetal thrombotic vasculopathy: the clinical significance of extensive avascular villi. Hum Pathol 1995;26(1):80–5.

[65] Bonduel M, Sciuccati G, Hepner M, et al. Prethrombotic disorders in children with arterial ischemic stroke and sinovenous thrombosis. Arch Neurol 1999;56(8):967–71.

[66] deVeber G, Monagle P, Chan A, et al. Prothrombotic disorders in infants and children with cerebral thromboembolism. Arch Neurol 1998;55(12):1539–43.

[67] Barnes C, deVeber G. Prothrombotic abnormalities in childhood ischaemic stroke. Thromb Res 2005 [Epub ahead of print].

[68] Gunther G, Junker R, Strater R, et al. Symptomatic ischemic stroke in full-term neonates: role of acquired and genetic prothrombotic risk factors. Stroke 2000;31(10):2437–41.

[69] Lynch JK, Nelson KB, Curry CJ, et al. Cerebrovascular disorders in children with the factor V Leiden mutation. J Child Neurol 2001;16(10):735–44.

[70] Nowak-Goettl U, von Eckardstein A, Junder R, et al. Lipoprotein (a) and genetic polymorphisms of MTHFR TT677, factor V G1691A, and prothrombin G20210A are risk factors of spontaneous ischaemic stroke in childhood. Thromb Haemost 1999;Suppl:1538a.

[71] Lao TT, Yin JA, Yuen PM. Coagulation and anticoagulation systems in newborns: correlation with their mothers at delivery. Lower levels of anticoagulants and fibrinolytic activity in the newborn. Gynecol Obstet Invest 1990;29(3):181–4.

[72] Young G, Manco-Johnson M, Gill JC, et al. Clinical manifestations of the prothrombin G20210A mutation in children: a pediatric coagulation consortium study. J Thromb Haemost 2003;1(5):958–62.

[73] Nelson KB, Dambrosia JM, Grether JK, et al. Neonatal cytokines and coagulation factors in children with cerebral palsy. Ann Neurol 1998;44(4):665–75.

[74] Hartfield DS, Lowry NJ, Keene DL, et al. Iron deficiency: a cause of stroke in infants and children. Pediatr Neurol 1997;16(1):50–3.

[75] Sebire G, Tabarki B, Saunders DE, et al. Cerebral venous sinus thrombosis in children: risk factors, presentation, diagnosis and outcome. Brain 2005;128(Pt 3):477–89.

[76] Miller G, Mamourian AC, Tesman JR, et al. Long-term MRI changes in brain after pediatric open heart surgery. J Child Neurol 1994;9(4):390–7.

[77] Pellicer A, Cabanas F, Garcia-Alix A, et al. Stroke in neonates with cardiac right-to-left shunt. Brain Dev 1992;14(6):381–5.

[78] Kirkham FJ. Recognition and prevention of neurological complications in pediatric cardiac surgery. Pediatr Cardiol 1998;19(4):331–45.

[79] Kirkham FJ, Prengler M, Hewes DK, et al. Risk factors for arterial ischemic stroke in children. J Child Neurol 2000;15(5):299–307.

[80] Menache CC, du Plessis AJ, Wessel DL, et al. Current incidence of acute neurologic complications after open-heart operations in children. Ann Thorac Surg 2002;73(6):1752–8.

[81] Domi T, Edgell D, McCrindle BW, et al. Frequency and predictors of vaso-occlusive strokes associated with congenital heart disease. Ann Neurol 2002;52(3S):S129–33.

[82] Monagle P, Karl TR. Thromboembolic problems after the Fontan operation. Semin Thorac Cardiovasc Surg Pediatr Cardiovasc Surg Annu 2002;5:36–47.

[83] Lynch JK. Cerebrovascular disorders in children. Curr Neurol Neurosci Rep 2004;4(2):129–38.

[84] Golomb M, Dick P, MacGregor D, et al. Neonatal arterial ischemic stroke and sinovenous thrombosis are more commonly diagnosed in males. Stroke 2003;34(1):288.

[85] Bhattacharya JJ, Luo CB, Alvarez H, et al. PHACES syndrome: a review of eight previously unreported cases with late arterial occlusions. Neuroradiology 2004;46(3):227–33.

[86] Pascual-Castroviejo I, Pascual-Pascual SI. Congenital vascular malformations in childhood. Semin Pediatr Neurol 2002;9(4):254–73.

[87] Nelson KB, Dambrosia JM, Iovannisci DM, et al. Genetic polymorphisms and cerebral palsy in very preterm infants. Pediatr Res 2005;57(4):494–9.

[88] Croen LA, Grether JK, Curry CJ, et al. Congenital abnormalities among children with cerebral palsy: more evidence for prenatal antecedents. J Pediatr 2001;138(6):804–10.

[89] Heier LA, Carpanzano CR, Mast J, et al. Maternal cocaine abuse: the spectrum of radiologic abnormalities in the neonatal CNS. AJNR Am J Neuroradiol 1991;12(5):951–6.

[90] Lequin MH, Peeters EA, Holscher HC, et al. Arterial infarction caused by carotid artery dissection in the neonate. Eur J Paediatr Neurol 2004;8(3):155–60.

[91] King WJ, Mackay M, Sirnick A. Shaken baby syndrome in Canada: clinical characteristics and outcomes of hospital cases. CMAJ 2003;168(2):155–9.

[92] Badawi N, Felix JF, Kurinczuk JJ, et al. Cerebral palsy following term newborn encephalopathy: a population-based study. Dev Med Child Neurol 2005;47(5):293–8.

[93] Rothman SM. Stroke in children: Freud's first analysis. Lancet 2002;360(9345):1526–7.

[94] Hagberg B, Hagberg G, Beckung E, et al. Changing panorama of cerebral palsy in Sweden. VIII. Prevalence and origin in the birth year period 1991–94. Acta Paediatr 2001;90(3):271–7.

[95] deVeber G, MacGregor D, Curtis R, et al. Neurologic outcome in survivors of childhood arterial ischemic stroke and sinovenous thrombosis. J Child Neurol 2000;15(5):316–24.

[96] Mercuri E, Barnett A, Rutherford M, et al. Neonatal cerebral infarction and neuromotor outcome at school age. Pediatrics 2004;113(1 Pt 1):95–100.

[97] Lee J, Croen LA, Lindan C, et al. Predictors of outcome in perinatal arterial stroke: a population-based study. Ann Neurol 2005;58(2):303–8.

[98] Mercuri E, Rutherford M, Cowan F, et al. Early prognostic indicators of outcome in infants with neonatal cerebral infarction: a clinical, electroencephalogram, and magnetic resonance imaging study. Pediatrics 1999;103(1):39–46.

[99] Golomb MR, deVeber GA, MacGregor DL, et al. Independent walking after neonatal arterial ischemic stroke and sinovenous thrombosis. J Child Neurol 2003;18(8):530–6.

[100] Bax M, Goldstein M, Rosenbaum P, et al. Proposed definition and classification of cerebral palsy, April 2005. Dev Med Child Neurol 2005;47(8):571–6.

[101] Boardman JP, Ganesan V, Rutherford MA, et al. Magnetic resonance image correlates of hemiparesis after neonatal and childhood middle cerebral artery stroke. Pediatrics 2005;115(2):321–6.

[102] Taylor TN, Davis PH, Torner JC, et al. Lifetime cost of stroke in the United States. Stroke 1996;27(9):1459–66.

[103] Mercuri E, Anker S, Guzzetta A, et al. Neonatal cerebral infarction and visual function at school age. Arch Dis Child Fetal Neonatal Ed 2003;88(6):F487–91.

[104] Ganesan V, Ng V, Chong WK, et al. Lesion volume, lesion location, and outcome after middle cerebral artery territory stroke. Arch Dis Child 1999;81(4):295–300.

[105] Mercuri E, Cowan F, Gupte G, et al. Prothrombotic disorders and abnormal neurodevelopmental outcome in infants with neonatal cerebral infarction. Pediatrics 2001;107(6):1400–4.

[106] Goldenberg NA, Knapp-Clevenger R, Manco-Johnson MJ. Elevated plasma factor VIII and D-dimer levels as predictors of poor outcomes of thrombosis in children. N Engl J Med 2004;351(11):1081–8.

[107] de Vries LS, van der GJ, van Haastert IC, et al. Prediction of outcome in new-born infants with arterial ischaemic stroke using diffusion-weighted magnetic resonance imaging. Neuropediatrics 2005;36(1):12–20.

[108] Bouza H, Dubowitz LM, Rutherford M, et al. Prediction of outcome in children with congenital hemiplegia: a magnetic resonance imaging study. Neuropediatrics 1994;25(2):60–6.

[109] Ganesan V, Hogan A, Shack N, et al. Outcome after ischaemic stroke in childhood. Dev Med Child Neurol 2000;42(7):455–61.

[110] Lansing AE, Max JE, Delis DC, et al. Verbal learning and memory after childhood stroke. J Int Neuropsychol Soc 2004;10(5):742–52.

[111] Ward NS, Cohen LG. Mechanisms underlying recovery of motor function after stroke. Arch Neurol 2004;61(12):1844–8.

[112] Paediatric Stroke Working Group. Stroke in childhood: clinical guidelines for diagnosis, management and rehabilitation. London: Royal College of Physicians of London; 2004.

[113] Monagle P, Chan A, Massicotte P, et al. Antithrombotic therapy in children: the Seventh ACCP Conference on Antithrombotic and Thrombolytic Therapy. Chest 2004;126(3 Suppl):645–87.

[114] deVeber G, Chan A, Monagle P, et al. Anticoagulation therapy in pediatric patients with sinovenous thrombosis: a cohort study. Arch Neurol 1998;55(12):1533–7.

[115] Hutchison JS, Ichord R, Guerguerian AM, et al. Cerebrovascular disorders. Semin Pediatr Neurol 2004;11(2):139–46.

[116] Mesples B, Plaisant F, Fontaine RH, et al. Pathophysiology of neonatal brain lesions: lessons from animal models of excitotoxicity. Acta Paediatr 2005;94(2):185–90.

[117] Ashwal S, Pearce WJ. Animal models of neonatal stroke. Curr Opin Pediatr 2001;13(6):506–16.

[118] Becker K. Intensive care unit management of the stroke patient. Neurol Clin 2000;18(2):439–54.

[119] Yager JY, Armstrong EA, Jaharus C, et al. Preventing hyperthermia decreases brain damage following neonatal hypoxic-ischemic seizures. Brain Res 2004;1011(1):48–57.

[120] Wirrell EC, Armstrong EA, Osman LD, et al. Prolonged seizures exacerbate perinatal hypoxic-ischemic brain damage. Pediatr Res 2001;50(4):445–54.

[121] Higgins RD. Hypoxic ischemic encephalopathy and hypothermia: a critical look. Obstet Gynecol 2005;106(6):1385–7.

[122] Taub E, Ramey SL, DeLuca S, et al. Efficacy of constraint-induced movement therapy for children with cerebral palsy with asymmetric motor impairment. Pediatrics 2004;113(2):305–12.

[123] Ferriero DM. Neonatal brain injury. N Engl J Med 2004;351:1985–95.

ELSEVIER
SAUNDERS

CLINICS IN
PERINATOLOGY

Clin Perinatol 33 (2006) 387–410

Hyperbilirubinemia and Kernicterus

Steven M. Shapiro, MD[a],*, Vinod K. Bhutani, MD[b], Lois Johnson, MD[c]

[a]Division of Child Neurology, Department of Neurology,
Virginia Commonwealth University Medical Center, Virginia Commonwealth University, Box 980211,
MCV Station, Richmond, VA 23298-0211, USA
[b]Departments of Neonatal-Developmental Medicine and Pediatrics,
Lucile Packard Children's Hospital, Stanford University, Stanford, CA, USA
[c]Department of Pediatrics, Pennsylvania Hospital, University of Pennsylvania School of Medicine,
Philadelphia, PA, USA

Before the mid-1960s and recognition of the central role of hyperbilirubinemia in its causation, kernicterus was primarily the result of Rhesus (RH) isoimmunization. Soon after, it was recognized as also occurring secondary to other blood group incompatibilities, prematurity, complicating illnesses (infection, hypoxia, respiratory distress) and liver enzyme abnormalities, most notably in Crigler-Najjar disease. Subsequent to the use of exchange transfusion for rapid reduction of the body bilirubin load and for removal of sensitized red blood cells, the availability of RHOgam to prevent RH disease, and the liberal use of phototherapy to minimize hyperbilirubinemia, the incidence of athetoid cerebral palsy (CP) decreased dramatically in developed countries from an estimated 6% of all cases of CP and 20% of those in the athetoid category [1–3]. Kernicterus in term and near term infants became so rare that no case was reported in the North American and European literature during the 1970s and early 1980s, and most practicing doctors and nurses had never seen a case. Not surprisingly the importance of close bilirubin monitoring and justification of the widespread use of preventive phototherapy began to be questioned, especially in healthy term infants but also in those born prematurely [4–6]. The advent of early postnatal hospital discharge, coupled with this decreased concern about the clinical importance of bilirubin as a toxic agent, coincided with a re-emergence of kernicterus as a recognized public health problem [7–11]. Concomitantly, the extent and

---

* Corresponding author.
E-mail address: sshapiro@vcu.edu (S.M. Shapiro).

0095-5108/06/$ – see front matter © 2006 Elsevier Inc. All rights reserved.
doi:10.1016/j.clp.2006.03.010   *perinatology.theclinics.com*

spectrum of posticteric brain damage in premature and term infants who were born at the turn of the 21st century is demanding definition and clarification. Development of additional rehabilitative techniques and treatments coupled with outreach education and funding of supportive facilities are high-priority needs.

As noted in the 1960s and still true today, posticteric encephalopathy is one of the few entities in the group of disorders known as cerebral palsy in which there is excellent correlation between etiology, pathogenesis, and clinical symptomatology [12]. This correlation was advanced greatly by the work of Ahdab-Barmada and Moossy during the benzyl alcohol epidemic of kernicterus in premature infants [13,14]. Drs. Ahdab-Barmada's and Moossy's painstaking study identified the distinctly different pathologic lesions that are caused by hypoxic— as opposed to bilirubin—cellular injury. Studies in the homozygous Gunn rat, the animal counterpart of Crigler-Najjar syndrome in humans, also contributed in major ways to this clarification [15–24].

As proposed by Perlstein [12] many years ago, the natural history and varied but distinctive patterns of sequelae following icteric encephalopathy represent "clinical aggregates in a continuation of syndromes." Descriptions of the range of these interactive syndromes and insights into their long-term effects on the quality of life among survivors provide insights into our need for research on 1. the patterns of disability as related to severity and location of insult in different infant populations and geographic locations, 2. the effect of central nervous system (CNS) maturation from infancy to adolescence on these patterns of disability, 3. the modification of disability and life expectancy by enhanced rehabilitative techniques (eg, computerized communication technologies) and medical/surgical interventions (eg, Nissan fundal plication, delivery of nutrition by indwelling gastronomy tubes, botulinum toxin [Botox] injections, automated intrathecal delivery of baclofen by way of indwelling baclofen pumps, and programmed cochlear implantation devices), 4. the use and ongoing development of diagnostic techniques (eg, sophisticated MRI) and objective definition of the emerging entity of posticteric auditory neuropathy/auditory dys-synchrony (AN/AD) using auditory brainstem responses (ABRs), cochlear microphonics, and otoacoustic emissions (OAEs), and 5. the relationship of perceptual and auditory deficits, including subtle degrees of compromise, to learning and behavioral disabilities during the school and adult years.

In Perlstein's [12] 1960 monograph and the chapter on kernicterus in the most recent edition (2001) of Volpe's [2] textbook on neonatal neurology, the possibility of major predominance of one site of damage over another in the auditory or extrapyramidal category, with or without other distinctive compromise of ophthalmologic, gastrointestinal, or visual perceptual function, is described. Diagnostic decisions and planning for ongoing educational and care needs rest on clarification of these issues. Perlstein [12] noted, for example, that motor involvement can range from the severe to so mild as to be virtually unrecognizable except under the broad descriptive terms of being "awkward" or "clumsy." Nevertheless, he believed that the absence of any athetosis or other forms of "extrapyramidal" dyskinesia might make the diagnosis of posticteric encephalopathy dubious if not untenable. With the availability of newer techniques this may no longer be true. More recently, Volpe [2] reviewed the literature and suggested that impairment of auditory function is the most consistent abnormality that is associated with chronic postkernicteric bilirubin encephalopathy, especially in premature infants, and that the auditory pathways constitute the most sensitive neural system to bilirubin injury. The authors have seen patients with impairment of auditory function without athetosis or an associated movement disorder. This has obvious importance for speech, language, and learning difficulties when the child reaches school age.

Ongoing study of infants who are enrolled in the voluntary kernicterus registry for healthy term and near-term babies and the registry for sick and preterm infants should help to clarify these and other issues. Early reports of this work include information on diagnostic categories, extent of sequelae, and problems with the routine management of neonatal hyperbilirubinemia that are pertinent to this article [25]. Pertinent also is the report from this database of four instances of apparent complete reversal of alarming acute-stage bilirubin encephalopathy of late moderate to early advanced stage severity by prompt and aggressive treatment [8]. Severity was defined as in the bilirubin-induced neurologic dysfunction (BIND) score [26,27] and the three stages of acute brain damage that were described by Volpe [2]. Reversal at this level of acute-stage damage has not been described in the past. The importance of emergency treatment to minimize, and occasionally completely reverse, advanced signs of acute damage is emphasized. Also emphasized is the need for effective bilirubin reduction strategies to prevent their occurrence in the first place.

This article describes new findings concerning the basic science of bilirubin neurotoxicity, new considerations of the definition of clinical kernicterus, and new and useful tools to diagnose kernicterus in older children, and discusses treatments for kernicterus beyond the newborn period and why proper diagnosis is important.

Basic science: how bilirubin damages the brain

Important determinants of neuronal injury by bilirubin are the concentrations of unconjugated bilirubin (UCB) and free bilirubin (Bf), the concentration of serum albumin and its ability to bind UCB, the concentration of hydrogen ion (pH), and neuronal susceptibility. A recent review by Wennberg and colleagues [28] seeks to evaluate the sensitivity and specificity of total serum bilirubin (TSB) and Bf as predictors of risk for bilirubin neurotoxicity and kernicterus. It concludes that although there is insufficient published data to define these sensitivities and specificities precisely, available laboratory and clinical evidence indicate that Bf is better than TSB (and UCB) in discriminating risk for neurotoxicity in patients who have severe hyperbilirubinemia.

The blood–brain barrier, also known as the blood–brain interface (BBI), is not a barrier to Bf. This interface consists of capillary endothelium and astrocytic foot processes, which exclude large molecules from the CNS, transport some substances into the CNS, and pump some substances out of the CNS [29]. Although there is no blood–brain barrier to Bf, the BBI and the chorioid plexus (the blood–cerebrospinal fluid interface) may pump Bf out of the CNS. Specific transporters for bilirubin may exist in the BBI [29], and may protect the CNS from exposure to excessive levels of UCB.

Windows of developmental susceptibility to bilirubin toxicity exist for certain CNS structures. A discrete 24-hour interval of phototherapy protects jaundiced infant Gunn rats from cerebellar atrophy on the seventh postnatal day of life [30]; the authors find that cerebellar neurons that are undergoing early differentiation at the time of bilirubin exposure are highly susceptible to bilirubin neurotoxicity and cell death, whereas slightly more or slightly less mature cells may show only transient changes [18]. The authors hypothesize that the developmental time of exposure to excess bilirubin is an important determinant of the specific pattern of neurologic damage. Because auditory pathways mature earlier than do motor pathways, it is reasonable to postulate that patterns of damage in premature infants may differ from those in term infants.

Intracellular calcium homeostasis

The authors believe that bilirubin acts by impairing intracellular calcium homeostasis, the principal mechanism of neuronal cell death in models of global ischemia [31] and increased neuronal excitability [32,33]. In neurons, calcium-binding proteins (CBPs) buffer and maintain extremely low intracellular levels of calcium, but transient increases in intracellular free calcium function as a second messenger system and stimulate many enzyme types [34], including the abundant calcium and calmodulin-dependent protein kinase II (CaMKII) [35], which has multiple substrates and regulates neurotransmitter release, calcium-regulated ion conductances, and neuroskeletal dynamics [34]. Decreased CaMKII activity is a feature of many models of selective neuronal toxicity, such as ischemia [31], as well as models of increased neuronal excitability and toxicity [36] and epilepsy [33,37,38]; it also can trigger programmed cell death (apoptosis). The authors showed that bilirubin inhibits CaMKII in vitro [39], that its developmental expression is impaired in jj Gunn rats [40], and that there is a selective decrease in expression of CBPs in the CNS [24,41]. There is evidence for [42–44] and against [45] the hypothesis that bilirubin increases intracellular calcium damage through an excitotoxic, n-methyl-d-aspartate (NMDA)-dependent mechanism. Preliminary data from animal experiments with an NMDA-channel blocker do not support this hypothesis (S.M. Shapiro, MD, unpublished data).

Role of multi-drug resistance-associated protein 1

There is recent evidence that bilirubin is removed from cells by way of multidrug resistance-associated protein 1 (MRP1), a member of the multidrug resistance-associated protein subfamily of ATP-binding cassette transporters

[46,47]. MRP1 transports bilirubin with an affinity that is 10 times greater than that of other substrates, such as leukotrienes [47]. Therefore, MRP1 may represent a mechanism by which bilirubin is removed from the CNS and excreted into the blood stream.

Apoptosis

Purified bilirubin with Bf concentration as low as 160 nM can induce apoptosis in cultured rat brain neurons [48,49]. Bilirubin triggers the release of cytochrome c from mitochondria with caspase-3 activation and cleavage of poly (ADP-ribose) polymerase, which confirms the role of one of the pathways that underlies induction of apoptosis [50]. Apoptotic changes are found in cerebellum [51,52] and brainstem of jaundiced Gunn rats [17], and in the basal ganglia of kernicteric human infants, and account for the prominent signs of bilirubin neurotoxicity in each.

The authors' overall hypothesis is that prolonged exposure of neurons to bilirubin causes cell death, and that the developmental stage of the neuron determines whether the cell can handle the bilirubin load. Whether the cell can handle the increased bilirubin load may depend on the expression of MRP1 that pumps bilirubin out of cells [46]. The authors hypothesize that expression is low or that the protein is less active in the areas of the brain that are most susceptible to hyperbilirubinemia, such as the brainstem auditory structures.

Neuropathology of kernicterus

Any explanation of how bilirubin damages the brain eventually must account for the selectivity of bilirubin toxicity (ie, the propensity for bilirubin to damage specific brain regions and not others).

The clinical expression of classic kernicterus corresponds to the selective neuropathology of kernicterus. The movement disorders (dystonia, athetosis, and sometimes spasticity) correspond to lesions in the basal ganglia, specifically the globus pallidus and the subthalamic nucleus, cerebellum, and brainstem nuclei that are related to trance tone and vestibular function. The auditory dysfunction (AN/AD [see later discussion], hearing loss, deafness) is associated with lesions of the auditory brainstem nuclei, and the oculomotor impairment is associated with damage to brainstem ocular nuclei.

In human autopsy studies, the globus pallidus pars externa (GPe) and interna (GPi), substantia nigra reticulata, subthalmic nucleus (STN), and less consistently, brainstem auditory structures, oculomotor nuclei, the hippocampus, and the cerebellum were affected selectively in cases of kernicterus without appreciable involvement of the striatum and thalamus [16,20,53–56]. In most cases, GPe and GPi show similar moderate to marked loss of neurons, demyelination, and prominent gliosis [14,55,57,58]. The pathologic alterations in STN are similar, but generally have been less severe. Unfortunately, good

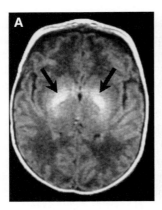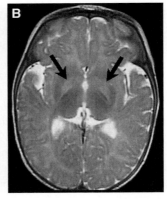

Fig. 1. Axial MRI scans showing bilateral hyperintense lesions in the globus pallidus in axial projections (*arrows*). (*A*) T1-weighted axial image of a 6-day-old, 37-week gestation boy with peak total bilirubin of 34.6 mg/dL. At age 7, this child was highly intelligent but moderately to severely disabled with dystonic, athetoid kernicteric CP; he ambulates with a walker. (*From* Shapiro SM. Bilirubin toxicity in the developing nervous system. Pediatric Neurology 2003;29:414; with permission.) (*B*) Axial T2-weighted MRI of a 2-year-old who has classic dystonic kernicterus. Note the increased intensity of the globus pallidus bilaterally (shown with arrows and dotted line on right side only). There were no abnormalities noted in brainstem or cerebellum.

clinical correlations between the degree of dystonia and athetoid features and the extent of the pathologic findings are lacking. In line with the autopsy findings, MRI studies of kernicterus demonstrate remarkably selective patterns of injury to GPe and GPi in children (see below and Fig. 1) [59].

Autopsy studies of infants who had classic kernicterus [55,60,61], and premature, low birth weight infants who had "low-bilirubin kernicterus" [14] showed central auditory pathology, with involvement of brainstem auditory structures, including the dorsal and ventral cochlear nuclei, superior olivary complex, and nuclei of the lateral lemniscus and inferior colliculus, but no significant abnormalities of the eighth nerve [60] or inner ear structures [62,63].

New clinical concepts and tools relating to kernicterus

The auditory system

The auditory brainstem response

Evoked potentials are highly sensitive to neuronal conduction delays, desynchronization, and loss of cells that occur in several pathologic conditions that involve brain injury, metabolic disorders, and demyelination [64–66]. The ABRs, also known as brainstem auditory evoked potentials (BAEPs) or responses (BAERs), are electrical potentials that are evoked by auditory stimulation and recorded noninvasively from the scalp. A series of peaks and trough (waves) can be distinguished from the background electrical activity (electroencephalogram) by averaging the response to many stimuli, which arise from neural generators in the auditory nerve and brainstem fiber tracts and nuclei [67–70]. Each ABR wave is generated by a small population of synchronously firing neurons, and reflects the activation of specific, temporally overlapping anatomic regions of the brainstem. The time between ABR wave peaks reflects the time that it takes for nerve impulses to travel from one anatomic location to another. Changes in the neural pathways cause delayed or abnormal conduction of impulses and manifest as increased interwave intervals (ie, the times between specific ABR waves). Desynchronization or loss of nerve cell activity also produces changes in amplitudes and morphology of the ABR waves. Thus, alterations of interwave interval or wave amplitude may reflect neuronal dysfunction.

ABRs, first described in 1967 [71] but not widely recognized until 1970 [72] were studied first in older children and adults who had chronic kernicteric bilirubin encephalopathy [73,74]. Abnormal function of the auditory nerve and the brainstem were found in patients from whom normal cochlear microphonic recordings were obtained [73]. Today, this would be diagnosed as AN/AD (see later discussion). In hyperbilirubinemic human newborns, increases in interwave intervals (the time between ABR peaks, a measure of central auditory function) and decreases in amplitudes were found [73,75–77]. These abnormalities were reversed when exchange transfusions were used to treat hyperbilirubinemia [77–79]. ABR changes correlate significantly with serum levels of total and Bf in the newborn period [76] and at follow-up [80].

Hyperbilirubinemic jj Gunn rats have functional abnormalities of the CNS as measured with ABRs [23,81,82]. Their ABRs have prolongation of interwave intervals that are equivalent to the conduction delays to the pons (wave III) and the midbrain (wave V) and reduced amplitudes of the ABR waves from these same brainstem areas in humans [23,81]. In more severely affected animals, all waves, including wave I from the auditory nerve, are lost. These abnormalities correlate with the known sites of bilirubin damage in the auditory brainstem pathways [17,19,83,84], specifically in the cochlear nuclei and other, lower brainstem (pontine) nuclei. Acute ABR abnormalities are reversible, at least in part [85,86]. Another test of central auditory function, binaural interaction as measured with ABR binaural difference waves [87], is abnormal in this model [88], and relates to neuropathologic damage to the superior olivary complex, an area of the lower brainstem (pons) that is involved with interaural processing of sound [14,17,84]. The use of noninvasive electrophysiologic measures, such as ABRs in human infants, may predict the onset of conditions that lead to brain damage, guide preventative therapies, and help to pinpoint the role of bilirubin encephalopathy in the development of hearing loss and later identification of central auditory processing disorders.

Auditory neuropathy/auditory dyssynchrony

This clinical entity, defined as the presence of normal OAEs and the absence of ABRs [89,90], affects about 1 in 400 newborns [91]. Stein and colleagues [92]

initially described a series of children who had AN after documented hyperbilirubinemia, which raised the possibility of an association between bilirubin neurotoxicity and AN/AD; this was confirmed by subsequent reports [91,93–97].
Often, but not always, AN/AD is associated with hearing loss and deafness. The
authors believe that AN/AD is the auditory damage that occurs with kernicterus.
Severe AN/AD usually is associated with deafness. Without the ABR, first
described in 1967 [71] and first applied to children with hearing loss secondary to
hyperbilirubinemia in 1979 [73], the distinction between deafness that is due to
AN/AD and other causes could not be made. Mild AN/AD may not be associated
with hearing loss, and thus, audiograms are normal, yet auditory processing is
not. The authors suspect that difficulties with speech perception (eg, hearing in
noisy situations, on the telephone, or in some classroom environments) may
underlie learning disorders, such as dyslexia or auditory memory problems, and
that central auditory processing disorders may be misdiagnosed as attention
deficit disorders.

In 1996, patients were described with hearing impairment, normal evoked
OAEs (a test of the integrity of the mechanical structure of the inner ear), and
absent or abnormal ABRs; the term "auditory neuropathy" was coined [90]. The
authors and other investigators prefer the term "auditory neuropathy/auditory
dyssynchrony" to describe the condition better and to reflect the concern that the
term "neuropathy" is inappropriate for pathologies that may affect only central
auditory pathways [98–100]. The pathophysiology of AN/AD involves inner hair
cells, spiral ganglion cells or their processes in the auditory portion of the
eighth nerve, or the auditory brainstem, any or all of which, in theory, could
preserve OAEs and cochlear microphonic responses while producing severely
abnormal ABRs.

Absent ABRs and normal cochlear microphonic responses (obtained from the
outer hair cells of the inner ear) were described in 1979 in children who had hearing loss that was due to hyperbilirubinemia [73]. This article, which came 12 years
after the first published description of the ABR [71], may be the first report of
the as yet unnamed AN/AD syndrome. Numerous recent studies have identified
significant hyperbilirubinemia as a risk factor or cause of AN/AD; patients who
have AN/AD secondary to hyperbilirubinemia may represent a unique subset of
patients who have AN/AD.

AN/AD prevalence in more than 5000 children who were assessed in an "at-
risk" screening program was 0.23%; it was 11% in a group of children who had
permanent hearing deficits [91]. Although 68% of patients who have AN/AD
have a complicated perinatal course [101], one third of children have no identifiable risk factors. Notably, a history of hyperbilirubinemia and prematurity is
found in more than half of patients who have AN/AD [101].

With the increased recognition of AD/AN through neonatal programs that
use ABRs or automatic ABR screening, the number of diagnosed cases of
AD/AN is likely to increase. A recent report of universal screening found that
24% of 477 graduates from a regional perinatal center neonatal ICU fit the
AN/AD profile of absent ABRs and present OAEs [102]. Of the possible risk

factors that were assessed (gender, gestational age, ototoxic drug regimen, low birth weight, hyperbilirubinemia, hydrocephalus, low Apgar score, anoxia, respiratory distress syndrome, pulmonary hypertension, intraventricular hemorrhage, multiple birth, seizure activity, and family history), only hyperbilirubinemia and administration of vancomycin or furosemide were more frequent in the group that had AN/AD.

The authors have seen less severe cases of hyperbilirubinemia that result in isolated AN/AD ([103] and S.M. Shapiro, unpublished data). Findings in the jaundiced Gunn rat parallel those that are found in children who have bilirubin-induced AN/AD [104]; these emphasize that the auditory pathology in children who have AN/AD may be in the brainstem, the spiral ganglia and auditory nerve, or both. Further studies are needed to strengthen and formalize this preliminary study.

When the perceptual abilities of children who have AN/AD are compared with normal children and those who have sensorineural hearing loss, the differences mostly are related to temporal abnormalities. Children who have AN/AD have a severe disruption in the temporal coding of speech and an inability to cope with the dynamics of speech [105]. The low threshold of activation and high spontaneous discharge rate of large-diameter axons that innervate inner hair cells in the cochlea [106] are electrophysiologic properties that are ideally suited for the temporal coding of auditory information, particularly as it relates to neural synchrony and temporally-dependent auditory events (eg, speech comprehension) [107].

Cochlear implants were approved for use in children in 1990. Subsequently, their use was shown to benefit children who have AN/AD [108,109]. The authors are aware of several children who have AN/AD and classic and auditory-predominant kernicterus who benefited from cochlear implantation. With the continued expansion of the indications of cochlear implantation, early diagnosis of AN/AD becomes more crucial to help determine which children will be good candidates for this surgical treatment of deafness; it is generally held that the earlier it is done, the better the result.

The neuromotor system: disorders of movement and tone

Dystonia is characterized by excessive and sustained contractions of opposing muscles. Early in the course of most forms of dystonia, abnormal muscle activation occurs, principally during voluntary movements, and is confined mostly to activated sets of muscles. With more severe disease, the contractions tend to become more constant and involve muscle groups that are not activated voluntarily (so-called "overflow contractions"). Often, painful muscle cramps are present in more severe forms of kernicterus; in the most severe form cramps are only relieved by intrathecal baclofen. Some mild, subtle cases of predominantly auditory kernicterus have included infrequent, but dramatic and painful, episodes of muscle cramps during infancy and early childhood. Incoordination of sucking, swallowing, gastrointestinal motility, and oculomotor motility disturbances, including strabismus and paresis of upward gaze, are other dystonic neuromotor signs.

In children dystonia has been defined as a movement disorder in which involuntary sustained or intermittent muscle contractions cause twisting and repetitive movements, abnormal postures, or both. Dystonia is common in infants and children who have kernicterus, although it may be hard to recognize in infants. The absence of velocity in dystonia distinguishes dystonia from spasticity.

Regardless of the type of dystonia, groups of EMG burst periods of 1 to 6.5 cycles/s are characteristic [110–112]. The EMG activity is typified by prolonged spasms that are separated by short silent periods and brief (< 500 milliseconds) myoclonic-like bursts. These bursts or spasms often present in rhythmic sequences [110].

Autopsy studies in human cases of kernicterus showed extensive neuronal loss in GPi and GPe, and typically less dramatic loss in STN, but correlations between dystonia and other extrapyramidal symptoms and the degree of preagonal neuronal loss have not been defined adequately.

Neuroimaging

MRIs in the authors' human patients have had the remarkably similar findings of abnormal intensity in the globus pallidus (GP) (see Fig. 1) and the subthalamic nucleus. Although similar changes have been reported only infrequently in STN, the STN is more difficult to visualize with standard MRI protocols.

Beginning in 1994, MRI abnormalities in GP and the STN in kernicterus have been described in the literature; these are largely single case reports that demonstrate abnormalities of the GP, and occasionally, the STN [57,113–130].

In autopsy studies, abnormalities also were reported in hippocampus; putamen; thalamus; cranial nerve nuclei III, IV, VI, and VIII; dentate nuclei; and cerebellar flocculi. Some of these abnormalities are too small to be seen on MRI; some abnormalities (eg, those in the putamen) may have been from concomitant hypoxic-ischemic brain injury because the babies died in an era before the widespread use of respirators to treat respiratory disorders of newborns.

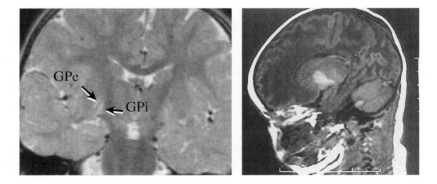

Fig. 2. T2-weighted MRI from a 1-Tesla magnet showing increased signal in coronal (*left*) and sagittal (*right*) views. Note the GPe and GPi can be distinguished in the coronal view.

Preliminary results from a retrospective analysis of 40 MRIs from 23 patients who were born between 1988 and July 2003 with clinically defined kernicterus showed that the GP was abnormal bilaterally in 20 individuals (87%), and that the STN was abnormal in 8 (35%; see Fig. 1, Fig. 2). The clinical severity of disease ranged from mild to severe, with a full range of classic, auditory-predominant, and neuromotor-predominant kernicterus. Gestational age at birth ranged from 33.5 weeks to 40 weeks, and peak total bilirubin ranged from 19.3 mg/dL to 47 mg/dL. The small number of identified abnormalities in the STN may have been largely attributable to limitations in visualizing this small nucleus. Other basal ganglia structures were normal except for 1 child who had an abnormal caudate and had concomitant hypoxia-ischemia encephalopathy (HIE), and 3 other children who had clinical and MRI evidence of periventricular leukomalacia, ventriculomegaly, and increased subarachnoid spaces. These findings also corresponded to the concomitant clinical findings of HIE. These latter patients emphasize the clinical usefulness of MRI in establishing other etiologies of CP or other coexistent conditions.

Clinical syndromes of kernicterus

Bilirubin neurotoxicity produces selective damage of the CNS. Clinical symptoms of classic, chronic bilirubin encephalopathy (kernicterus) in humans correlate with specific pathologic findings. The classic sequelae of excessive neonatal hyperbilirubinemia is a tetrad of athetoid CP, deafness or hearing loss, impairment of upward gaze, and enamel dysplasia of the primary teeth; they correspond to pathologic lesions in the GP, subthalamic nucleus, and auditory and oculomotor brainstem nuclei. Other areas that are damaged classically by bilirubin are the cerebellum, particularly the Purkinje cells, and the hippocampus, which is affected in CA-2, a different locus than in other disorders (eg, hypoxia-ischemia and epilepsy). Gastrointestinal problems, including suck and swallowing disturbances, reflux, and constipation, occur commonly.

Acute bilirubin encephalopathy

In neonates who have acute bilirubin toxicity symptomatology begins with lethargy and decreased feeding, and progresses to variable or fluctuating tone (hypo- and hypertonia), high-pitched cry, retrocollis and opisthotonus, impairment of upward gaze (setting sun sign), fever, seizures, and death. Laboratory studies show absent or abnormal ABRs [79,80,131], which are reversible with double-volume exchange transfusion [78,132]. MRIs show bilateral hyperintense lesions in the GP [59,117,121,124,128] on T1-weighted images as soon as 1 day after peak TSB (S.M. Shapiro, unpublished data). The authors consider significant neonatal hyperbilirubinemia with signs of encephalopathy to be a neurologic emergency that should be treated immediately, because outcome is related, in part, to the duration of exposure to excessive bilirubin. The authors' anecdotal evidence suggests that exchange transfusion may, in part, reverse neurotoxicity. While awaiting blood for exchange transfusion, intense photo-therapy (eg, a double bank of phototherapy lamps overhead as close to the infant as possible with or without spotlights, plus intense light from below), and gavage feedings with preferably elemental formula [133] to promote fecal excretion of bilirubin are recommended.

Mistakes in treatment frequently encountered in reviewing neonatal records of children later diagnosed with kernicterus include:

1. No knowledge that the distance of the lights from the baby is important— the closer the better
2. No knowledge that oral feeding helps to promote bilirubin excretion—the baby is made NPO
3. Belief that the bilirubin level "cannot be that high" leads to unnecessary delays in treatment
4. Other investigations (eg, sepsis work-ups, lumbar punctures, echocardio-gram) lead to unnecessary delays in initiating phototherapy or ex-change transfusions
5. Babies with very high TSB and conjugated bilirubin levels are not treated because of fear of "bronze baby" syndrome
6. Surgical treatment of other urgent, life-threatening illnesses (eg, cardiac conditions or necrotizing endocarditis with perforation) leads to discon-tinuing phototherapy in the operating and recovery rooms
7. That opinion that because the bilirubin level is so high and the baby is so encephalopathic that it is too late to treat

The authors strongly believe that it is never too late to treat acute, symptomatic bilirubin encephalopathy, because the duration of excessive hyperbilirubinemia is related to outcome [134,135]. They also believe that the faster and the more aggressive the treatment, the more reversible and better the outcome.

Chronic bilirubin encephalopathy

The clinical features of bilirubin encephalopathy range from deafness and severe athetoid CP, seizures, or death from kernicterus, to subtle cognitive dis-turbances. The most extreme brain injury—classic kernicterus—produces extra-pyramidal abnormalities, especially dystonia, athetosis, and less frequently, spasticity; hearing loss or deafness that is due primarily to AN/AD; gaze abnor-malities, especially impairment of upward gaze but including other oculomotor pareses (eg, strabismus); and enamel hypoplasia of deciduous (baby) teeth [1,2,12]. Intellect usually is within the normal range. Seizures may occur with acute, severe neonatal encephalopathy, and usually resolve over several weeks. Paroxysmal movement disorders that are diagnosed as seizures and treated with antiepileptic medications have been reported by parents in some patients who have classic kernicterus. Whether these represent an increased incidence of epilepsy or the misidentification of paroxysmal movement disorders as epilepsy remains to be determined; appropriate electroencephalogram (EEG) and video EEG monitoring should illuminate this issue, especially because some movement disorders (eg, paroxysmal dyskinesias) are responsive to small doses of anti-epileptic medications, such as carbamazepine (Tegretol).

Subtle bilirubin encephalopathy is associated with less severe injury, learning disabilities, mild neurologic abnormalities [134,136–140], isolated neural hearing loss [141,142], and AN [91,94]. The extent to which subtle bilirubin encepha-lopathy contributes to the prevalence of learning disabilities, central auditory processing disorders, and hearing loss in the population is not known because it is difficult to relate peak TSB levels—which do not necessarily reflect brain tissue exposure to bilirubin—in newborns to disabilities that may be discovered years later.

Subtypes of clinical kernicterus may exist, including auditory-predominant and motor-predominant kernicterus, and the pattern of involvement may relate to factors, such as gestational age and amount and duration of hyperbilirubinemia. In a preliminary review of 18 cases of kernicterus, auditory-predominant symp-toms (ie, AN/AD with no or minimal motor involvement) were seen in four children, three of whom were born at up to 34 weeks' gestation with peak total bilirubin levels of up to 24 mg/dL [143]. Because the auditory system develops earlier than the extrapyramidal motor control pathways, the authors hypothesize that early exposure to bilirubin toxicity during development may affect the auditory system preferentially.

Subtle kernicterus

Prospective controlled studies have revealed cognitive and neurologic impair-ment in children with elevated levels of unbound bilirubin in the newborn period [134,138,144]. Large studies of healthy, term newborns, such as the National Collaborative Perinatal project [139,140,145], found associations between "low levels" of hyperbilirubinemia that ordinarily would not be treated and subtle cognitive sequelae. There is concern that moderate degrees of hyperbilirubinemia in healthy term neonates may not be safe for the brain [146]. Although deafness is a feature of classic kernicterus, the authors' studies [141] and those of other investigators [135,147] showed an association between moderate to severe sen-sorineural hearing loss and central auditory dysfunction and elevated biliru-bin levels in the newborn in the apparent absence of other manifestations of kernicterus. The amount and duration of hyperbilirubinemia are risk factors [135,141]. Some evidence suggests that the development of sensorineural loss associated with hyperbilirubinemia may be delayed and progressive [125].

New definitions of kernicterus

The authors classify clinical symptoms by severity (mild, moderate, severe) and localization (isolated, mixed, classic) using objective criteria, as presented last year by one of us (S.M.S.) at a National Institutes of Health–National Institute of Child Health and Development conference [143]. Taken together, these factors permit formulation of a more detailed picture of kernicterus, and perhaps a larger spectrum of kernicterus (BIND).

Severity. From the authors' experience and that of other investigators, the severity of kernicterus varies widely from mild to severe in children and adults. The authors previously suggested definitions for categorizing the range of severity of kernicterus [103], which they now believe underemphasizes the wide spectrum of the true disability and does not account for the fact that the degree of handicap may change with age and maturation. Further, their classification of severity applies to the usually most disabling neuromotor features of kernicterus and does not consider the effect of treating the most profound auditory disability—AN/AD plus deafness—with cochlear implantation (see later discussion). Subtly to mildly affected individuals remain high functioning, with little to no functional disability, but may have significant learning disabilities; subtle movement disorders, especially under stressful conditions; and occasional muscle cramps. Moderately affected individuals have more prominent dystonia, perhaps with athetoid movements, but eventually are able to talk with reasonable clarity, feed themselves, and ambulate unassisted, although awkwardly and with poor stability. Severely affected individuals have a more disabling dystonia and are nonambulatory, ambulate only with assistance (eg, a walker), or ambulate independently for limited periods with great difficulty, usually after years of depending on a walker. Their speech is dysarthric and hardly understandable. Profoundly affected individuals are invariably wheelchair-bound, and do not speak or speak only with great difficulty. They have severe auditory dysfunction or deafness, and have totally disabling dystonia, often with frequent or constant painful muscle cramps.

The degree of handicap may change with age and maturation, but the change is within limits and is not dramatic. Individuals may move between, but do not skip, categories (eg, change from profound to moderate or from severe to mild).

The severity of auditory symptoms often correlates with the severity of the neuromotor symptoms, but discrepancies may occur. Both AN/AD and hearing loss may vary in severity. AN/AD varies from a mild, subtle central auditory processing disorder to a severe disorder with persistent, absent ABRs and deafness. Hearing loss may vary from none to profound, and can appear variable with time. The severities of the AN/AD and hearing loss are usually similar but are sometimes discrepant.

Localization. The localization varies from patient to patient. Isolated kernicterus describes symptoms that are limited to one system (eg, auditory without movement disorder, or vice versa); however, strictly isolated kernicterus is not seen, but can be classified as mixed—auditory predominant or motor predominant. Preliminary evidence suggests that auditory-predominant kernicterus is more likely to occur in prematurely born infants [143].

Diagnosis of kernicterus

Too often, parents are told that the diagnosis of kernicterus can be made only at autopsy. Although technically correct—because the original condition was defined pathologically and refers to yellow coloration of the deep nuclei of the brain, and the correct term is "bilirubin encephalopathy"—the statement is foolish, upsetting to parents, and suggests a lack of understanding that kernicterus can be diagnosed clinically, and that characteristic lesions can be imaged with MRI. It is as incorrect as refusing to use the term "cerebral palsy" when talking to parents, because the correct term is "static encephalopathy," and saying that "CP can be diagnosed only at autopsy."

In the newborn period and beyond, kernicterus is diagnosed by a combination of history, physical examination, and laboratory tests. In all cases there should be a history of jaundice, and it is hoped that there is laboratory confirmation of an increased serum bilirubin level, the significance of which is modified by duration and risk factors. Important history is whether bilirubin encephalopathy was present or if the child was symptomatic neurologically in any way at the time of the hyperbilirubinemia. Special attention should be paid to tone; hypertonia, hypotonia, or variability of tone from increased to decreased is particularly significant. Setting sun sign, with the sclera visible below the upper eyelid, is characteristic during acute bilirubin encephalopathy, although it is not unique to bilirubin toxicity.

An ABR that is taken soon after the suspected exposure is most helpful, because absent or abnormal ABRs may improve with time. Although improvement in ABR is a good sign, it does not mean that the auditory system has returned to normal. The ABR tests only a small subpopulation of neurons in the ascending auditory system, and even if all dysfunctional neurons recover completely, their dysfunction could disrupt normal neurodevelopmental processes and lead to suboptimal or deviant development. One mistake is confusing the two types of newborn hearing screening. An automated ABR (AABR) is a crude, pass/fail ABR that is often abnormal with severe kernicterus and an absent ABR; however, AABR can be normal in milder kernicterus when ABR is abnormal but not absent. Regardless, OAEs will be normal, even when ABRs and AABRs are absent. An MRI scan of the brain with an abnormal GP—with or without an abnormal STN—and without other significant abnormalities is nearly pathognomonic of kernicterus. Initially, within the first few days after the insult, the T1-weighted scans show hyperintensity. Weeks or months later, T2-weighted images become hyperintense, and T1-weighted images become normo- or hypointense. Head CT and ultrasound are of no use in the diagnosis of kernicterus.

Examination in older children and adults often involves determining whether CP or neurodevelopmental problems are due to neonatal hyperbilirubinemia. To determine whether neurodevelopmental problems are due to hyperbilirubinemia, the authors consider history, physical examination, MRI, and ABR. Important in the history is the amount and duration of hyperbilirubinemia; other risk factors, such as sepsis, acidosis, Rh disease, history of neonatal neurologic signs or symptoms (eg, abnormal tone, cry, posturing, abnormal eye movements or positions) at the time of or following hyperbilirubinemia; and history of dental enamel dysplasia. A history of muscle cramps or delayed gross or fine motor development or speech is sought. Inconsistency of hearing or sound localization in a young child raises the suspicion of a subtle AN/AD. A history of past or present sucking and swallowing dysfunction, gastroesophageal reflux, constipation, and failure to thrive often can be obtained.

On examination, athetosis (slow writhing movements), dystonia (abnormal tone, fixed postures, cocontraction of agonist and antagonist muscles), variable hypo/hypertonia, spasticity, ataxia, incoordination, impaired upgaze, staining or flaking of deciduous teeth (enamel hypoplasia), dysarthria, hearing impairment, or difficulty localizing sound may be found. Improvement of impaired upward gaze has been described, but it is difficult to examine upward gaze in older infants and young children who have learned to turn their heads to compensate for gaze pareses.

The MRI may show abnormal signal in GP or STN, but a normal MRI does not exclude the diagnosis. Abnormal MRIs may or may not improve with time. Few other etiologies cause discrete bilateral lesions in GP and STN, and most of these are metabolic conditions with a different history and onset (eg, glutaric aciduria with a sudden onset of encephalopathy or abnormal movements during an acute febrile illness or episode of vomiting). In addition, MRIs in these conditions usually show more extensive areas of damage. MRIs with other lesions in putamen and cortex or with periventricular leukomalacia may occur in children who have other conditions or with "kernicterus plus syndrome"(ie, kernicterus plus other neonatal encephalopathies, such as hypoxic-ischemia, stroke, encephalitis, intraventricular hemorrhage).

The ABR may be absent or abnormal with an increase of conduction time between waves I and III and I and V. The cochlear microphonic response, which can be obtained at the time of ABR testing, should be present even in the absence of ABR neural waves (I through V). Occasionally, "giant" cochlear microphonic responses may occur and be mistaken for ABR waves, but they can be distinguished by the fact that they do not change their latencies with intensity and they phase reverse with phase reversal of the click stimulus. ABRs may or may not improve with time. OAEs, initially normal, may disappear with time. A full audiology evaluation usually is advisable. As with MRI, an abnormal ABR in the presence of AN/AD is consistent with bilirubin neurotoxicity, but a normal ABR does not rule out kernicterus.

Treatment of kernicterus

Therapies

Physical, occupational, and speech therapy evaluations can be helpful. Some audiologists consider "cued speech," a combination of speech lip reading and hand signals, to be helpful to develop literacy. Certain therapy techniques seem to work better with kernicterus than with other types of CP. Because intelligence usually is normal, cooperation with therapy may be better than expected usually. Aids, such as reverse walkers, have been helpful to parents. If reading problems develop, an auditory processing problem may prevent the child from being able to hear the phonemic content of speech, and thus, be unable to decode how letter combinations represent speech sounds. Tailored education programs, such as the Wilson Reading Program, are geared to having the child memorize the 46 phonemes in the English language to compensate for not hearing these sounds normally [148,149] (for more information visit www.ecs.org/clearing house/19/01/1901.htm or www.wilsonlanguage.com).

Medical treatments

Treatment is undertaken often to improve dystonia, which can manifest as irritability in infants. First, gastroesophageal reflux should be excluded or treated. Benzodiazepines, such as diazepam, are beneficial. Artane, gradually building up to high dosages, has been recommended by some investigators. Often, baclofen is tried if benzodiazepine is unsuccessful. Gastrointestinal problems should be evaluated with barium swallow and consultation with a pediatric gastroenterologist. Supplemental feeding in children who are not gaining weight often is beneficial.

Surgical treatments

Some of the most encouraging treatments for moderate to severe kernicterus are surgical, including gastrostomy tubes and Nisson fundoplication to treat gastroesophageal reflux, and sometimes feeding or gastrostomy tubes to supplement feeding. Most children who have classic or motor-predominant kernicterus are thin because of their movement disorder–induced increased caloric requirements, coupled with the abnormal sucking and swallowing that are due to their dystonia and hyperkinetic movement disorder. Fixed contractures do not seem to occur as frequently as in CP from other causes, and orthopedic surgery is discouraged in favor of medication and Botox injections. With severe dystonia and muscle cramps, intrathecal baclofen pumps have been successful when medication has failed.

Cochlear implantation has been used in about a dozen children who have AN/AD and deafness that is due to kernicterus. Although the use of a cochlear implant seems paradoxic with AN/AD, especially when the lesions are proximal to the device, it works. The success of cochlear implantation for AN/AD is well documented in the literature [108,109,150], although these studies did not include clear cases of kernicterus. The authors have experienced dramatically positive results with examination or parent reporting of cochlear implantation in about a half dozen children who had kernicterus. There is some urgency in diagnosing AN/AD properly early in life because if cochlear implantation is to be considered, the earlier the better. Most implants are being done at 1 year of age or younger.

Finally, deep brain stimulation has been considered and tried in one or two patients who have kernicterus. This technology is promising because the condition is static and, in severe cases, even small improvements in function may have a large impact on quality of life. Unfortunately, current knowledge does not provide the answer to where to put the stimulators.

References

[1] Byers RK, Paine RS, Crothers B. Extrapyramidal cerebral palsy with hearing loss following erythroblastosis. Pediatrics 1955;15:248–54.

[2] Volpe JJ. Bilirubin and brain injury. In: Volpe JJ, editor. Neurology of the newborn. 3rd edition. Philadelphia: W.B. Saunders; 2001. p. 490–514.

[3] Larroche JC. Kernicterus. In: Vinken P, Bruyn GW, editors. Handbook of clinical neurology, vol. 6. Amsterdam: North-Holland; 1968. p. 491–515.

[4] Watchko JF, Oski FA. Bilirubin 20 mg/dL = vigintiphobia. Pediatrics 1983;71(4):660–3.

[5] Newman TB, Maisels MJ. Evaluation and treatment of jaundice in the term newborn: a kinder, gentler approach. Pediatrics 1992;89(5):809–18.

[6] Watchko JF, Oski FA. Kernicterus in preterm newborns: past, present, and future. Pediatrics 1992;90(5):707–15.

[7] Brown AK, Johnson L. Loss of concern about jaundice and the reemergence of kernicterus in full term infants in the era of managed care. In: Fanaroff AA, Klaus M, editors. Yearbook of neonatal and perinatal medicine. St. Louis (MO): Mosby Yearbook; 1996. p. xvii–xxviii.

[8] Johnson LH, Bhutani VK, Brown AK. System-based approach to management of neonatal jaundice and prevention of kernicterus. J Pediatr 2002;140(4):396–403.

[9] Bhutani VK, Johnson LH, Maisels MJ, et al. Kernicterus: epidemiological strategies for its prevention through systems-based approaches. J Perinatol 2004;24(10):650–62.

[10] Maisels MJ, Newman TB. Kernicterus in otherwise healthy, breast-fed term newborns. Pediatrics 1995;96(4 Pt 1):730–3.

[11] JCAHO issues warning on kernicterus danger. Hosp Peer Rev 2001;26(7):100–1.

[12] Perlstein MA. The late clinical syndrome of posticteric encephalopathy. Pediatr Clin North Am 1960;7:665–87.

[13] Ahdab-Barmada M. Kernicterus in the premature neonate. J Perinatol 1987;7(2):149–52.

[14] Ahdab-Barmada M, Moossy J. The neuropathology of kernicterus in the premature neonate: diagnostic problems. J Neuropathol Exp Neurol 1984;43:45–56.

[15] Johnson L, Sarmiento F, Blanc WA, et al. Kernicterus in rats with an inherited deficiency of glucuronyl transferase. Am J Dis Child 1959;97:591–608.

[16] Blanc WA, Johnson L. Studies on kernicterus; relationship with sulfonamide intoxication, report on kernicterus in rats with glucuronyl transferase deficiency and review of pathogenesis. J Neuropathol Exp Neurol 1959;18:165–89.

[17] Conlee JW, Shapiro SM. Morphological changes in the cochlear nucleus and nucleus of the trapezoid body in Gunn rat pups. Hear Res 1991;57(1):23–30.

[18] Conlee JW, Shapiro SM. Development of cerebellar hypoplasia in jaundiced Gunn rats treated with sulfadimethoxine: a quantitative light microscopic analysis. Acta Neuropathol (Berl) 1997; 93:450–60.

[19] Jew JY, Williams TH. Ultrastructural aspects of bilirubin encephalopathy in cochlear nuclei of the Gunn rat. J Anat 1977;124:599–614.

[20] Rose AL, Wisniewski H. Acute bilirubin encephalopathy induced with sulfadimethoxine in Gunn rats. J Neuropathol Exp Neurol 1979;38:152–65.

[21] Roy Chowdhury N, Gross F, Moscioni AD, et al. Isolation of multiple normal and functionally defective forms of uridine diphosphate-glucuronosyltransferase from inbred Gunn rats. J Clin Invest 1987;79(2):327–34.

[22] Schutta HS, Johnson L. Clinical signs and morphologic abnormalities in Gunn rats treated with sulfadimethoxine. J Pediatr 1969;75:1070–9.

[23] Shapiro SM, Hecox KE. Developmental studies of brainstem auditory evoked potentials in jaundiced Gunn rats. Brain Res 1988;469(1–2):147–57.

[24] Spencer RF, Shaia WT, Gleason AT, et al. Changes in calcium-binding protein expression in the auditory brainstem nuclei of the jaundiced Gunn rat. Hear Res 2002;171(1–2):129–41.

[25] Johnson L, Brown AK. A pilot registry for acute and chronic kernicterus in term and near-term infants. Pediatrics 1999;104(3):736.

[26] Johnson L, Brown AK, Bhutani VK. BIND-A clinical score for bilirubin induced neurologic dysfunction in newborns. Pediatrics 1999;104(3 Part 3):746–7.

[27] Bhutani VK, Johnson LH, Caren R. Acute bilirubin encephalopathy in healthy term and near-term newborns. Contemp Pediatr 2005;22:57–74.

[28] Wennberg RP, Ahlfors CE, Bhutani VK, et al. Toward understanding kernicterus: a challenge to improve the management of jaundiced newborns. Pediatrics 2006;117:474–85.

[29] Ostrow JD, Pascolo L, Brites D, et al. Molecular basis of bilirubin-induced neurotoxicity. Trends Mol Med 2004;10(2):65–70.

[30] Keino H, Sata H, Semba R, et al. Mode of prevention by phototherapy of cerebellar hypoplasia in new Sprague-Dawley strain of jaundiced Gunn rats. Pediatr Neurosci 1985;12:145–50.

[31] Churn SB, Taft WC, DeLorenzo RJ. Effect of ischemia on multifunction calcium/calmodulin-dependent protein kinase II in the gerbil. Stroke 1990;21(Suppl III):112–26.

[32] Wasterlain CG, Farber DB. Kindling alters the calcium/calmodulin-dependent phosphorylation of synaptic membrane proteins in rat hippocampus. Proc Natl Acad Sci U S A 1984;81:1253–7.

[33] Perlin JB, Churn SB, Lothman EW, et al. Loss of type II calcium/calmodulin-dependent kinase activity correlates with stages of development of electrographic seizures in status epilepticus in rat. Epilepsy Res 1992;11:111–8.

[34] Greengard P. Neuronal phosphoproteins. Mediators of signal transduction. Mol Neurobiol 1987;1:51–119.

[35] Braun AP, Schulman H. The multifunctional calcium/calmodulin-dependent protein kinase: from form to function. Annu Rev Physiol 1995;57:417–45.

[36] Malinow R, Schulman H, Tsien RW. Inhibition of postsynaptic PKC or CaMKII block induction but not expression of LTP. Science 1989;245:862–6.

[37] Churn SB, Kochan LD, DeLorenzo RJ. Chronic inhibition of Ca(2+)/calmodulin kinase II activity in the pilocarpine model of epilepsy. Brain Res 2000;875(1–2):66–77.

[38] Kochan LD, Churn SB, Omojokun O, et al. Status epilepticus results in an N-methyl-D-aspartate receptor-dependent inhibition of Ca2+/calmodulin-dependent kinase II activity in the rat. Neuroscience 2000;95(3):735–43.

[39] Churn SB. Multifunctional calcium and calmodulin-dependent kinase II in neuronal function and disease. Adv Neuroimmunol 1995;5(3):241–59.

[40] Conlee JW, Shapiro SM, Churn SB. Expression of the alpha and beta subunits of Ca2+/calmodulin kinase II in the cerebellum of jaundiced Gunn rats during development: a quantitative light microscopic analysis. Acta Neuropathol (Berl) 2000;99(4):393–401.

[41] Shaia WT, Shapiro SM, Heller AJ, et al. Immunohistochemical localization of calcium-binding proteins in the brainstem vestibular nuclei of the jaundiced Gunn rat. Hear Res 2002;173(1–2):82–90.

[42] Hoffman DJ, Zanelli SA, Kubin J, et al. The in vivo effect of bilirubin on the N-methyl-D-aspartate receptor/ion channel complex in the brains of newborn piglets. Pediatr Res 1996;40(6):804–8.

[43] McDonald JW, Shapiro SM, Silverstein FS, et al. Role of glutamate receptor-mediated excitotoxicity in bilirubin-induced brain injury in the Gunn rat model. Exp Neurol 1998;150(1):21–9.

[44] Grojean S, Koziel V, Vert P, et al. Bilirubin induces apoptosis via activation of NMDA receptors in developing rat brain neurons. Exp Neurol 2000;166(2):334–41.

[45] Warr O, Mort D, Attwell D. Bilirubin does not modulate ionotropic glutamate receptors or glutamate transporters. Brain Res 2000;879(1–2):13–6.

[46] Ostrow JD, Pascolo L, Shapiro SM, et al. New concepts of bilirubin encephalopathy. Eur J Clin Invest 2003;33(11):988–97.

[47] Rigato I, Pascolo L, Fernetti C, et al. The human multidrug-resistance-associated protein MRP1 mediates ATP-dependent transport of unconjugated bilirubin. Biochem J 2004;383(Pt 2): 335–41.

[48] Silva RF, Rodrigues CM, Brites D. Bilirubin-induced apoptosis in cultured rat neural cells is aggravated by chenodeoxycholic acid but prevented by ursodeoxycholic acid. J Hepatol 2001; 34(3):402–8.

[49] Rodrigues CMP, Sola S, Brites D. Bilirubin induces apoptosis via the mitochondrial pathway in developing rat brain neurons. Hepatology 2002;35:1186–95.

[50] Hanko E, Hansen TW, Almaas R, et al. Bilirubin induces apoptosis and necrosis in human NT2-N neurons. Pediatr Res 2005;57(2):179–84.

[51] Schutta HS, Johnson L. Bilirubin encephalopathy in the Gunn rat. A fine structure study of the cerebellar cortex. J Neuropathol Exp Neurol 1967;26:377–96.

[52] Yamamura H, Takagishi Y. Cerebellar hypoplasia in the hyperbilirubinemic Gunn rat: morphological aspects. Nagoya J Med Sci 1993;55(1–4):11–21.

[53] Kumada S, Hayashi M, Umitsu R, et al. Neuropathology of the dentate nucleus in developmental disorders. Acta Neuropathol (Berl) 1997;94(1):36–41.

[54] Ahdab-Barmada M, Moossy J. Kernicterus reexamined. Pediatrics 1983;71(3):463–4.

[55] Haymaker W, Margles C, Pentschew A. Pathology of kernicterus and posticteric encephalopathy. In: Swinyard CA, editor. Kernicterus and its importance in cerebral palsy. Springfield (IL): Charles C. Thomas; 1961. p. 21–229.

[56] Johnson L, Garcia ML, Figueroa E, et al. Kernicterus in rats lacking glucuronyl transferase. Am J Dis Child 1961;101:322–49.

[57] Claireaux AE. Pathology of human kernicterus. Montreal (Canada): University of Toronto Press; 1961.

[58] Malamud N. Pathogenesis of kernicterus in the light of its sequelae. In: Swinyard CA, editor. Kernicterus and its importance in cerebral palsy. Springfield (IL): Charles C. Thomas; 1961. p. 230–46.

[59] Johnston MV, Hoon Jr AH. Possible mechanisms in infants for selective basal ganglia damage from asphyxia, kernicterus, or mitochondrial encephalopathies. J Child Neurol 2000;15(9): 588–91.

[60] Dublin W. Neurological lesions in erythroblastosis fetalis in relation to nuclear deafness. Am J Clin Path 1951;21:935–9.

[61] Dublin W. Fundamentals of sensorineural auditory pathology. Springfield (IL): Charles C. Thomas; 1976.

[62] Gerrard J. Nuclear jaundice and deafness. J Laryngol Otol 1952;66:39–46.

[63] Kelemen G. Erythroblastosis fetalis. Pathologic report on the hearing organs of a newborn infant. AMA Arch Otolaryngol 1956;63:392–8.

[64] Hecox KE, Cone B, Blaw ME. Brainstem auditory evoked response in the diagnosis of pediatric neurologic diseases. Neurology 1981;31:832–9.

[65] Starr A. Sensory evoked potentials in clinical disorders of the nervous system. Annu Rev Neurosci 1978;1:103–27.

[66] Greenberg RP, Ducker TB. Evoked potentials in the clinical neurologies. J Neurosurg 1982; 56:1–18.

[67] Huang C-M, Buchwald JS. Interpretation of the vertex short-latency acoustic response: a study of single neurons in the brain stem. Brain Res 1977;137:291–303.

[68] Jewett DL, Romano MN. Neonatal development of auditory system potentials averaged from the scalp of rat and cat. Brain Res 1972;36:101–15.

[69] Melcher JR, Guinan Jr JJ, Knudson IM, et al. Generators of the brainstem auditory evoked potential in cat. II. Correlating lesion sites with waveform changes. Hear Res 1996;93(1–2): 28–51.

[70] Starr A, Hamilton AE. Correlation between confirmed sites of neurological lesions and abnormalities of far field auditory brainstem responses. Electroenceph Clin Neurophysiol 1976;41: 595–608.

[71] Sohmer H, Feinmesser M. Cochlear action potentials recorded from the external ear in man. Ann Otol Rhinol Laryngol 1967;76(2):427–35.

[72] Jewett DL, Romano MN, Williston JS. Human auditory evoked potentials: possible brain stem components detected on the scalp. Science 1970;167(924):1517–8.

[73] Chisin R, Perlman M, Sohmer H. Cochlear and brain stem responses in hearing loss following neonatal hyperbilirubinemia. Ann Otol 1979;88:352–7.

[74] Kaga K, Kitazumi E, Kodama K. Auditory brain stem responses of kernicterus infants. Int J Ped Otorhinolaryngol 1979;1:255–94.

[75] Lenhardt ML, McArtor R, Bryant B. Effects of neonatal hyperbilirubinemia on the brainstem electrical response. J Pediatr 1984;104:281–4.

[76] Nakamura H, Takada S, Shimabuku R, et al. Auditory nerve and brainstem responses in newborn infants with hyperbilirubinemia. Pediatrics 1985;75:703–8.

[77] Perlman M, Fainmesser P, Sohmer H, et al. Auditory nerve-brainstem evoked responses in hyperbilirubinemic neonates. Pediatrics 1983;72:658–64.

[78] Nwaesei CG, Van Aerde J, Boyden M, et al. Changes in auditory brainstem responses in hyperbilirubinemic infants before and after exchange transfusion. Pediatrics 1984;74(5):800–3.

[79] Wennberg RP, Ahlfors CE, Bickers R, et al. Abnormal auditory brainstem response in a newborn infant with hyperbilirubinemia: improvement with exchange transfusion. J Pediatr 1982;100(4):624–6.

[80] Funato M, Tamai H, Shimada S, et al. Vigitiphobia, unbound bilirubin, and auditory brainstem responses. Pediatrics 1994;93(1):50–3.

[81] Shapiro SM, Hecox KE. Brain stem auditory evoked potentials in jaundiced Gunn rats. Ann Otol Rhinol Laryngol 1989;98(4 Pt 1):308–17.

[82] Uziel A, Marot M, Pujol R. The Gunn rat: an experimental model for central deafness. Acta Otolaryngol 1983;95:651–6.

[83] Jew JY, Sandquist D. CNS changes in hyperbilirubinemia. Functional implications. Arch Neurol 1979;36:149–54.

[84] Shapiro SM, Conlee JW. Brainstem auditory evoked potentials correlate with morphological changes in Gunn rat pups. Hear Res 1991;57(1):16–22.

[85] Shapiro SM. Acute brainstem auditory evoked potential abnormalities in jaundiced Gunn rats given sulfonamide. Pediatr Res 1988;23(3):306–10.

[86] Shapiro SM. Reversible brainstem auditory evoked potential abnormalities in jaundiced Gunn rats given sulfonamide. Pediatr Res 1993;34(5):629–33.

[87] Dobie RA. Binaural interaction in brainstem-evoked responses. Arch Otolaryngol 1979;105: 391–8.

[88] Shapiro SM. Binaural effects in brainstem auditory evoked potentials of jaundiced rats. Hear Res 1991;53:41–8.

[89] Deltenre P, Mansbach AL, Bozet C, et al. Auditory neuropathy: a report on three cases with early onsets and major neonatal illnesses. Electroencephalogr Clin Neurophysiol 1997;104(1): 17–22.

[90] Starr A, Picton TW, Sininger Y, et al. Auditory neuropathy. Brain 1996;119(Pt 3):741–53.

[91] Rance G, Beer DE, Cone-Wesson B, et al. Clinical findings for a group of infants and young children with auditory neuropathy. Ear Hear 1999;20(3):238–52.

[92] Stein LK, McGee T, Tremblay K, et al. Auditory neuropathy associated with elevated bilirubin levels. Abstracts of the Twentieth Midwinter Research Meeting, Association for Research in Otolaryngology, St. Petersberg Beach, Florida, February 2–6, 1997.

[93] Morant Ventura A, Orts Alborch M, Garcia Callejo J, et al. [Auditory neuropathies in infants]. Acta Otorrinolaringol Esp 2000;51(6):530–4 [in Spanish].

[94] Simmons JL, Beauchaine KL. Auditory neuropathy: case study with hyperbilirubinemia. J Am Acad Audiol 2000;11(6):337–47.

[95] Tapia MC, Almenar Latorre A, Lirola M, et al. [Auditory neuropathy]. An Esp Pediatr 2000; 53(5):399–404 [in Spanish].

[96] Tapia MC, Lirola A, Moro M, et al. [Auditory neuropathy in childhood]. Acta Otorrinolaringol Esp 2000;51(6):482–9 [in Spanish].

[97] Yilmaz Y, Degirmenci S, Akdas F, et al. Prognostic value of auditory brainstem response for neurologic outcome in patients with neonatal indirect hyperbilirubinemia. J Child Neurol 2001; 16(10):772–5.

[98] Berlin CI, Hood L, Rose K. On renaming auditory neuropathy as auditory dys-synchrony. Auditory Today 2002;13(1):15–7.

[99] Berlin CI, Morlet T, Hood LJ. Auditory neuropathy/dyssynchrony: its diagnosis and management. Pediatr Clin North Am 2003;50(2):331–40.

[100] Rapin I, Gravel J. "Auditory neuropathy": physiologic and pathologic evidence calls for more diagnostic specificity. Int J Pediatr Otorhinolaryngol 2003;67(7):707–28.

[101] Madden C, Rutter M, Hilbert L, et al. Clinical and audiological features in auditory neuropathy. Arch Otolaryngol Head Neck Surg 2002;128(9):1026–30.

[102] Berg AL, Spitzer JB, Towers HM, et al. Newborn hearing screening in the NICU: profile of failed auditory brainstem response/passed otoacoustic emission. Pediatrics 2005;116(4):933–8.

[103] Shapiro SM. Definition of the clinical spectrum of kernicterus and bilirubin-induced neurologic dysfunction (BIND). J Perinatol 2005;25(1):54–9.

[104] Shaia WT, Shapiro SM, Spencer RF. The jaundiced Gunn rat model of auditory neuropathy/dyssynchrony. Laryngoscope 2005;115(12):2167–73.

[105] Rance G, Cone-Wesson B, Wunderlich J, et al. Speech perception and cortical event related potentials in children with auditory neuropathy. Ear Hear 2002;23(3):239–53.

[106] Merchan-Perez A, Liberman MC. Ultrastructural differences among afferent synapses on cochlear hair cells: correlations with spontaneous discharge rate. J Comp Neurol 1996;371(2): 208–21.

[107] Kraus N, Ozdamar O, Stein L, Reed N. Absent auditory brain stem response: peripheral hearing loss or brain stem dysfunction? Laryngoscope 1984;94(3):400–6.

[108] Shallop JK, Peterson A, Facer GW, et al. Cochlear implants in five cases of auditory neuropathy: postoperative findings and progress. Laryngoscope 2001;111(4 Pt 1):555–62.

[109] Peterson A, Shallop J, Driscoll C, et al. Outcomes of cochlear implantation in children with auditory neuropathy. J Am Acad Audiol 2003;14(4):188–201.

[110] Yanagisawa N, Goto A. Dystonia musculorum deformans. Analysis with electromyography. J Neurol Sci 1971;13(1):39–65.

[111] Benecke R, Rothwell JC, Dick JP, et al. Simple and complex movements off and on treatment in patients with Parkinson's disease. J Neurol Neurosurg Psychiatry 1987;50(3):296–303.

[112] Cohen LG, Hallett M. Hand cramps: clinical features and electromyographic patterns in a focal dystonia. Neurology 1988;38:1005–12.

[113] Aramideh M, Devriese PP, Ongerboer de Visser BW, et al. [Blepharospasm; results of treatment with botulin]. Ned Tijdschr Geneeskd 1993;137(30):1509–12 [in Dutch].

[114] Gourley GR. Bilirubin metabolism and kernicterus. Adv Pediatr 1997;44:173–229.

[115] Govaert P, Lequin M, Swarte R, et al. Changes in globus pallidus with (pre)term kernicterus. Pediatrics 2003;112(6 Pt 1):1256–63.

[116] Harris MC, Bernbaum JC, Polin JR, et al. Developmental follow-up of breastfed term and near-term infants with marked hyperbilirubinemia. Pediatrics 2001;107(5):1075–80.

[117] Martich-Kriss V, Kollias SS, Ball Jr WS. MR findings in kernicterus. AJNR Am J Neuroradiol 1995;16(4 Suppl):819–21.

[118] Ozates M, Acar M, Basak F. [Cranial MRI findings in epileptic children]. Tani Girisim Radyol 2003;9(4):427–31 [in Turkish].

[119] Shah Z, Chawla A, Patkar D, et al. MRI in kernicterus. Australas Radiol 2003;47(1):55–7.

[120] Steinborn M, Seelos KC, Heuck A, et al. MR findings in a patient with kernicterus. Eur Radiol 1999;9(9):1913–5.

[121] Sugama S, Soeda A, Eto Y. Magnetic resonance imaging in three children with kernicterus. Pediatr Neurol 2001;25(4):328–31.

[122] Yokochi K. Magnetic resonance imaging in children with kernicterus. Acta Paediatr 1995; 84(8):937–9.

[123] Yilmaz Y, Ekinci G. Thalamic involvement in a patient with kernicterus. Eur Radiol 2002; 12(7):1837–9.

[124] Yilmaz Y, Alper G, Kilicoglu G, et al. Magnetic resonance imaging findings in patients with severe neonatal indirect hyperbilirubinemia. J Child Neurol 2001;16(6):452–5.

[125] Worley G, Erwin CW, Goldstein RF, et al. Delayed development of sensorineural hearing loss after neonatal hyperbilirubinemia: a case report with brain magnetic resonance imaging. Dev Med Child Neurol 1996;38(3):271–7.

[126] Newman TB, Maisels MJ. Magnetic resonance imaging and kernicterus. Pediatrics 2002; 109(3):555.

[127] Okumura A, Hayakawa F, Kato T, et al. Preterm infants with athetoid cerebral palsy: kernicterus? Arch Dis Child Fetal Neonatal Ed 2001;84(2):F136–7.

[128] Penn AA, Enzmann DR, Hahn JS, et al. Kernicterus in a full term infant. Pediatrics 1994; 93(6 Pt1):1003–6.

[129] Straver B, Hassing MB, van der Knaap MS, et al. [Kernicterus in a full-term male infant a few days old]. Ned Tijdschr Geneeskd 2002;146(19):909–13 [in Dutch].

[130] Tabarki B, Khalifa M, Yacoub M, et al. Cerebellar symptoms heralding bilirubin encephalopathy in Crigler-Najjar syndrome. Pediatr Neurol 2002;27(3):234–6.

[131] Amin SB, Ahlfors C, Orlando MS, et al. Bilirubin and serial auditory brainstem responses in premature infants. Pediatrics 2001;107(4):664–70.

[132] Wennberg R. Bilirubin transport and toxicity. Mead Johnson Symp Perinat Dev Med 1982;19: 25–31.

[133] Gourley GR, Kreamer B, Cohnen M, et al. Neonatal jaundice and diet. Arch Pediatr Adolesc Med 1999;153(9):1002–3.

[134] Johnson L, Boggs TR. Bilirubin-dependent brain damage: incidence and indications for treatment. In: Odell GB, Schaffer R, Sionpoulous AP, editors. Phototherapy in the newborn: an overview. Washington DC: National Academy of Sciences; 1974. p. 122–49.

[135] de Vries LS, Lary S, Dubowitz LMS. Relationship of serum bilirubin levels to ototoxicity and deafness in high-risk, low birth-weight infants. Pediatrics 1985;76(3):351–4.

[136] Hyman CB, Keaster J, Hanson V, et al. CNS abnormalities after neonatal hemolytic disease or hyperbilirubinemia. A prospective study of 405 patients. Am J Dis Child 1969;117:395–405.

[137] Naeye RL. Amniotic fluid infections, neonatal hyperbilirubinemia and psychomotor impairment. Pediatrics 1978;62:497–503.

[138] Odell GB, Storey GN, Rosenberg LA. Studies in kernicterus III. The saturation of serum proteins with bilirubin during neonatal life and its relationship to brain damage at five years. J Pediatr 1970;76:12–21.

[139] Rubin RA, Balow B, Fisch RO. Neonatal serum bilirubin levels related to cognitive development at ages 4 through 7 years. J Pediatr 1979;94(4):601–4.

[140] Scheidt PC. Toxicity to bilirubin in neonates: infant development during first year in relation to maximal neonatal serum bilirubin concentration. J Pediatr 1977;92:292–7.

[141] Bergman I, Hirsch RP, Fria TJ, et al. Cause of hearing loss in the high-risk premature infant. J Pediatr 1985;106(1):95–101.

[142] Salamy A, Eldredge L, Tooley WH. Neonatal status and hearing loss in high-risk infants. J Pediatr 1989;114(5):847–52.

[143] Shapiro SM, Daymont MJ. Patterns of kernicterus related to neonatal hyperbilirubinemia and gestational age. Pediatr Res 2003;53(4 Part 2):398A–9A.

[144] Oktay R, Satar M, Atici A. The risk of bilirubin encephalopathy in neonatal hyperbilirubinemia. Turk J Pediatr 1996;38(2):199–204.

[145] Wennberg RP, Thaler MM. Influence of intravenous nutrients on bilirubin transport. I. Amino acid solutions. Pediatr Res 1977;11:163–7.

[146] Soorani-Lunsing I, Woltil HA, Hadders-Algra M. Are moderate degrees of hyperbilirubinemia in healthy term neonates really safe for the brain? Pediatr Res 2001;50(6):701–5.

[147] de Vries LS, Lary S, Whitelaw AG, et al. Relationship of serum bilirubin levels and hearing impairment in newborn infants. Early Hum Dev 1987;15(5):269–77.

[148] Wilson BA. Wilson Reading System. 3rd edition. Oxford (MA): Wilson Language Training; 1996.

[149] Wilson Reading System. Denver (CO): Education Commission of the States; 2002.

[150] Madden C, Hilbert L, Rutter M, et al. Pediatric cochlear implantation in auditory neuropathy. Otol Neurotol 2002;23(2):163–8.

CLINICS IN
PERINATOLOGY

Clin Perinatol 33 (2006) 411–479

Neurometabolic Diseases in the Newborn

James J. Filiano, MD

*Department of Pediatric Medicine, Dartmouth Medical School Children's Hospital at
Dartmouth Hitchcock Medical Center, One Medical Center Drive, Lebanon, NH 03756-0001, USA*

This article is designed to be a basic introduction to neurometabolic diseases (ie, inheritable inborn errors of metabolism, genetic disorders of developmental neural topography, degenerative disorders of neural function) that present in the neonate. It is intended to assist those who provide primary care for newborns by helping them to recognize signs and symptoms that signify neurometabolic disease; teaching them how and when to initiate a neurometabolic diagnostic sequence; and helping neurologists and pediatricians to interface with geneticists and metabolists. This article does not discuss the neuroanatomy and physiology of clinical findings of neurometabolic disease in detail. It does not discuss endocrine or renal disorders that affect electrolyte or glucose metabolism nor myopathies. This article is intended to inform general newborn care practitioners, not metabolists. Therefore, pathways and concepts are presented in a simplified manner for deliberate educational purposes. As a consequence of that intent, this article does not discuss intricate details of biochemical pathophysiology, genetic diagnosis, and metabolic management, nor does it analyze each individual disorder of organic acids, amino acids, the urea cycle, or peroxisomal and mitochondrial diseases. Each such topic deserves an article of its own for detailed discussion to assist expert managers of those diseases. Detailed expositions of treatments are described in more thorough manner elsewhere [1–9]. Instead, this article focuses on the approach to diagnosis for the general newborn practitioner.

There are many ways to organize this article. Traditional ways include listing the diseases based on the abnormal metabolite that is found in urine or blood (eg, aminoaciduria or urea cycle defect), which organelle is defective (eg, mitochondrial, peroxisomal, lysosomal, or Golgi apparatus diseases), which part of the neuraxis is involved (eg, the childhood dementias or leukodystrophies), or the

E-mail address: james.j.filiano@hitchcock.org

age of presentation [3]. These are reasonable organizing approaches, depending on the diagnostic starting point (eg, neuropathologist, neurologist, metabolic geneticist or general pediatrician). Each has its merit and each has its flaw. The primary flaw is that neurometabolic diseases usually have multisystem effects, and evolve over time to affect different parts of the neuraxis. For example, organic acidopathies can cause dementia, lactic acidosis, leukodystrophy, and epilepsy at different times in the same patient. Therefore, no one-dimensional organization plan is adequate.

This article incorporates elements of all of those organization approaches, in an overlapping, multidimensional way. It starts by choosing the basic food groups to extract from the universe of neurometabolic disease two parts: diseases of small molecules (intermediary metabolism) and diseases of large molecules (eg, storage diseases). This keeps the reader's focus simultaneously on the etiology of characteristic symptoms, and on a framework for management in the simplest and most familiar chemical reference frame we know—food. Next, this article incorporates other traditional categories of disease because they have the merit of being recognizable and part of the standard literature [5–7]. Of necessity, some disorders are listed in more than one category. For example, elevated levels of abnormal organic acids (including lactic acid) can be derived from diseases of fatty acid oxidation, protein metabolism, or mitochondrial dysfunction, because the pathways of intermediary metabolism are interwoven so intricately.

For efficiency, this article is constructed of many expanded lists and tables. This is done so that each paragraph does not become an unreadable collection of biochemical and clinicopathologic data. Instead, the paragraphs are designed to impart concepts, and the tables are designed to impart correlations and facts efficiently. Read the paragraphs, but save the tables for rapid reference, or to compare and contrast diseases.

General aspects of the diagnostic process

Why pursue a neurometabolic diagnosis?

These are important diseases because they usually are severely debilitating. Often they can be treated effectively if diagnosed early. Diagnosis can be difficult to make quickly, because presenting symptoms are protean, not specific, and may not be obvious until permanent damage has occurred. Diagnostic tests for neurometabolic diseases usually are sent away to specialty laboratories, so that results do not return promptly. These factors are why newborn screening is so important for this category of disease; however, many of these diseases have not been added to government authorized newborn screens. Clinicians sometimes dismiss this category of diseases as being too rare to warrant committing aspects of these diseases to memory. Although each individual disease is rare, this collective class of diseases is not rare among the causes of neurologic impairment in pediatrics. It will benefit our patients for all of us to become familiar with the modes of presentation of each subcategory of rare neurometabolic diseases, and to initiate the diagnostic and therapeutic sequence when one of these disorders is considered.

When should one pursue diagnosis of a possible neurometabolic disease?

Neurometabolic disease can cause many symptoms. As a result, neurometabolic disease, as an etiologic class, can be on the differential diagnosis for every undiagnosed disease. Usually, it should be at the bottom of the differential diagnosis list, because each neurometabolic disorder is rare. Neurometabolic etiology should be pursued with vigor when the patient's illness is associated with any of the following unexplained clues (Box 1).

The first of these characteristics is intrinsic to the diagnostic technique of "exclusion." This remains the first task of diagnosis, because every other characteristic in Box 1 can be caused by more common etiologies, such as trauma, infection, autoimmune disease, or malignancy. Because the more common disorders are more probable (by definition) it is efficient, and therefore prudent, to pursue the common disorders first, and exclude them if they are not present. Occasionally, there are physical examination findings that point strongly to a specific diagnosis, such as coarsening of facial features in lysosomal storage diseases, alopecia with trichorhexis nodosa in argininosuccinic aciduria, or external ophthalmoplegia in mitochondrial disease. Sometimes, there will be a particular diad, triad, or tetrad of findings that establishes a diagnosis, such as cataplexy plus loss of upgaze in Neimann-Pick disease type C; intractable epilepsy plus alopecia plus severe diaper dermatitis in biotinidase deficiency; or

---

Box 1. Neurometabolic diagnosis clues from medical history

Common etiologies excluded
Family history of similar symptoms or of metabolic disease
Growth failure, especially with recurrent vomiting
Developmental delay
Intractable, severe symptoms
Recurrent, unexplained neurologic events
Progressively degenerating course
Recurrent apparent severe infections, without infectious
    agent identified
Movement disorder
Myoclonus
"Cerebral palsy" without prenatal or perinatal difficulties
A feature in the patient's history or physical examination that is
    pathognomonic for a particular disease

trismus plus strabismus plus retrocolis in neonatal Gaucher's disease. These clustered findings add so much to improve the efficiency of our diagnostic pursuit that they are discussed more later.

Usually, and unfortunately, our diagnostic efforts are not aided by such fortuitous pathognomonic findings. Instead, a diagnosis is made by judicious and cross-correlated laboratory investigations, sometimes over a protracted time course. This reality does not please the patient or family, our colleagues who await our input, or the third-party payers and hospital business managers. The best that we can do is to be attuned to clues of history and examination, while mindful of cost, but aware that the cost of missing a treatable or familial disease in terms of human suffering, medical charges, and other fees is usually greater than the expense of a well-paced laboratory investigation. It may be most prudent to exclude treatable disorders first, while pursuing, simultaneously, some of the more common untreatable disorders that fit the patient's symptoms. Patients may benefit from us explaining to them how long it may be to make a full diagnosis, because they need courage to continue the diagnostic process. This is especially true at the emotional time when a baby is born with unexpected neurologic symptoms.

The idea to pursue neurometabolic disease may come readily if there is an older sibling or other family member with neurologic disease. If there is no such family history, then it is useful to keep in mind that neurometabolic disease may masquerade as an acute or recurrent infection, or with unexplained low Apgar scores. If an infectious agent is not identified, the symptoms may be attributed to "a viral syndrome." That presumptive diagnosis usually is correct, because viral infections are common, after all. If, however, the clinical course of a "viral syndrome" or other infectious syndrome, such as pneumonia, is unusually severe or prolonged in the patient or her siblings, then it may be prudent to consider a neurometabolic explanation. For example, parents may say "He gets the same viral illnesses as the other children, but the illnesses affect him much worse, last much longer, and he vomits and just won't eat." Similarly, parents may report, "He had low Apgar scores that were not explained, and he was slow to feed for days after birth." Astute clinicians may take such comments about prolonged infections or unexplained low Apgar scores as clues to consider that the patient may have a disorder of fatty acid, organic acid, amino acid, or urea cycle metabolism. Such disorders are treatable, but, if not identified and treated early, they cause developmental delay and future cognitive and motor impairment, and may cause a fatal Reye-like illness. Unfortunately, it is difficult for even gifted clinicians to recall and apply the usefulness of these subtle clues, because so many patients have viral illnesses and mildly low Apgar scores; common things are common, as the adage says with truth.

Those two scenarios above highlight an important general feature of inborn errors of metabolism: the symptoms and laboratory abnormalities may worsen dramatically when the patient is stressed by any combination of birth, fasting, protein load, infection, surgery, exercise, and sometimes, menstrual periods. The common features of these stressors are that they cause catabolism, or drive a combination of impaired metabolic, mitochondrial, endocrine, or inflammatory pathways. This phenomenon can assist our efforts to make a diagnosis by using these circumstances as "stress testing" that occurs naturally (as in the case of infection) or under our control (as when we perform newborn metabolic screening after feeding). Sometimes the patient may have an infection at the time of neurometabolic presentation, but that infection may be the trigger for catabolism that makes an underlying metabolic disease manifest for the first time. In this situation a usually mild infectious agent may cause a patient who has a neurometabolic disease to have a severe illness, whereas the same infectious agent might manifest as an otherwise mild infection in a normal host. Alternatively, the patient may have a mild, but persistent, acidosis substantially after the acute infection is treated and the patient's hemodynamic state has normalized.

Box 2 lists a diagnostic sequence that is convenient for a medical care provider who is pursuing a neurometabolic diagnosis. It uses a "biochemical modification" of the principles that are used in diagnosing other classes of neurologic disorders. Although it is listed in sequence, logistics usually requires a sequential overlap of our thinking and testing.

Using symptoms and physical signs is one way to classify neurometabolic diseases [3]. It is a time-tested aid to diagnosis, which used to be called pathognomy. It helps us to assess probabilities as to the location of the lesion in the neuraxis, and this can help us to focus our laboratory investigations. Many diseases can produce the same symptoms and signs, however, and there is much overlap among disease categories; therefore, this method of classification can

---

Box 2. Diagnostic sequence to identify a neurometabolic disorder

Where is the predominant lesion?
  Central or peripheral nervous system or both?
  White matter or gray matter or both?
  Brain or spinal cord or both?
  Disorder of small molecules or large molecules?
  In which food group is the involved pathway?
What pathognomonic clues are found in history or physical examination?
Do the symptoms fit a common, nonmetabolic etiology?
Screen for an abnormal metabolite in a tissue or body fluid (chemical or genetic test, MRI or spectroscopy, microscopy: light or electron)
Confirm the diagnosis by testing for a defect in a specific enzyme or gene (leukocytes, fibroblasts, chorionic villi, amniotic fluid).
Restart the sequence if no diagnosis is found, mindful of circumstances that cause false positive and false negative results

Table 1
Pathognomy: using signs and symptoms to facilitate diagnosis

Signs and symptoms	Diagnosis
Growth failure	Too nonspecific to be a definitive clue, but points toward an underlying systemic defect
Dysmorphic features	Chromosomal and subtelomeric disorders; peroxisomal disorders; 7-dehydrocholesterol reductase deficiency
Coarsened features	Lysosomal storage diseases (eg, mucopolysaccharidoses and oligosaccharidoses); coarsening results from "organomegaly" of the ground substance of cartilage and bone
Cataracts	Galactosemia; Marinesco-Sjögren syndrome (sometimes in mitochondrial neurodegeneration with ataxia and retinitis pigmentosa), storage diseases, lipidoses with retinitis pigmentosa
Keyser Fleisher rings	Wilson disease
Retinitis pigmentosa	Mitochondrial disease, ceroid lipofuscinosis, lipidoses, metachromatic leukodystrophy; others
Optic pallor	Mitochondrial or peroxisomal disease; lipidoses; others
Cherry red macula	Lipidoses
Hepatomegaly	Organic acidopathies and urea cycle defects; fatty acid oxidation disorders with or without cardiomyopathy; mitochondrial disorders with or without cardiomyopathy; peroxisomal disorders; storage diseases (lysosomal and nonlysosomal). (The association of coarse features and organomegaly raises the probability that the patient has a storage disease. Hepatomegaly with acidosis may imply a disorder of small molecules; hepatomegaly with profound hypoglycemia may imply glycogen storage disease.)
Skin lesions	Eczema or alopecia in biotinidase deficiency; angiokeratoma in several lipidoses, such as Fabry disease; lipid deposits in Farber disease and cerebrotendinous xanthomatosis; café au lait in neurofibromatosis and congenital disorders of glycoprotein synthesis; ash leaf spots and chagrin patch in tuberous sclerosis; jaundice in hepatopathy; hyper-pigmentation in adrenoleukodystrophy and some urea cycle defects; contractures, trismus, retrocolis found in infantile Gaucher disease, lipodystrophy, wide spaced nipples, severe hypotonia or seizures or coagulopathy in congenital disorders of glycoprotein synthesis (Golgi apparatus disorders); ichthyosis in ceroid lipofuscinosis
Alopecia	With eczema in biotinidase deficiency; with trichorhexis nodosa in argininosuccinate lyase deficiency; with acrodermatitis enteropathica in zinc deficiency; pili torti with severe seizures and developmental stagnation in Menke disease; thallium exposure; porphyria
Dark hair with blond roots	With painful myopathy and pale nail beds in selenium deficiency
Hypospadius	With 2–3 syndactyly in 7-dehydrocholesterol reductase deficiency; chromosomal and subtelomeric abnormalities; endocrine defects
Unusual odor	Small molecule diseases; see separate list
Renal acidosis	Mitochondrial diseases and organic acidopathies; Lowe syndrome
Self-injurious behavior	Lesch-Nyhan hyperuricemia; Smith-Magenis syndrome
Dementia	With psychosis may imply leukodystrophy; with seizures may imply gray matter disease; with chorea may imply mitochondrial disease or Huntington chorea; with spasticity or blindness may imply storage diseases or ceroid lipofuscinosis

(continued on next page)

Table 1 (*continued*)

Signs and symptoms	Diagnosis
Epilepsy	Gray matter disease: all small molecule diseases (including mitochondrial and peroxisomal diseases); ceroid lipofuscinosis; storage diseases; Glut-1 and folate transporter and pyridoxine defects; Rett syndrome; ARX and neuroligand gene defects; chromosomal and subtelomeric diseases; repetitive nucleotide expansion gene defects in myoclonic epilepsies
Retinal blindness	Gray matter diseases more than leukodystrophies; mitochondrial and peroxisomal diseases; ceroid lipofuscinosis; lipidoses; oligosaccharidoses
Loss of upgaze	With cataplexy and hepatomegaly +/− seizures in Neimann-Pick disease type C; with deafness and choreoathetosis in kernicteris
Lateral gaze paresis	With hepatomegaly in Gaucher disease type III; without hepatomegaly in mitochondrial defects
Movement disorders	Basal ganglion and cerebellar disorders: all small molecule diseases, especially mitochondrial diseases, cerebral folate deficiency, and disorders of neurotransmitters and neoptorin defects, kernicteris, neurodegeneration with brain iron deposition, expansion gene defects, creatine deficiency
Central ataxia	Small molecule diseases, especially mitochondrial diseases; leukodystrophies; storage diseases; nucleotide expansion gene defects
Spasticity	Leukodystrophies more often than gray matter diseases; peroxisomal diseases; arginase deficiency; spinocerebellar degeneration gene defects
Neuropathy	Peroxisomal disease more often than mitochondrial disease; selenium toxicity; late metachromatic leukodystrophy and late Krabbe disease; inherited neuropathies from nucleotide repeat gene defects
Myopathy/ cardiomyopathy	Disorders of fatty acid oxidation; mitochondrial oxidation/phosphorylation defects; taurine deficiency

Modified from: Lockman LA. Coma. In: Swaiman K, editor. The practice of pediatric neurology. St. Louis (MO): Mosby; 1982. p. 150.

have low diagnostic specificity. Individual neurometabolic diseases can be multisystem, or affect many cell types in the neuraxis. This limits the value of diagnosis that is based on neuraxial location. Therefore, classification that is based on symptoms has only modest and partial usefulness. That usefulness is valid, nonetheless, because some of the clues add efficiency to our investigations.

Using the diagnostic approach of pathognomy and relative probabilities, the following are simple points to start the neurometabolic sequence:

Metabolic acidosis may imply the patient has a small molecule disease

Hypoglycemia without ketones may imply the patient has a disorder of fatty acid oxidation

Organomegaly with coarse features, may imply the patient has a storage disease

Organomegaly without coarse features can be caused by storage and non-storage disease

Severe spasticity, ataxia, and, later, peripheral neuropathy may imply the patient has a white matter disease, rather than a gray matter disease

Seizures may imply the patient has a gray matter disease rather than a white matter disease

Table 2
Clues to the cause of coma from the physical examination

Site	Finding	Disease
Head	Contusion	Trauma, coagulopathy
	Vasodilation	Sagittal sinus thrombosis
Neck	Rigid	Meningitis, encephalitis, subarachnoid hemorrhage, neck or throat inflammation, pneumonia
	Enlarged thyroid	Myxedema, thyrotoxicosis
Eyes	Chemosis	Cavernous sinus thrombosis
	Periorbital ecchymosis	Blow out orbital fracture, periorbital and cavernous sinus parameningeal infection
	Subhyaloid blood	Subarachnoid hemorrhage
	Vasospasm	Hypertensive encephalopathy
	Retinal hemorrhages	Shaken-impact syndrome
Ears	Hemorrhage	Basilar skull fracture
	Otitis media	Brain abscess, lateral sinus thrombosis
Nose	CSF rhinorrhea	Basilar skull fracture
Mouth	Scarred tongue	Seizure disorder
	Pigmentation	Addison disease
	Lead lines	Lead intoxication
Odors	Acetone	Diabetes mellitus
	Alcohol	Ingestion
	Almond	Cyanide poisoning
	Cabbage	Methioninemia, tyrosinemia
	Feculent	Hepatic encephalopathy (fetor hepaticus)
	Fishy	Trimethylaminuria
	Fruity	Diabetic ketoacidosis
	Garlic	Selenium/paraldehyde/arsenic toxicity; also part of fetor hepaticus
	Hops	Oasthouse disease (methionine malabsorption)
	Maple syrup	Maple syrup urine disease (branched chain ketoaciduria)
	Mouse urine	Phenylketonuria
	Musty	Glycine
	Sweaty feet	Glutaric acuria (II), isovalericacidemia
	Swimming pool	Hawkinsism (tyrosyluria, 5-oxoprolinuria, hydroxy-cyclohexylacetic acid)
	Tomcat urine	Methylcrotonyl acidemia or multiple carboxylase deficiency
	Uremia	Renal failure
Heart	Murmur	Endocarditis, cerebral embolism/abscess
Lung	Rales	Heart failure, pneumonia, systemic inflammatory response syndrome
Abdomen	Hepatomegaly	Leukemia, hepatic failure, storage disease, heart failure
	Vomiting	Organic acidemia, galactosemia, hyperglycinemia, β-keto-thiolase deficiencies
Limbs	Fracture	Trauma, fat embolism
	Ecchymosis	Trauma, coagulopathy
Skin	Ash leaf spots	Neurophakomatoses with seizures
	Butterfly rash	Lupus, tuberous sclerosis
	Café au lait	Neurofibromatosis with seizures
	Cyanosis	Hypoxia, congenital heart disease with cerebral embolism/abscess
	Desquamation	Vitamin A toxicity, scarlatina, Toxic shock syndrome

(continued on next page)

Table 2 (*continued*)

Site	Finding	Disease
Skin	Dry	Dehydration, myxedema, adrenal insufficiency
	Erythema	Carbon monoxide, atropine/mercury toxicity
	Periungual fibroma	Tuberous sclerosis with seizures
	Petechiae/Purpura	Sepsis, endocarditis, trauma Hemolytic-uremic syndrome, Henoch-Schoenlein purpura, thrombocytopenia
	Hyperpigmentation	Addison disease
	Splinter hemorrhages	Endocarditis, hypoparathyroidism
	Uremic frost	Uremia
	Wet	Syncope
	Needle tracks	Addiction, chronic disease, abuse/neglect, risk for HIV

Abbreviation: CSF, cerebrospinal fluid.
Modified from: Lockman LA. Coma. In: Swaiman K, editor. The practice of pediatric neurology. St. Louis (MO): Mosby; 1982. p. 150.

These "rules of thumb" are only starting probabilities. They can be misleading, so caution should be exercised. For example, small molecule diseases can cause hepatomegaly, and large molecule diseases can cause acidosis. Similarly, white matter diseases can present with seizures, and some neurometabolic diseases can affect combinations of white and gray matter, or cause central and peripheral neuraxial disease.

Tables 1 and 2 relate signs to specific diseases. Much of the tables are not directly relevant to neonatal diagnosis; however, they might be a helpful background for the clinician who may use the information in questioning parents about family history, or in providing prognostic information after a neurometabolic diagnosis is made.

Small molecule diseases

The disorders of small molecules are so named because the diseases are characterized by the accumulation of a small toxic molecule, or the deficiency of a small molecule whose presence is vital for health. These disorders are important because of all of the neurometabolic diseases, they are most likely to be rapidly fatal. They also are most likely to be treated successfully by dietary management [1,2,5]. In the neonatal period their clinical presentations may include low Apgar scores, marked hypotonia, vomiting or poor suck, seizures, coma or neonatal Reye-like syndrome (sometimes recurrent), and unexplained jaundice. The patients may be born with intrauterine growth retardation, but this is not common because the infant's metabolism may be protected in utero. Later, they are likely to suffer growth failure, often with feeding difficulties or vomiting. Whether or not the infant escaped the earlier symptoms, eventually, patients who have small molecule disease are likely to suffer any combination of developmental delay, mental retardation, movement disorder, or intermittent ataxia added to their previous symptoms. Those are the general clinical characteristics of small molecule diseases, but individual disorders may have unique clinical features; for example, nonketotic hyperglycinemia often presents as refractory hiccups.

It is convenient to subclassify the small molecule disorders according to the relevant food group that is most likely to be the origin of the abnormal metabolites (Box 3). Classifying the small molecule diseases by dysfunctional food group is convenient because it reminds us of the metabolites for which we must screen, and whose nutrient intake we must manage (by regulating diet or intravenous intake).

A cardinal feature of disorders of small molecules is that an enzyme in a pathway of intermediary metabolism is defective—by genotype, nutritional/vitamin deficiency, or toxic insult. This takes the general form of $A \rightarrow B \rightarrow// \rightarrow C$, where each letter represents a metabolite, each arrow represents an enzymatic reaction, and $\rightarrow// \rightarrow$ represents the dysfunctional enzymatic step. This produces two immediate outcomes: metabolite B (and perhaps its precursor) accumulates, and there is a deficiency of metabolite C, which cannot be synthesized because of the dysfunctional enzymatic step. The accumulated metabolite B may be toxic, or

---

Box 3. Classification of small molecule diseases

Sugars and energy metabolism
    Galactosemia (and galactosurias)
    Fructosemia (and fructosuria, and pentosuria)
    Glut-1 cerebral transporter defect
    Cerebral creatine metabolism defects
    Mitochondrial disorders of the electron transport chain
Proteins (+ heme and porphyrin) metabolism
    Amino acid and organic acid disorders
    Urea cycle defects (amino acid disorders
       causing hyperammonemia)
    Disorders of glutathione metabolism
    The porphyrias
Fat metabolism
    Disorders of fatty acid oxidation, with abnormal organic acids
    Disorders of cholesterol metabolism
Disorders of purine, pyrimidine, and uric acid metabolism
Nutrient defects
    Vitamin deficiencies
    Cerebral folate deficiency
    Metal metabolism defects (especially copper and selenium)
    Deficiencies of other micronutrients
Toxins (including excess of vitamins or other micronutrients)

its precursor or one of its breakdown products may be toxic; that may cause symptoms. The body will be deficient in metabolite C and its breakdown products, and that, too, may cause symptoms. The general approach to diagnosis of diseases of small molecules is to find the increased concentration of a diagnostic unmetabolized biochemical marker (metabolite B), and to confirm the diagnosis by proving the presence of a deficient enzyme or defective gene. The general approach to treatment is to minimize the dietary supply of substance B (or A), supplement the deficient substance C, or provide high doses of a vitamin that catalyzes the step from B to C.

The newborn care provider usually is not responsible for treating these diseases without the direction of geneticists and metabolists, unless the patient is far from such resources; however, a neonatal or neurologic specialist may be one of the first to see the patient in consultation from a primary care provider. It may be useful for clinicians to consider the diagnostic possibility of disorders of small molecules to recommend proper screening laboratory studies. These studies are best obtained simultaneously with a workup for infection, inflammation, toxin, trauma, hemorrhage, and endocrine and other diseases. Additionally, it may be prudent for the clinician to recommend the rudiments of emergency stabilization for small molecule disorders (see later discussion). To aid in the rapid diagnosis, it is useful to keep in mind the laboratory hallmarks of disorders of small molecules: acidosis, hypoglycemia, or hyperammonemia at times of metabolic stress. Further clarification of a specific disorder requires a more detailed evaluation (Box 4).

Each urine test requires approximately 10 mL of urine, each in its own frozen aliquot. These have the greatest sensitivity when obtained promptly at the time of the patient's symptoms, before rehydration or prolonged treatment with dextrose. The results may be normal in a patient who has an "intermittent" form of a disease if the laboratory studies are obtained when the patient is no longer symptomatic. Therefore, if clinical suspicion is high that the patient has a disorder of small molecules, and tests done when the patient is not acutely ill return normal, however, the tests may become diagnostic if obtained at the next sign of acute illness. Thus, it may be prudent to obtain the urine at the time of acute illness, freeze it, store it, and send it for analysis later if other studies do not reveal a nonmetabolic diagnosis or if the patient has a marked acidosis. If, however, a diagnosis of a nonmetabolic diagnosis is made the frozen specimen can be thrown away. Usually, urine "screening" amino acids and organic acids are sufficient to make a presumptive diagnosis, although quantitative versions are superior. The quantitative form of the tests, and blood quantitative amino acids, are most indicated for following the course of dietary management or for clarifying a presumptive diagnosis.

Elevated blood lactate is a hallmark of disorders of the mitochondrial electron transport chain (oxidative/phosphorylation diseases; Ox/Phos diseases) although elevated lactate may not be observed in every patient who has Ox/Phos disease. Lactate accumulates because of the inability of dysfunctional mitochondria to metabolize pyruvate that is generated from the breakdown of sugars (glycolysis);

Box 4. Diagnostic tests and queries for small molecule diseases

Any feeding intolerances (protein load intolerance in organic
    acidemias and urea cycle defects; fruit juices in fructosemia)?
Seizures or tremor in the morning (fasting hypoglycemia)?
Ravenous eater of sweets (disorder of fatty acid oxidation)?
Slow developmental progress, or loss of milestones?
Are there previous similar episodes, symptoms, or
    laboratory abnormalities?
Is family or ethnic history consistent with
    neurometabolic disease?
Does the patient show unique or salient physical findings?
Test urinalysis for ketones, sugars, pH
Rapid glucose test
Blood electrolytes (hyponatremia and acidosis often occur in
    small molecule diseases)
Blood ammonia (obtain from free-flowing blood, not a
    tourniqueted vessel)
Liver enzymes, bilirubin
Blood L-lactate (on ice)
Uric acid
Complete blood count (anemia and thrombocytopenia may
    be present)
Urine organic acid screen
Urine amino acid screen
Urine acylglycines
Blood acylcarnitine profile
Blood filter paper newborn screen (especially the newer
    "expanded" screens)
Specific vitamin levels, if indicated
Chromosomes and subtelomeric studies, especially if patient is
    dysmorphic, or if sex chromosome polyploidy is suspected
Heavy metal studies in blood or urine, if indicated (eg, selenium
    if there are blond hair roots in otherwise dark hair plus painful
    myopathy; thallium if alopecia is present; lead if anemia with
    basophilic stippling or lead lines on plain roentgenograms)
Plain roentgenograms when appropriate (eg, patellar calcifi-
    cation in neonatal peroxisomal disease; dysostosis multiplex
    (beaked vertebrae, distal extremities) in storage disease;
    adrenal calcification in Wolman disease)
Lumbar puncture for cerebrospinal fluid specimens
Cells, protein, glucose, VDRL test

CSF L-lactate (may be abnormal in mitochondrial disease even if blood lactate is normal)

CSF Amino acids (may be abnormal even if blood and urine amino acids are normal)

CSF Neurotransmitter metabolites and neopterin profile if spasticity, tremor, or dystonia

CSF 3-methyltetrahydrofolate if seizures and motor signs are not explained by earlier studies

Cerebral imaging

Electrophysiology (encephalogram or nerve/muscle studies) if indicated

Urine orotic acid should be added to tests of amino and organic acids if there is hyperammonemia. This test clarifies the specific subtype of urea cycle defect.

Blood pyruvate can be added if blood L-lactate is elevated. If pyruvate is elevated, it implies that the disorder is in the early phases of the electron transport chain, and less likely the result of sepsis or dehydration.

however, in addition to the electron transport chain, many other biochemical reactions take place, at least in part, in the mitochondria. As a result, disorders of small molecules may make mitochondrial function inefficient and increase blood lactate or ammonia, as an epiphenomenon, even if the defective enzyme is not strictly part of the electron transport chain or urea cycle. Therefore, elevated blood lactate can be found in many diseases of small molecules. It is helpful, therefore, to obtain simultaneous, correlated laboratory studies at the time of the acute illness to clarify the diagnosis; if possible, it is best not to rely on a single test, such as L-lactate. This is demonstrated in Fig. 1, which depicts a simplified view of the expansive role of mitochondria in intermediary metabolism.

The pivotal role of mitochondria is due to a great extent to the importance of energy metabolism for living things. (That is only part of the function of each mitochondrion; see later discussion.) When mitochondrial energetics and the urea cycle fail, many pathways and many tissues are disrupted. One symptomatic outcome is the combination of hepatic and cerebral failure in the presence of lactic acidemia with or without hyperammonemia. In the neonate, this syndrome has several names, including "overwhelming neonatal metabolic coma". In older children, it sometimes takes the form of what has been called the Reye-like syndrome.

The Reye syndrome and the Reye-like syndrome may not be unique, independent diseases. Rather, the Reye syndrome has been shown, in some cases, to be a presentation of several treatable neurometabolic disorders of small molecules. This was first recognized several decades ago when patients who had classic Reye syndrome were shown to have urea cycle defects in a state of catabolic

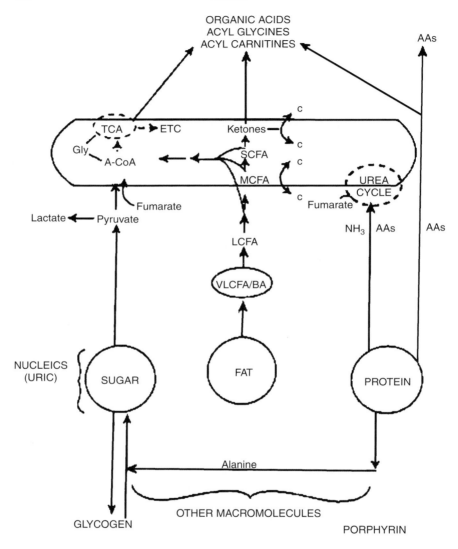

Fig. 1. Role of mitochondria in intermediary metabolism. AAs, amino acids; A-CoA, acetyl CoEnzyme A; BA, bile acids; c, carnitine; ETC, electron transport chain; Gly, glycine; LCFA, long-chain fatty acids; MCFA, medium-chain fatty acids; NH_3, ammonia; nucleics, nucleic acids; SCFA, short-chain fatty acids; TCA, tricarboxylic acid cycle; VLCFA, very long–chain fatty acids.

decompensation. This hepatocerebral dysfunction syndrome has been reported in the setting of several other small molecule diseases, most of which involve impairment of mitochondrial function. It is noteworthy that salicylic acid (aspirin), the use of which was associated with Reye's epidemiologic analysis of the syndrome, can uncouple oxidative phosphorylation. To accommodate this

---

Box 5. Causes of the Reye-like syndrome

Urea cycle defects
    Ornithine transcarbamylase deficiency (X-linked:
        males > females)
    Argininosuccinic acid synthase deficiency (homozygote
        and heterozygote)
    Acetyl glutamate synthetase deficiency
    Citrullinemia
    Triple H-syndrome (hyperornithinemia-
        hyperammonemia-homocitrullinuria)
    Lysinuric protein intolerance
Organic acidemias
    3-methylcrotonyl CoA carboxylase
    Glutaric aciduria type I
    Methylmalonic aciduria
    Propionic aciduria
    Isovaleric acidemia
    Biotinidase deficiency
Disorders of fatty acid oxidation and ketogenesis
    Medium chain acyl CoA dehydrogenase deficiency
    Long chain acyl CoA dehydrogenase deficiency
    Long chain hydroxy-acyl CoA dehydrogenase deficiency
    Short chain acyl CoA dehydrogenase deficiency (not a
        definitively confirmed cause)
    Multiple acyl CoA dehydrogenase deficiency
    3-hydroxy-3-methylglutaryl CoA lyase deficiency
    3-ketoacyl CoA thiolase deficiency (not a definitively
        confirmed cause)
Carnitine metabolism defects
    Carnitine palmitoyl transferase I (CPT I) deficiency
    CPT II deficiency
    CPT translocase deficiency
*Mitochondrial electron transport chain defects and pyruvate
    carboxylase deficiency*
Wilson disease
Carbohydrate metabolism disorders
    Fructosemia
    Fructose diphosphatase deficiency
Glycogen storage disorders
Alpha-1-antitrypsin deficiency

new information, some metabolists prefer the term "Reye-like syndrome" to encompass classic Reye syndrome and hepatocerebral complications of metabolic disease. Symptoms can present late in the course of a viral syndrome, and may be made more likely to occur by the use of salicylate. Symptoms start with irritability, followed by stupor and then coma, hyperammonemia and fatty liver usually are present, and death or severe disability from cerebral edema and herniation can occur. Known or suspected causes of the Reye-like syndrome, and those that "mimic" it, are listed in Box 5.

Neonatal jaundice can be associated with neurologic disorders. Other than the important issue of applying the guidelines for phototherapy to prevent kernicterus, it is also valuable to pursue underlying causes of neonatal jaundice, including neurometabolic causes (Box 6).

Treatment of small molecule diseases

Early diagnosis, especially through newborn screening, is a mainstay of effective management. A complete exposition of treatments for all of these disorders is beyond the scope of this article; however, the general approach may be instructive (Box 7).

Effective therapy is available for many organic and amino acidopathies, urea cycle defects, and galactosemia. In some cases, treatment with a specific vitamin alone may be effective. For example, some cases of biotinidase deficiency and multiple carboxylase deficiency can be treated effectively with biotin supplementation alone. There are also rare forms of thiamine-dependent branched-chain ketoaciduria (maple syrup urine disease) that respond to thiamine alone. Usually, treatment for small molecule diseases is more involved than the fortuitous circumstance of a vitamin-responsive disease.

Box 6. Causes of neonatal jaundice

Hemolysis
Neonatal hemochromatosis
α-1 Antitrypsin deficiency
Crigler-Najjar, Alagille, and Gilbert syndromes
Wilson disease
Galactosemia
Fructosemia (rare, because neonates usually are not exposed
  to fructose)
Tyrosinemia
Organic acidemias (eg, propionic acidemia)
Urea cycle defects
Biliary atresia

Box 7. General treatments for disorders of small molecules

Avoid catabolism if possible (eg, fasting, infections, surgery without dextrose)

Avoid introducing the unmetabolized nutrient (metabolite B in the paradigm, above; eg, avoid excessive protein intake in urea cycle defects)

Supply the vitamin/cofactor for the deficient enzyme

Supply the missing metabolite to bypass the metabolic block (metabolite C; eg, arginine in some of the urea cycle defects)

Remove toxic metabolites (eg, chelation in Wilson disease; careful use of intestinal cathartics in organic acidemias and urea cycle defects to minimize production of unmetabolized toxins, such as propionic acid, from gut bacteria)

Avoid toxic drugs if possible (eg, barbiturates in porphyria)

Provide general medical and neurologic therapies (eg, cardio-respiratory support, anticonvulsants, mannitol in Reye-like syndrome)

Genetic counseling and family planning

Psychosocial interventions

Enzyme replacement (if available; eg, some storage diseases)

Bone marrow transplant (if effective)

Gene replacement (experimental)

Phototherapy or dialysis when indicated

Referral to additional consultants, including nutrition, when feasible

---

An instructive example of therapy that involves all three aspects of small molecule enzyme dysfunction is found with disorders of the pyruvate dehydrogenase complex. Pyruvate dehydrogenase is a key enzyme in the use of pyruvate for energy metabolism at the beginning of the electron transport chain. Pyruvate dehydrogenase complex uses thiamine and lipoic acid in its processes. Pyruvate dehydrogenase function can be impaired by one of three mechanisms: (1) mutations in genes that are involved in synthesis or assembly of its protein subunits; (2) thiamine deficiency; or (3) accumulation of a toxin, such as acetaldehyde, which is a breakdown product of ethanol and is toxic to the pyruvate dehydrogenase complex. Recall that small molecule diseases take the general form: $A \rightarrow B \rightarrow // \rightarrow C$; where each letter represents a metabolite, each arrow represents an enzymatic reaction, and $\rightarrow // \rightarrow$ represents the dysfunctional enzymatic step. The general approach to treatment of small molecule diseases is to minimize the dietary supply of substances B (or A), supplement the deficient substance C, or provide high doses of a vitamin that catalyzes the step from B to C. If the defective enzyme is pyruvate dehydrogenase (whether from gene mutation, cofactor deficiency, or toxin), symptoms may be improved by four steps: (1) minimize excessive sugar intake (the source of pyruvate); (2) provide thiamine and lipoic acid supplementation; (3) avoid alcohol or other drugs that are toxic to pyruvate dehydrogenase; and (4) use the ketogenic diet to provide energy substrate that bypasses dependence on pyruvate to drive the electron transport chain.

Patients who have urea cycle defects develop hyperammonemia and symptoms after a high protein load, because the urea cycle facilitates the excretion of nitrogen during protein metabolism. Treating urea cycle defects may require limiting protein intake to just the patient's basal needs; no greater, but also not less, because insufficient protein causes the body to catabolize muscle to salvage essential amino acids. This essential amino acid recycling during "negative nitrogen balance" liberates other amino acids. When these amino acids are metabolized they release nitrogen that forms ammonia, which cannot be removed efficiently in a patient who has a urea cycle defect. Clinicians also can replace insufficient arginine or citrulline to restore the ability of the urea cycle to remove ammonia in some urea cycle defects. In addition, phenylbutyrate or phenylacetate may be given; these combine with excessive toxic metabolites to form harmless byproducts that are excreted in the urine. If a patient who has a urea cycle defect develops the Reye-like syndrome, vigorous urgent therapy is indicated, which may include management of increased intracranial pressure, cardiorespiratory stabilization, and sometimes, dialysis.

When possible, it is prudent to tailor treatment to the needs of the individual patient and the managing institution. For example, newborns need not be counseled to avoid alcohol. Use of dialysis may be replaced with exchange transfusion, if that is what is best for a particular infant. Often, breastfeeding may be done by strict measurement of pumped breast milk so that protein intake can be regulated. Nutrition and genetic consultation is indicated.

Disorders of sugar metabolism (not storage)

The common pathogenic mechanism in these disorders is disruption of enzymes that are involved in the metabolism and use of a simple sugar, pyruvate, or the energy currencies of NADH/NADPH, ATP, or phosphocreatine. These disorders are summarized in Table 3, which lists each disease name, its clinical and laboratory hallmark features, enzyme defect, gene defect, general prognosis, and basic treatment.

Additional entities deserve mention. Galactosuria can occur from impaired galactokinase or epimerase enzymes. Galactosuria is detected by the same newborn screening techniques as is galactosemia; patients may be asymptomatic or develop cataracts or pseudotumor cerebri. Fructosuria (also called essential fructosuria) is a benign disorder that is characterized by excessive fructose in urine after ingesting foods that are high in fructose or sucrose. The fructose may be detected by test of urine reducing substances. It is caused by deficiency of

Table 3
Small molecule disorders of sugar metabolism

Disease name	Galactosemia	Fructosemia (hereditary fructose intolerance)	Glut-1 transporter defect	Cerebral creatine defect	Mitochondrial disorders of electron transport
Enzyme defect	Galactose-1-phosphate uridyl transferase; several variants	Hepatic fructose –1-phosphate aldolase.	Cerebral glut-1 transporter	Guanidino acetate-methyl-transferase	See separate section
Clinical features	Congenital hepatomegaly, jaundice, vomiting, neonatal sepsis, failure to thrive, microcephaly or infantile pseudotumor cerebri, hypoglycemia, acidosis, thrombocytopenia, urinary reducing substances, renal Fanconi syndrome, seizures; later cataracts, mental retardation, speech dyspraxia, hypergonadotropic hypogonadism	Symptoms after ingestion of fructose or sucrose: hypoglycemia, tremor, disorientation, vomiting, +/– convulsions and coma. Chronic growth failure, vomiting, jaundice, hepatomegaly, proteinuria, aminoaciduria. Severe in infants; mild later because patients develop aversion to sweets	Intractable epilepsy, mental retardation, other neurologic signs. Phenobarbital may worsen these seizures.	Neonates +/– hypotonia and seizures; developmental delay; later extrapyramidal movement disorder	See separate section
Hallmark laboratory findings	Urine-reducing substances (galactosuria) and galactitol; blood galactose	Fructosuria; +/– fructosemia, hypoglycemia, amino aciduria, hypophosphatemia, hypokalemia, hyperuricemia.	Low CSF glucose (< 40 mg/dL)	Low creatinine in serum, CSF, urine, brain MR spectroscopy. High urine guanidino acetate.	See separate section
Genetics	9p13, recessive	Autosomal recessive and autosomal dominant forms	Autosomal recessive	Autosomal recessive	See separate section
Treatment	Galactose-free diet and ophthalmologic, endocrine, and educational assistance	Avoidance of foods with fructose and sucrose; IV glucose during crisis	Ketogenic diet	Creatine monohydrate	See separate section
Prognosis	Good, with diet and support	Normal if sucrose and fructose are withheld; may be fatal if continued	Good if treated early, otherwise mental impairment	Amelioration on treatment	See separate section

Abbreviations: +/–, with or without; CSF, cerebrospinal fluid; IV, intravenous; MR, magnetic resonance.

liver fructokinase and does not produce the clinical symptoms of fructosemia. Pentosuria is a benign disorder that is characterized by excretion of urinary L-xylulose, and is common in the Jewish population. Remember that testing urine with the glucose oxidase method (used for diabetes mellitus) will not detect galactose, fructose, or other reducing substances.

The Glut-1 transporter defect causes a low concentration of glucose in the cerebrospinal fluid (CSF), which results in intractable epilepsy and mental retardation, among other symptoms. Phenobarbital can worsen the seizures. Noting that the CSF glucose is one third of the serum level confirms the diagnosis. The ketogenic diet may be the best current remedy, perhaps by forcing cerebral metabolism to shift away from glucose as the preferred energy source.

Mitochondrial diseases

This rich collection of disorders can be subdivided into several groups (Box 8) [6,10,11]. Mitochondrial disease is associated commonly with disorders of pyruvate metabolism and the electron transport chain, so they are included in this section on disorders of sugar metabolism because pyruvate is the end-product of sugar metabolism, and the beginning of the electron transport chain; however, the mitochondrion is involved in more functions than just the vital function of energy metabolism. It has been stated that oxidative phosphorylation may involve less than 10% of the role of the mitochondrion. Other aspects of its role in energy metabolism involve pyruvate metabolism and fatty acid β-oxidation such that there is valid reason to include mitochondrial disease among diseases of fat metabolism. Its other roles in intermediary metabolism include free radical detoxification, the citric acid cycle, the carnitine shuttle, the urea cycle, sterol and sex hormone synthesis, pyrimidine synthesis (dihydroorotate dehydrogenase involved in orotic aciduria), heme synthesis (by way of δ-amino levulinic acid synthetase), and even neurotransmitter metabolism. In the last 2 decades there has been a blossoming of molecular genetic diagnostic techniques. These have been used to identify electron transport chain disorders that are encoded in the maternally inherited mitochondrial genome. This has been a "celebrity marriage" of clinical and basic science that, in clinical literature, has overshadowed the importance of other roles of the mitochondrion. The other pathways usually are discussed among other classes of diseases, such as urea cycle defects and organic acidopathies. For the sake of completeness and order, they are listed separately. Usually, they are characterized by various degrees of acidosis (lactate or pyruvic and other organic or dicarboxylic acids), developmental delays, seizures, motor dysfunction, and dysfunction of other organ systems, especially liver, kidney, and blood cells. Virtually all can present with some symptoms and signs in the neonatal period, although the full manifestation of certain syndromes depends on maturity, and some patients do not present until adulthood.

Disorders of fatty acid oxidation often present as follows: short-chain acyl CoA dehydrogenase deficiency as cyclic vomiting; 3-ketothiolase as cyclic vomiting and migraine; medium-chain acyl CoA dehydrogenase as seizures with

---

Box 8. Mitochondrial disease subgroups

Enzyme defects in fatty acid oxidation

    CoA deficiency
    Carnitine palmitoyl transferase I
    Carnitine palmitoyl transferase II
    Carnitine uptake defect
    Carnitine depletion (from exogenous or endogenous toxins;
        eg, valproate toxicity, organic acidopathy, or starvation)
    Electron transfer flavoprotein (Complex II)
    Very long–chain acyl or hydroxy acyl CoA dehydrogenase
    Long-chain 3-OH-acyl CoA dehydrogenase
    Medium-chain acyl CoA dehydrogenase
    Short-chain acyl CoA dehydrogenase
    3-OH-acyl CoA dehydrogenase
    Enoyl-CoA hydratase
    3-keto thiolase deficiency

Enzyme defects in pyruvate metabolism

    Monocarboxylase translocase
    Pyruvate carboxylase complex
    Pyruvate dehydrogenase complex
    Phosphoenolpyruvate carboxykinase

Enzyme defects in the citric acid cycle

    Fumarase
    α-Ketoglutarate dehydrogenase

---

fasting (morning) hypoketotic hypoglycemia, apparent life-threatening events, and sudden infant death.

Long-chain disorders of fat oxidation present as acute fatty liver with or without rhabdomyolysis. Most can present with intermittent lethargy, coma, cardiomyopathy, the Reye-like syndrome, and retinopathy.

Disorders of carnitine metabolism can present as cramps, rhabdomyolysis, acute fatty liver, myopathy, the Reye-like syndrome, and developmental delay.

Disorders of the Ox/Phos electron transport chain are caused by a defective enzyme complex, deficient cofactor of electron transport, or mitochondrial depletion (Box 9). Simplistically, electrons that are derived from pyruvate (from sugar) enter the chain preferentially through complex I; electrons from lipids enter preferentially by way of complex II. Thiamine and lipoic acid are cofactors for

---

Box 9. Some syndromes of oxidative phosphorylation disorders

MELAS (myopathy, encephalopathy, lactic acidosis, stroke-
  like episodes)
MERRF (myoclonus, epilepsy, with ragged red fibers)
NARP (neurodegeneration, ataxia, retinitis pigmentosa)
MNGIE (myopathy, neuropathy, gastrointestinal disorder,
  encephalopathy; nuclear DNA thymidine
  phosphorylase deficiency)
HEADD (hypotonia, epilepsy, autism, with developmental delay)
HAM (Hearing loss, ataxia, myoclonus)
Luft (hypermetabolic uncoupling of oxidative phosphorylation)
Leigh (subacute necrotizing encephalomyelopathy)
Kearns-Sayre (chronic progressive external ophthalmoplegia)
Barth (X-linked cardiomyopathy and leucopoenia)
Pearson (bone marrow depression, pancreatic dysfunction)
LHON (Leber hereditary optic neuropathy)
Dystonia +/− LHON
Childhood diabetes +/− deafness
DIDMOAD (diabetes insipidus, diabetes mellitus, optic atrophy,
  deafness = Wolfram syndrome)
Deafness +/− aminoglycoside ototoxicity
Fatal neonatal cardiomyopathy
Myopathy
Hackett-Tarlow (juvenile mitochondrial myopathy)
Cardiomyopathy (hypertrophic, dilated, histiocytoid,
  or fibroelastosis)
Alpers
Menke +/− (X-linked copper deficiency → secondary
  cytochrome C dysfunction; ATPase 7a, Xq12)

---

pyruvate dehydrogenase/complex I. Riboflavin is a cofactor that is involved in complex II. The hallmark of these disorders is high body fluid lactate or a lactate/pyruvate ratio of more than 20. The simplified electron transport pathway is:

$$\text{Pyruvate dehydrogenase/complex I} \;\rightarrow\; \text{CoQ} \;\leftarrow\; \text{complex II}$$
$$\downarrow$$
$$\text{Complex III} \;\rightarrow\; \text{cytochrome C}$$
$$\downarrow$$
$$\text{Complex IV/V}$$

In general, disorders of the mitochondria, whether of the electron transport chain or not, usually are multisystem disorders with slow, intermittently accelerated degeneration. Some can progress so slowly as to be virtually static. They often are worsened during times of metabolic stress, such as during febrile illnesses. Mitochondrial diseases can be considered as rare causes for a variety of common symptoms. In the newborn, mitochondrial Ox/Phos diseases mimic hypoxic/ischemic encephalomalacia, or present with any combination of the following symptoms: intrauterine growth retardation, hypotonia, seizures, apnea, cardiomyopathy, difficulties feeding and swallowing, lactic acidosis, sideroblastic anemia, or hepatopathy. Box 10 lists some of the most frequent presenting symptoms.

Other characteristics of mitochondrial Ox/Phos disease include necrosis in any tissue caused by acute or subacute energy deficiency; acidotic disruption of intermediary metabolism (lactic, uric, organic, amino, ammonia); symptoms triggered by catabolism or cytokinesis (eg, infection, birth); and vulnerability to drug toxicity (chloramphenicol, valproate, adriamycin, aminoglycoside).

Mitochondrial diseases can be inherited by any inheritance pattern, not just from maternally inherited mitochondrial genome inheritance. Mitochondrial genome maternal inheritance accounts for only 5% of mitochondrial disease that presents in pediatrics; however, 30% of adults who present with mitochondrial Ox/Phos disease get it from maternal inheritance. Nuclear genome autosomal recessive inheritance is the most common form of inheritance of Ox/Phos disease, including causes of decreased mitochondrial number (from impaired mitochondrial replication) [6]. Autosomal dominant inheritance is less common, but has been found in some forms of progressive external ophthalmoplegia that are associated with nuclear gene deletions. X-linked dominant disease is found in Barth syndrome. Disordered intergenomic communication has been observed in cases of defects in nuclear DNA control of mitochondrial DNA repair.

Mitochondrial genome inheritance refers to diseases that are caused by deletions or mutations of the circular genome that is found in mitochondria, rather than Mendelian inheritance of nuclear chromosomes. Usually, there are approximately six different mitochondrial genomes in the oocyte, and each type is found in several copies. When the sperm unites with the egg, the mitochondria in the sperm's tail fall away or are destroyed by the oocyte; usually, only the egg's mitochondria survive. (In some animals, and in rare situations in humans, sperm mitochondria may enter the fertilized egg.)

As the fertilized egg replicates, multiple copies of each mitochondrial genome "segregate" randomly into different offspring cells. This process is called "replicative segregation." It is believed that at least 75% of the mitochondria in a cell must be defective for the cell to be defective and produce symptoms. This means that any offspring cell's function in which at least 75% of its mitochondrial genome is defective will be a dysfunctional cell, and thus will convey symptoms in the person. For example, if most of the defective mitochondria segregated into muscle, the patient will have a myopathy. Replicative segregation causes some cells to accumulate mutant mitochondrial genome, and others to have limited mutant copies; this is called heteroplasmy. This heteroplasmy ac-

---

Box 10. Systemic and neurologic signs of mitochondrial disease:

Systemic signs
  Cardiomyopathy +/− cardiac pre-excitation and
    other dysrhythmias
  Esophageal dysmotility
  Intestinal dysmotility
  Fanconi nephropathy
  Acute fatty liver
  Reye-like syndrome
  Pancreatitis
  Hypoparathyroidism
  Childhood diabetes
  Multiple autoimmune endocrinopathies
  Blood dyscrasias, pancytopenia
Neurologic signs
  Microcephaly
  Apnea
  Developmental delay
  Complicated migraine
  Retinitis pigmentosa
  Hearing loss
  Stroke-like episodes
  Parkinsonian symptoms
  Ataxia
  Chorea
  Epilepsy
  Myoclonic epilepsy
  Dorsal column dysfunction (in Leigh syndrome)
  Spinocerebellar degeneration
  Neuropathy/leukodystrophy
  Myopathy
  Hypotonia
  Hepatocerebral complications

---

counts for variable presentation of diseases, such that one mitochondrial mutation or deletion can cause myopathy in one person and encephalomyopathy with neurodegeneration in another person, sometimes even within the same family. For example, a mutation at site 3243 can cause the Kearns-Sayre symptom in one person, NARP (neurodegeneration, ataxia, retinitis pigmentosa) in another, and MELAS (myopathy, encephalopathy, lactic acidosis, strokelike episodes) in a third. Conversely, the Leigh syndrome can be caused by defects of complex I, cytochrome oxidase, mutations at 3243, or large-scale mutations. The determining feature is not which mutation causes the cellular dysfunction, but, rather, which cell has inherited dysfunctional oxidative phosphorylation enzymes.

Another cause of variability lies in age-dependent tissue energy requirements. For example, the basal ganglia are at risk for acute or subacute necrosis in childhood, but only for slow deterioration in adulthood. An additional cause of vulnerability is that some patients incur external stressors, whereas other children are fortunate to avoid them. For example, a patient who is treated with aminoglycosides for an infection may suffer profound hearing loss even at levels that usually are not considered toxic, whereas his sibling, with the same mitochondrial genome but who is not exposed to aminoglycosides, may not lose hearing (see the paragraph on "triple-risk model of disease").

To confirm a diagnosis of most mitochondrial diseases, other than Ox/Phos diseases (eg, a disorder of fatty acid oxidation), the clinician need only demonstrate an enzyme dysfunction or a gene defect that matches the clinical syndrome of the patient. Confirming the diagnosis of a mitochondrial Ox/Phos disease is made more difficult by heteroplasmy. That is because heteroplasmy creates a situation whereby a disease may not be present even if a mitochondrial mutation is present; disease is only present if there is sufficient mutation load ($>75\%$ of the cells involved). Therefore, for Ox/Phos diseases the standard for definitive diagnosis is high. It requires clinicians to prove the presence of enzyme defect (usually in muscle) plus an appropriate gene defect, or enzyme defect plus definitive histologic findings in muscle or other tissues, or appropriate gene defect plus definitive histologic findings.

Because of this high standard for diagnosis, to enter into the "diagnostic sequence" (see above), one must first screen for more common disease. After that, one may initiate a diagnostic workup for mitochondrial disease if the patient has any one of the following criteria:

A characteristic mitochondrial disease syndrome;
Maternal lineage disease (only found in some disorders of
 oxidative phosphorylation);
Lactate elevation (with or without pyruvate) in blood, urine, or CSF;
The combination of multisystem disease (three or more organs), common
 diseases excluded, and recurrent paroxysmal or progressive disease.

Tests for non-Ox/Phos mitochondrial disorders can be included when testing for other disorders of small molecules. If these are normal, one can pursue Ox/Phos diseases more invasively. Before obtaining a muscle biopsy, the studies in Box 11 are helpful to indicate that a mitochondrial Ox/Phos disease may be present.

It may be helpful to consult ophthalmology, genetics, cardiology, clinical pharmacology, nutrition, or rehabilitation services. Swallowing studies may be helpful.

Box 11. Diagnostic tests in oxidative phosphorylation diseases

Blood mitochondrial mutations and deletions (abnormal in < 35%
    of confirmed cases of Ox/Phos diseases)
CSF L-lactate and alanine elevation (from CSF amino acids)
MRI to look for lesions of Leigh syndrome or MELAS syndrome
Magnetic resonance spectroscopy looking for a lactate peak and
    inversion at affected area
Urine organic acids & amino acids, urine orotic acid, and blood
    ammonia when ill
Urine methylglutaconic acid elevation
Skin biopsy (electron transport chain and other enzymes)
ECG (pre-excitation; conduction block)
Fanconi nephropathy
Liver biopsy if symptoms are appropriate
Muscle biopsy, even if creatine kinase and electromyogram are
    normal (microscopy, genome, and enzyme analysis; fresh
    specimens are much more reliable than flash frozen specimens)

Several fallacious clinical pearls exist regarding mitochondrial diseases, and
these must be addressed directly.

Not all Ox/Phos disorders cause elevated blood lactate; some patients have
    elevated CSF lactate with a normal blood lactate.
Not all Ox/Phos disorders follow maternal inheritance; rather, of 100 proteins
    that are involved in oxidative phosphorylation, only 13 proteins, 22tRNA,
    and 2riboRNA are derived from the mitochondrial (nonnuclear) genome.
Not all disorders fit a characteristic syndrome.
Not all mitochondrial Ox/Phos myopathies manifest with histologic abnor-
    malities, such as ragged red fibers, initially. These ragged red fibers are rare
    in children who are younger than 4 years old, even those who have pro-
    nounced multisystem dysfunction.
Not all mitochondrial disorders require muscle biopsy; only the Ox/Phos dis-
    orders that present without the triad of characteristic syndrome, abnormal
    blood mitochondrial mutations, and maternal lineage disease may require it.
Collectively, Ox/Phos and non-Ox/Phos mitochondrial diseases are not rare,
    although each is rare, individually.
Not all mitochondrial disorders cause noticeable degeneration.
The mitochondrial genome defect does not necessarily predict the syndrome,
    and the syndrome does not predict the genome defect.

Treatment for mitochondrial disease follows the same pattern as that for all
diseases of small molecules (ie, replace the defective metabolite, avoid the precursors of the toxic metabolites, provide vitamins that improve the function of the

dysfunctional enzyme, and provide symptom relief for affected organs) [5,6]. For disorders of fatty acid oxidation, the treatment is to arrange the dietary intake of selected fats that bypass the oxidation block. For example, in disorders of long-chain oxidation (long chain acyl CoA dehydrogenase deficiency) treatment requires supplying medium-chain fats, and avoiding long-chain fats. Nocturnal cornstarch has been recommended to treat disorders of fatty acid oxidation to ameliorate early morning hypoglycemia. Ox/Phos disorders are difficult to treat. Treatment has emphasized the use of vitamins to facilitate electron transport. Thiamine, riboflavin, and lipoic acid are used in cases of defects of electron transport complexes I and II and pyruvate dehydrogenase deficiency. The keto-genic diet has been recommended to treat pyruvate dehydrogenase deficiency. Co-enzyme Q (ubiquinone) and carnitine have been recommended for the treatment of all Ox/Phos disorders. Dichloroacetate has been recommended for severe lactic acidosis. Idebenone and vitamin K have been recommended. Vitamins C and E also have been recommended, on general grounds because they are free radical scavengers, but current data show that high dosages of vitamin E are associated with increased cardiac risk. There are some data to indicate that arginine supplementation may help to prevent infarctions in MELAS. There are scant data to confirm that any of these treatments are effective in most patients who have Ox/Phos disease, although there have been small studies of patients who seemed to have dramatic improvement. There is theoretical reason to believe that in cases of mitochondrial disease associated with elevated methylglutaconic acid, supplementation with pantothenic acid (vitamin B5) might reduce the level of methylglutaconic acid; this may have no impact on symptoms, however.

There are a few drugs that can exacerbate symptoms in mitochondrial diseases and these may be best avoided, when possible. These include aminoglycosides, valproate, chloramphenicol, doxorubicin, phenobarbital, salicylate, azothiaprine, ifosfamide, simvastatin, and pravastatin.

Diseases of protein metabolism

Diseases of protein metabolism can be subdivided into organic acidopathies, urea cycle defects, aminoacidopathies, and disorders of glutathione metabolism [5,6]. The porphyrias are added to this category for mnemonic value; they are derived from the breakdown of proteins that contain the heme/porphyrin moiety. This is a convenient separation, but is artificial because there is much overlap and some disorders present with abnormal amino and organic acids. The glutathione disorders can be considered forms of aminoacidopathies. In disorders of protein metabolism, some metabolic steps occur in the mitochondria and some occur in the cytosol. These diseases share the common, but variable, feature of protein intolerance: symptoms and laboratory abnormalities worsen with protein load. Treatment of disorders of protein metabolism usually involves feeding with formulas that are restricted in specific amino acids for each specific disease. Breast-feeding usually is stopped or modified. These diseases also share a tendency to cause various degrees of neonatal or infant growth failure, feeding intolerance

Table 4
Disorders of protein metabolism that cause abnormal urine organic acids

Disease	Propionic acidemia	MMA	MMA & homocystinuria (Cbl C,D)	Multiple carboxylase deficiency (two types)
Enzyme defect	Propionyl CoA carboxylase	Methylmalonyl CoA mutase. Several variations.	Methylmalonyl CoA mutase & methionine synthase.	Holocarboxylase synthase propionyl CoA carboxylase, 3-methylcrotonyl-CoA and pyruvate carboxylase or biotinidase
Clinical features	Recurrent ketosis, acidosis, dehydration, Reye, osteoporsis, rash.	Recurrent hypotonia ketoacidosis, dehydration, Reye, hepatomegaly, monilia, growth failure. Later: osteoporosis, chorea, seizures, ataxia, tremor, mental impairment.	Recurrent hypotonia ketoacidosis, dehydration, Reye, hepatomegaly, monilia, growth failure. Later osteoporosis, mental impairment, chorea, seizures, ataxia, tremor.	Infantile red scaly rash, alopecia, cyclic vomiting, coma, Reye. Same as PPA, MMA, Cbl disorders. Stupor, hypotonia, hydrocephalus, ataxia. Deafness, blindness, seizures in biotinidase defect.
Hallmark laboratory findings	High propionic, glycine, methylcitrate, tiglylglycine, neutropenia, thrombocytopenia, hyponatremia, ammonia. "Ketones" in urine. Spongioform brain.	High glycine, MMA, neutropenia, thrombocytopenia, megaloblastic anemia, hypersegmented polys +/− ammonia, homocystine, cystathionine. "Ketones" in urine. Spongy brain.	High glycine, MMA, neutropenia thrombocytopenia, megaloblastic anemia, hypersegmented granulocytes. "Ketones" in urine +/− ammonia, homocystine, cystathionine. MRI T2 lesion in basal ganglion hemispheres.	Lactate, methylcitrate, 3-methylcrotonylglycine, 3-OH-isovaleric, ammonia; urine "ketones" Abnormal EEG. Spongioform brain.
Genetics	Autosomal recessive	Chromosome 6 recessive	Autosomal recessive	Autosomal recessive
Treatment	Restrict methionine, threonine, valine, isoleucine. Add carnitine, metronidazole to clear bacteria; growth hormone. Reye management. Biotin for rash.	B12, +/− restrict isoleucine, threonine, methionine, valine. Add alanine and carnitine, metronidazole to clear bacteria, growth hormone. Reye therapy when needed.	Hydroxy-B12 or methyl B12 Rare restrict isoleucine, threonine, methionine, valine. Add alanine, carnitine, growth hormone. Reye therapy when needed.	Dramatic response to biotin. Prenatal biotin is helpful. Late biotin will not reverse loss of cranial nerve function.
Prognosis	Neonatal fatality if not treated promptly. Older age presentations good prognosis.	Good if treated early (newborn screen).	Unsatisfactory compared with other coblamin defects.	Good if treated early. Delays, dilated ventricles, deafness, blindness may stay.

Abbreviations: Cbl, cobalamin; EEG, electroencephalogram; IV, intravenous; MMA, methyl-malonic aciduria; PPA, propionic acidemia.

3-Methyl-crotonyl-glycinuria	Isovaleric acidemia	Glutaric aciduria I	Glutaric aciduria II	D-2-hydroxy-glutaric aciduria
3-methyl-crotonyl CoA carboxylase	Isovaleryl CoA dehydrogenase	Glutaryl CoA dehydrogenase	Electron transfer flavoprotein or its multiple acyl CoA dehydrogenase	D-2-hydroxy-glutaric acid dehydrogenase
Late infant Reye-like episodes, coma, growth failure, seizures, delays	Neonatal Reye. Sweaty feet locker room smell. Brain hemorrhage. Vomiting mimics pyloric stenosis or bowel obstruction. Intermittent pancreatitis, fatty liver. Delays, microcephaly ataxia, tremor, seizures.	Megalencephaly, acute infant or child-hood encephalitic-like crisis -> dystonia, degenerative spasticity ataxia, dyskinesia, seizures, profuse sweating. Cyclic vomiting.	Fatal neonatal acidosis, sweaty odor, dysmorphic. Later-onset vomiting hypoglycemia, lipid storage myopathy.	Macrocephaly, hypotonia, vomiting, seizures, delays, coarse features, later dystonia
Ketoacidosis hypoglycemia, ammonia, hepatopathy, 3-methyl-crotonyl-glycinuria, 3-OH-isovalerate, low free carnitine	Ketoacidosis hypo-glycemia, ammonia, hepatopathy, leuko-penia, thrombo-cytopenia, urine: isovalerylglycine, 3-OH-isovalerate, low free carnitine. Abnormal EEG. Spongioform brain.	MRI: wide operculum, Caudate/putamen signal. Mild acidosis. Spongy white matter. Mild fatty liver.	Lactate, glutaric, ethylmalonic, adipic, butyric, methyl-butyric, isobutyric, isovaleric. Hypoketotic hypo-glycemia, ammonia. Urea cycle inter-mediates in urine. Polycystic kidneys. Low carnitine.	D-2-hydroxyglutaric and oxoglutaric acids. Cerebral atrophy.
Autosomal recessive	Autosomal recessive	Autosomal recessive. Eg, Amish, Swedish, Ojibway.	Autosomal recessive	Autosomal recessive
Reduce intake of protein and leucine. Add carnitine. Reye therapy.	Reye therapy. Restrict dietary leucine. Add glycine and carnitine.	Restrict tryptophan and lysine. Add riboflavin, carnitine, baclofen; IV saline, and dextrose for cyclic vomiting.	Dextrose fluids, comfort care in fatal neonatal form. Restrict protein and fat. Add riboflavin, carnitine, glycine.	Unknown.
Can be normal	50% die in acute neonatal event. Normal if treated early.	Normal if early treatment.	Fatal in neonates; poor development if survival.	Poor development

(continued on next page)

Table 4 (*continued*)

Disease	L-2-hydroxy-glutaric aciduria	Ethylmalonic aciduria	3-hydroxy-isobutyric aciduria
Enzyme defect	Unknown	Unknown	Defective oxidation of valine and B-alanine.
Clinical features	Moderate delays, hypotonia, ataxia, tremor, seizures, neonatal apnea. Mild spasticity.	Slow neurodegeneration, petechiae, acrocyanosis, hypotonia with hyperreflexia, epicanthal folds, torturous retinal vessels. May die in childhood, pulmonary and brain edema	Recurrent ketoacidosis, cyclic vomiting, Russel-Silver growth failure, clinodactyly, hypospadius
Hallmark laboratory findings	L-2-hydroxy-glutaric acid. Cerebellar atrophy. White matter and caudate hypoplasia.	Ethylmalonic, lactic pyruvic acids; episodic acidosis, T2 basal ganglion lesions.	3-hydroxy-isobutyric, 2-ethyl-3-hydroxy-propionic, lactic acids, hypoglycemia. Severe have dysmorphic brains.
Genetics	Autosomal recessive	Autosomal recessive	?X-linked
Treatment	Unknown. Laboratory must distinguish D from L isomers for diagnosis.	Not known	Restrict valine. Add carnitine, growth hormone.
Prognosis	Moderately impaired.	Usually fatal	Good on treatment.

4-hydroxy-butyric aciduria	2-methyl-3-hydroxy-isobutyric aciduria	Malonic aciduria	2-oxo-adipic Aciduria
Succinic semialdehyde dehydrogenase	3-Oxo- thiolase = mitochondrial acetoacetyl CoA thiolase	Not known in cases of normal malonyl CoA decarboxylase	2-oxoadipic acid dehydrogenase
Mental impairment, hyperkinetic, intermittent lethargy, autism, hypotonia, motor delay, ataxia, hyporeflexia, seizures	Recurrent severe ketosis, cyclic vomiting	Global delay, growth failure, moniliasis, seizures, spasticity severe dystonia, myoclonic seizures	Varies from normal to growth impairment, infantile global delay, hypotonia, edema, seizures, ventricular dilation, ataxia, ichthyosis
Urine 4-hydroxy-butyric acid, cerebral atrophy	2-methyl-3-hydroxy-isobutyric aciduria, hyperglycemia Glycine may be high. T2 signal in basal ganglia.	Malonic acid, methylmalonic, 3-hydroxy-3-methyl glutaric, dicarboxylic, lactic acids, ammonia, +/− hypoglycemia. Progressive atrophy of cortex, white matter, and basal ganglia.	Aminoadipic acids; 2-oxoadipic acid
Autosomal recessive	11q22 recessive	Autosomal recessive or X-linked?	Autosomal recessive
Benzodiazepine, vigabatrin have been used.	Restrict isoleucine. Carnitine. IV resuscitation of emesis episodes.	Unclear. Support during episodes of ketoacidosis. Clonazepam, carnitine.	Not known. Q? lysine restriction. Acute acidosis management.
Mild to moderately impaired.	Good if treated.	Poor	Varies

and emesis, hepatopathy, anion gap metabolic acidosis, hypoglycemia, hyper-ammonemia, hyponatremia, moderate elevation of lactate, propensity to develop the Reye-like syndrome and myelinolysis during infectious or catabolic stress, hypotonia followed by movement disorder or seizures, and later, mental impairment. Many organic acidemias and amino acidemias have acute severe neo-natal, infantile, and childhood forms, as well as intermediate or intermittent forms, depending on the specific gene mutation or the degree of residual enzyme function. Table 4 lists features for each disorder that are particularly prominent or distinctive. General principles of treatment were discussed in the section entitled "Treatment of small molecule diseases." Cerebral intracranial pressure monitoring, mannitol therapy, cardiorespiratory stabilization, and other treatments may be helpful in the Reye-like syndrome. In contrast to the other disorders of protein metabolism, the porphyrias often are not affected by protein load, generally do not require amino acid restriction formulas, and may not cause the Reye-like syndrome.

Disorders of protein metabolism that cause abnormal urine organic acids have a tendency to present as potentially fatal Reye-like crisis in infancy, and are characterized by elevated excretion of organic and amino acids that are specific for each disease (Table 4). Some disorders are treated effectively with vitamin therapy alone, if diagnosed early. The neurologist may see the child for seizures, hypotonia, movement disorder, developmental delay, or coma.

Methylmalonic acidemia is the salient metabolic disturbance of a collection of defects of vitamin B12 (cobalamin) metabolism. Vitamin B12 undergoes modifications to function as a cofactor for methylation, in conjunction with folate. Some cobalamin defects are designated by their complementation group title, termed cobalamin defect A–G (eg, Cbl A, Cbl B). These include deficiencies of several enzymes and proteins: methylmalonyl CoA mutase (mutation 0, mutation −); adenosyltransferase (Cbl A); homocystinuria with methylmalonic acidemia (Cbl C, Cbl D); transcobalamin II; lysosomal B12 transporter (Cbl F); methionine synthetase (Cbl G); intrinsic factor (pernicious anemia); and infantile B12 deficiency (from breastfeeding vegan mother = "vegan child"). Depending on the variation, treatment may require cyano-, hydroxy-, or methylcobalamin, usually by frequent intramuscular injection, which is obtained by way of a compounding pharmacy. Patients may have delayed language development and have no convulsions and normal daytime EEG, but have nonconvulsive, slow spike wave status epilepticus during sleep; their language may improve abruptly when treated with anticonvulsants.

The "ketones" that are found by urine indicator strips in these disorders usually are ketoacids not normal ketones. Ketoaciduria serves as an early sign of organic acidopathy, and can be used to prompt the clinician to send urine organic and amino acids and to start presumptive therapy.

Glutaric aciduria II can be considered a disorder of metabolism of fatty acids more than a disorder of protein metabolism.

The methylglutaconic acidurias are disorders of leucine or mitochondrial metabolism (Table 5). There are three types, and a possible fourth type.

Table 5
Methylglutaconic acidurias

Disease	Type I	Type II (Barth syndrome)	Type III
Enzyme defect	3-methylglutaconyl CoA hydratase	Mitochondrial defect	Indirect marker of mitochondrial dysfunction; sometimes ATP synthase.
Clinical features	Speech delay. Global neurologic dysfunction.	Cardiomyopathy. Neutropenia and recurrent infections, growth failure, lipid myopathy.	Neurodegeneration, sometimes optic atrophy, mitochondrial cytopathies.
Hallmark laboratory findings	Fasting hypoglycemia, acidosis: 3-methylglutaconic, 3-methylglutaric, 3-hydroxyisovaleric.	3-methylglutaconic, 3-methylglutaric, neutropenia, low carnitine, hypertrophic ventricular fibroelastosis	+/− acidosis, +/− hypoglycemia, +/− sideroblastic anemia, (Pearson aplastic anemia), markers of disorders of oxidative phosphorylation
Genetics	Autosomal recessive	X-linked: Xq28; TAZ1/G4.5 gene	Autosomal recessive, and mitochondrial deletions.
Treatment	? restrict leucine, ? treat with pantothenic acid (Vitamin B5)	Restrict protein. Add carnitine and cholesterol. Heart transplant. ? treat with pantothenic acid (Vitamin B5)	Mitochondrial therapies. ? treat with pantothenic acid (Vitamin B5)
Prognosis	Mild impairment	Can be fatal	Variable

Urea cycle defects and hyperammonemias are characterized by their tendency to cause hyperammonemia, excessive excretion of urea cycle intermediates, and respiratory alkalosis (Table 6) [5]; however, many diseases cause hyperammonemia even if the defective enzyme is not in the urea cycle (eg, organic acidemias caused by dysfunctional enzymes within mitochondria, such as pyruvate carboxylase). Occasionally, disorders that cause excessive excretion of urea cycle intermediates may not cause hyperammonemia, such as hyperornithinemia with gyrate atrophy. In both situations, these disorders are listed in different sections of this article (Tables 6, 7).

Diseases of glutathione metabolism are a subset of aminoacidopathies because in these disorders there is an accumulation of individual amino acids, but they are listed here separately for educational convenience [6]. They are believed to follow autosomal recessive inheritance. They usually do not express their full features in the neonatal period. Pyroglutamic aciduria (5-oxoprolinuria) is caused by glutathione synthetase deficiency. It is associated with mental impairment, spasticity, ataxia, dysarthria, and intermittent acidosis and hemolytic anemia that are associated with febrile illnesses, and possibly with diaphragmatic hernia. When this enzyme defect is limited to red cells, there is intermittent hemolytic anemia and splenomegaly, but no 5-oxoprolinuria or neurologic signs. γ-Glutamylcysteine synthetase deficiency is associated with myopathy, peripheral neuropathy, spinocerebellar degeneration, intermittent hemolytic anemia, and

Table 6
Urea cycle defects and hyperammonemia

Disease	Orotic aciduria and hyperammonemia	Ornithinemia	Citrullinemia and orotic aciduria	Argininosuccinic aciduria	Argininemia	"HHH" syndrome	Lysinuric protein intolerance
Enzyme defect	Ornithine transcarbamylase	Carbamyl phosphate synthetase	Argininosuccinate synthetase.	Argininosuccinase.	Arginase.	Ornithine transport into mitoch	Transport of cationic amino acids
Clinical features	Male infantile or childhood Reye-like hyperammonemic crisis, coma, seizures, stroke-like episodes; affected girls	Neonatal hyperammonemic crisis.	Neonatal seizures, hyperammonemia with or without Reye-like crisis; cyclic vomiting, recurrent emesis, headache, tremor, ataxia, seizures, all intermittently. Short hair.	Same as argininosuccinate synthetase deficiency, but more hepatomegaly, trichorhexis nodosa.	Spastic quadriplegia. opisthotonos, microcephaly, seizures.	Intermittent emesis or Reye.	Growth failure, intermittent emesis, headache, diarrhea or Reye. Pulmonary fibrosis, nephritis, fractures, pancreatitis, liponecrosis, terminal liver failure
Hallmark laboratory findings	Elevated glutamine, alanine, orotic acid, ornithine; low citrulline in fluids. Respiratory alkalosis.	High Ornithine. Low citrulline, orotic acid, arginine and low BUN. Respiratory alkalosis	High citrulline, high orotic acid, low argininosuccinate	High argininosuccinate, glutamine, alanine, moderate citrulline	High arginine, cystine, lysine, ornithine, orotic acid, arginic acid	Hyper ornithine, ammonia, homocitrulline	Low lysine and other amino acids in blood; high urine lysine, ornithine, arginine. Anemia, leukopenia.

Genetics	X-linked; also affected girls	Autosomal recessive	Autosomal recessive	Autosomal recessive	Autosomal recessive	Autosomal recessive	Autosomal recessive
Treatment	Protein restriction, benzoate, phenylacetate, or phenylbutyrate, arginine, citrulline, pyridoxine, folate, IV dextrose; mannitol +/− dialysis may be necessary. Keep glutamine normal.	Same as OTC, plus N-carbamyl-glutamate	Same as OTC. Once stable, some may be managed with just arginine supplementation. Others need protein restriction.	Same as argininosuccinate synthetase deficiency	Low arginine diet. Add lysine, ornithine, benzoate.	Restrict protein, add lysine, add ornithine	Restrict protein. As for OTC, plus lysine, ornithine, arginine, citrulline, prednisolone for lungs.
Prognosis	Treatable, but potentially lethal acutely	Treatable, but potentially lethal acutely	Treatable, but potentially lethal acutely. 75% 10-year survival. Moderate mental impairment.	Same as argininosuccinate synthetase deficiency	Good amelioration	Good amelioration	Guarded

Abbreviation: IV, intravenous.

Table 7
Disorders of protein metabolism that cause abnormal urine amino acids (deficient tyrosine, excess phenylalanine and homocystine)

Disease	Phenylketonuria	Hyperphenylalaninemia	Homocystinuria type 1	Homocystinuria type 2
Enzyme defect	Phenylalanine hydroxylase and secondary: tyrosinase	GTP cyclohydrolase, or pyruvoyltetrahdro-bioperin or other defects of tetrahydro-biopterin metabolism.	Cystathionine synthase	N(5,10)-Methylene-tetrahydrofolate reductase
Clinical features	Blond hair, blue eyes, pale skin, eczema, infant vomiting, mousy odor, short, mental impairment hyperactivity, seizures, spasticity, tremor, athetosis	Microcephaly, hypotonia, growth impairment, mild vomiting, mental impairment, parkinsonian rigidity, dystonia, drooling, seizures.	Ectopia lentis, cataracts, glaucoma, detached retinae, vascular occlusions, malar flush, osteoporosis and bony dysplasia, aortic dilation, strokes, behavioral disturbances	Vascular occlusions, strokes, variable mental delay and psychosis, infantile spasms. Strokes may occur if additional risk factors.
Hallmark laboratory findings	Phenylalanine high. Tyrosine low.	Phenylalanine. Tyrosine low. Prolactin high.	Homocystine, methionine are high	Homocystine high. Methionine low or normal.
Genetics	12q recessive	Autosomal recessive	Autosomal recessive	Autosomal recessive
Treatment	Restrict phenylalanine lifelong. Add carnitine. Treat pregnant patients to protect fetus.	Tetrahydrobiopterin, folinic acid	Pyridoxine, folate, betaine.	Folate or folinic acid. with B12 to avoid spinal toxicity. Betaine and pyridoxine may help, but pyridoxine alone has caused deterioration.
Prognosis	Normal during treatment	Good if treated	Fair	Variable

Phenylalanine inhibits tyrosinase, causing the pale skin and hair in phenylalaninemias by interfering with melanin production. Genetic deficiency of tyrosinase itself, caused by several gene defects, causes albinism, translucent iris, retinal pallor, nystagmus, photophobia, and dysplastic optic chiasm. Tyrosinemias also benefit from reduction in dietary phenylalanine.

Abbreviations: CSF, cerebrospinal fluid; EEG, electroencephalogram; IV, intravenous.

Tyrosinemia type I (oculocutaneous) (Richner-Hanhart syndrome)	Tyrosinemia type II (hepatorenal)	Maple syrup urine disease (branched-chain oxoaciduria)	Nonketotic hyperglycinemia	Ornithinemia with gyrate atrophy
Tyrosine aminotransferase of cytosol, normal mitochondrial	Fumarylacetoacetate hydrolase	Branched-chain ketoacids dehydrogenase 4 protein complex: E1 α, E1 β, E2, thiamine/E3	Glycine cleavage 4 enzyme complex	Ornithine-5-aminotransferase
Painful keratitis with inflammation, lacrimation, photophobia, painful keratosis of hands and feet. Usually very mild mental impairment, but can be severe, with hyperactivity, self injury, seizures.	Liver failure, cirrhosis, hepatocellular carcinoma, rickets, cabbage odor, Reye-like crisis rare, painful peripheral neuropathy. Uncommon: myopathy, cardiomyopathy, behavioral disorder, self-injury, seizures.	Neonatal coma, hypotonia that leads to opisthotonus, seizures, delays, recurrent ataxia. Intemediate and intermittent forms also. Maple syrup odor of fluids and earwax if protein intake.	Severe neonatal coma, seizures, myoclonus, hiccups, hypotonia leads to spasticity, developmental stagnation. Rare mild and slow degenerative forms.	Gyrate atrophy of choroid and retina, mental impairment, renal impairment
Tyrosine high, its crystals cause the keratoses.	High tyrosine and α fetoprotein. Succinylacetone is diagnostic. Fanconi nephropathy (aminoaciduria, phosphaturia, glycosuria).	Branched-chain amino and oxo acids. Acidosis is not common. Brain edema, myelinolysis.	High CSF/plasma glycine ratio (> 0.06, normal = 0.02), EEG burst-suppression, spongiform white more than gray matter.	Ornithinemia but normal ammonia
16q22 recessive	15q23 recessive; French Canadians	E1α 19q13; E1β 6p21; E2 1p31; E3 7q31; all recessive.	Autosomal recessive	Autosomal recessive
Restrict tyrosine and phenylalanine, add etretinate.	Restrict tyrosine and phenylalanine. Use of NTBC reverses liver failure, and may prevent need for liver transplant.	Restrict leucine, isoleucine, valine. Add thiamine. Dialysis, exchange transfusion. IV dextrose & nonbranched-chain amino acids to overcome catabolism.	Benzoate, dextromethorphan, pyridoxine, anticonvulsants.	Restrict protein. Add lysine.
Excellent on treatment	Excellent on NTBC treatment	Excellent if treated early	Often fatal to neonate	Variable

generalized aminoaciduria; one patient had acute psychosis. 5-Oxoprolinase deficiency seems to be restricted to intestine and kidney and causes enterocolitis and urolithiasis. Glutathione peroxidase deficiency is associated with drug-induced hemolysis and platelet dysfunction. This is a selenium-dependent enzyme, and selenium deficiency impairs this enzyme and causes cardiomyopathy, painful skeletal myopathy, and blond roots of dark hair, among other symptoms. Glutathione disulfide reductase deficiency causes hemolysis.

The porphyrias are a collection of disorders characterized by abnormal heme metabolism, and excretion of porphyrins, which sometimes cause dark urine [6,8]. They can be divided into hepatic and erythropoietic subclasses. All symptoms are acute and intermittent or subacute. Neurologic signs include psychiatric changes from abnormal tryptophan metabolism and increased serotonin, Kluver-Bucy behavior, seizures, proximal or distal weakness and diaphragmatic weakness that can be mistaken for Guillain-Barré syndrome, sensory neuropathies, and seizures. Abdominal symptoms include pain, nausea, vomiting, diarrhea, and constipation. The intensity of abdominal symptoms can prompt surgical exploration. Some porphyrias produce photosensitive rash. Other less prominent symptoms include back or chest pain, hypertension, and tachycardia. Most patients have no symptoms unless triggered by menses, light exposure, or medications, including anticonvulsants, sedatives, antidepressants, and antibiotics that clinicians may prescribe for the presenting symptoms before the diagnosis of porphyria is made. Bromides are safe for treating seizures in this disorder. Given that several porphyrias are inherited with autosomal dominance, these are not very rare disorders; it may be prudent to test extended family members. Secondary porphyria occurs as an unexplained laboratory finding. Porphyria cutanea tarda may be the only porphyria that presents in infancy, and can do so as a light sensitive rash (Table 8).

Small molecule diseases of fat metabolism

It is convenient to separate this category into disorders of fatty acid β-oxidation and disorders of cholesterol metabolism. Disorders of fatty acid β-oxidation also can be placed in the category of organic acidemias, because poorly metabolized fats produce unusual organic acids (eg, adipic acid, sebacic acid, suberic acid, octenedioic acid). Some of these fatty acids may be toxic. The patient also may have a deficiency of appropriate fatty acids downstream from the enzyme defect, and also may have energy depletion, because as much as 60% of our energy needs may be fulfilled by fat in ordinary circumstances. The body compensates for lack of fat by increasing the usage of sugars; however, at times of fasting or energy need, the patient may develop nonketotic hypoglycemia. Strictly speaking, disorders of fatty acid oxidation are "mitochondrial diseases" because of the role that mitochondria have in fatty acid β-oxidation, although fatty acid oxidation is not a direct part of the electron transport chain. Disorders of fatty acid β-oxidation are discussed in more depth in the section on mitochondrial diseases.

Disorders of cholesterol metabolism

Disorders of cholesterol metabolism cause excess or deficiency of cholesterol and its precursors or metabolites. They cause neurologic symptoms by any combination of disrupting neuronal cell membranes, disrupting fetal cerebral development and myelin formation, or causing atheromata with subsequent ischemic complications. Excess cholesterol is present in familial hypercholesterolemia, and type I hyperlipoproteinemia. Types II through V hyperlipoproteinemia tend to present after childhood. Deficient cholesterol is found in mevalonic aciduria, Smith-Lemli-Opitz syndrome, abetalipoproteinemia, and cerebrotendinous xanthomatosis. Of the disorders in Table 9, only mevalonic aciduria and Smith-Lemli-Opitz syndrome present in newborns.

There are other, rarer disorders of cholesterol metabolism that are not listed in Table 9 that are useful to mention for completeness [6]. Hypobetalipoproteinemia and chylomicron retention disease are variants of abetalipoproteinemia and are caused by defects of posttranslational modification of Apo B. Tangier disease is a disorder of unknown cause characterized by very low high-density lipoprotein, apo A-I, and apo A-II in plasma, and is distinguished by tangerine-colored, lipid-filled histiocytes in many tissues, especially in rectal mucosa and tonsils. (Use the mnemonic of "tangerine tonsils of Tangier disease.") These findings, with hepatomegaly, can be present in the newborn. Autosomal recessive familial lecithin:cholesterol acyl transferase (LCAT) deficiency causes high levels of unesterified cholesterol in the plasma, and very low levels of esterified cholesterol. Foam cells may be noted in bone marrow, as in Niemann-Pick C disease, but there is no organomegaly as is found in Niemann-Pick disease. A variant of LCAT deficiency causes only corneal opacity, and is called "fish eye disease." Cholesterol is stored within cells in other diseases, such as in cholesterol ester storage disease and Wolman disease; these are listed and discussed under large molecule lipid storage diseases.

Disorders of purine and pyrimidine metabolism

These are important causes of developmental delay and spasticity. Some disorders of purine metabolism, especially adenosine deaminase deficiency, may have no neurologic symptoms [7,8]. Each disorder disrupts purine metabolism, but only some cause various degrees of hyperuricemia. Some variants of Lesch-Nyhan disease produce only mild elevation of uric acid levels in infancy—in a range that may be considered normal by adult standards (5 mg/dL)—and therefore, can be misdiagnosed. For the sake of thorough comparison and contrast, some disorders are shown in Table 10. The most important disorders for the neonatal care provider to recall are Lesch-Nyhan disease and adenosine deaminase deficiency. Lesch-Nyhan disease can present in the neonate as hypotonia and tiny stones that can be identified in a cloth diaper (rarely reported with modern diapers). Untreated, its outcome is severe spasticity, mental retardation, and severe self-injurious behavior. Adenosine deaminase deficiency causes

Table 8
The porphyrias

Disease	Acute intermittent (hepatic)	Coproporphyria (hepatic)	Variegate (hepatic)	Aminolevulinic aciduria (hepatic)	Cutanea tarda (hepatic)	Congenital (Gunther) (erythropoietic)	Protoporphyria (erythropoietic)
Enzyme defect	Porphobilinogen deaminase	Coproporphyrinogen oxidase	Protoporphyrinogen oxidase	Aminolevulinic dehydrase	Uroporphyrinogen decarboxylase	Uroporphyrinogen III cosynthase (isomerase)	Heme synthase (ferrochelatase)
Neurologic signs	3+	2+	2+	1–2+	0	0	0
Abdominal signs	3+	3+	3+	2–3+	0	0–1	2+
Rash (light and trauma)	0	1+	2+	0	2+ childhood	3+ disfiguring	2+
Hemolytic anemia	0–1	0–1	0–1	0–1	0–1	Infant, dark urine, 3+ hemolysis, splenomegaly, erythrodontia	Childhood, dark urine, 2+ hemolysis, splenomegaly, erythrodontia
Other	Teen, adult. Dark urine, back and chest pain. Acute psychosis.	Any age dark urine, back and chest pain	Dark urine, back and chest pain		Alopecia or hirsutism, hyper or hypopigmentation, mild elevated transaminases	Alopecia or hirsutism. Later disfigured face and fingers	Gall stones

Hallmark laboratory findings	Hyponatremia, urine aminolevulinic acid, porphobilinogen and enzyme	Urine and stool coproporphyrin	Plasma porphyrin fluorescence	Urine aminolevulinic acid and enzyme	Urine uroporphyrin III and enzyme	Uroporphyrin and coproporphyrin in urine, blood, and feces, and enzyme	Protoporphyrin in blood and feces, and enzyme
Genetics	11q23 dominant (Swedish)	Autosomal dominant	Autosomal dominant (South African)	Autosomal recessive	Autosomal dominant and sporadic	Autosomal recessive	18q dominant
Treatment	Avoid barbiturates, estrogens, etc. Add hematin, ?histrelin, ?hemin, ?zinc mesoporphyrin, other study drugs. Bromide for seizures. Saline and dextrose.	Avoid sun, barbiturates, estrogens, etc. Add ?histrelin, hemin, zinc mesoporphyrin. Bromide for seizures. Saline and dextrose.	Avoid sun, fasting, alcohol, drugs. Add ?histrelin, hemin, zinc mesoporphyrin. Bromide for seizures. Saline and dextrose.	Avoid sun, fasting, alcohol, drugs. Add hemin, zinc mesoporphyrin. Bromide for seizures. Saline and dextrose.	Avoid sun, alcohol, chlorinated hydrocarbons, iron, estrogens. Add hemin, zinc mesoporphyrin. Saline and dextrose.	Transfusion, splenectomy, hematin. Saline and dextrose. Avoid sun.	Avoid sun. Add beta-carotene, cholestyramine, ? L- cysteine. Saline and dextrose.

Table 9
Disorders of cholesterol metabolism

Disease	Familial hypercholesterolemia	Type I hyperlipoproteinemia	Cerebrotendinous xanthomatosis	Mevalonic aciduria	Smith Lemli Opitz	A/hypobeta-lipoproteinemia
Enzyme defect	At least four defects in LDL receptor synthesis and processing	Lipoprotein lipase or apolipoprotein C-II	Mitochondrial C27 steroid 26-hydrolase	Mevalonic acid kinase	7-dehydro-cholesterol reductase	Posttranslational modification of apo-B-100; several defects
Clinical features	Xanthomas, arcus senilis, multiorgan vascular disease. Homozygotes have xanthomas as children.	Infantile episodic abdominal pain, pancreatitis, eruptive xanthomas, hepatosplenomegaly, lipemia retinalis, scrotal swelling, some have anemia, leukopenia, or thrombocytopenia. Apolipoprotein C-II–deficient patients present late adolescence with abdominal pain or pancreatitis; sometimes with lupus, lymphoma, or histiocytosis, but none with xanthomas or hepatomegaly.	Childhood cognitive delays, sometimes mental deterioration; adolescent white matter degeneration and xanthomas of cholestanol in tendons, lungs, and brain, causing tendon pain, ataxia, and spasticity, with gray and white matter degeneration of brain and spinal cord	Growth failure and malabsorption, recurrent fever, hepatosplenomegaly, lymphadenopathy arthralgia, rash, psychomotor retardation, cataracts, ataxia.	Microcephaly, dysmorphic face, small jaw, cleft palate, 2, 3-syndactyly, hypospadius or ambiguous genitalia, Hirschprung obstipation, pyloric stenosis, hypotonia, mental retardation, behavioral disorder; seizures are not common	Childhood chronic diarrhea, vomiting, growth failure, oxalate stones, cardiomyopathy and myopathy, pigmentary retinopathy and visual impairment, nystagmus without cataracts, ataxia, head tremor, movement disorder, sensory neuropathy and dorsal column demyelination and hypotonia with Babinski sign

Hallmark laboratory findings	High LDL cholesterol	Creamy fasting plasma from high triglycerides and chylomicrons	High blood cholestanol. Low cholesterol.	Urine mevalonic acid; elevated plasma IgD, anemia, elevated creative kinase during febrile crises, low plasma ubiquinone	High blood 7-dehydro-cholesterol, low cholesterol	Acanthocytes, low vitamins A, E, and K (not D), low prothrombin, low ApoB and LDL cholesterol
Genetics	Chromosome 19 Dominant. Most common single-gene disease in humans	Autosomal recessive	Autosomal recessive	Autosomal recessive	Autsomal recessive	Autosomal recessive
Treatment	Liver transplant for homozygotes Binding resins, and HMG CoA reductase inhibitors, nicotinic acid and low-fat diet in heterozygotes	Dietary restriction of fats; vigilance for pancreatitis	Oral chenodeoxycholic acid; surgical removal of xanthomas in tendons; cataract removal, other	None known. Corticosteroids ameliorate febrile crises. HMG-CoA reductase inhibitors trigger rhabdomyolysis Vitamins A, D, E, and K?	High doses of cholesterol, often by way of egg yolks; symptom management	Vitamins A, E, and K; restrict long- and medium-chain triglycerides
Prognosis	Poor for homozygotes	Amelioration	Amelioration	Poor	Guarded	Amelioration

Abbreviations: HMG, 3-OH-3-methylglutaryl-coenzyme A; LDL, low-density lipoprotein.

Table 10
Disorders of purine and pyrimidine metabolism

Disease name	Lesch-Nyhan	Lesch-Nyhan variants	Phosphoribosylpyrophosphate synthetase excess	Adenylo-succinate lyase deficiency	Adenine phosphoribosyl transferase deficiency	Severe combined immune deficiency
Enzyme defect	HPRT	Variants of HPRT deficiency	Phosphoribosylpyrophosphate synthetase excess	Adenylosuccinate lyase	Adenine phosphoribosyl transferase.	Adenosine deaminase
Clinical features	Motor delay, spasticity, dystonia, chorea, athetosis, mental impairment, severe self-injury, tophi, gouty arthritis, urate and xanthine nephropathy.	Renal stones alone, or Lesch-Nyhan without self-injury, or mild spasticity and mental retardation	Hyperuricemia, uricosuria, hematuria, crystalluria and stone nephropathy, gouty arthritis, sensorineural deafness, variable mental impairment (rare absent lacrymal ducts, small teeth, hypospadius)	Developmental delay, autistic behavior, seizures	Renal calculi and crystalluria, hematuria +/− nephropathy in children, rarely brown spots on cloth diapers; normal neurodevelopment	Severe combined immune deficiency, diarrhea, pneumonia, moniliasis, skeletal defects
Hallmark laboratory findings	Hyperuricemia, uricosuria, and calculi 3 mg uric acid/mg creatinine	Serum uric acid >5 mg/dL	Elevated uric acid and oxypurines in urine and blood	Adenylosuccinate and succinylamino-imidazole carboxamide riboside in urine and CSF, uric acid normal	Crystalluria, 2,8-dihydroxy adenine in urine; uric acid normal	Enzyme or gene, deficient immune markers, uric acid normal

Genetics	Xq26 recessive	Xq26 recessive	X-linked, with some lyonization symptoms in girls	22q, recessive, some heterozygote effect	16q24 subtelomere; Japanese, recessive	ADA gene, autosomal recessive
Treatment	Allopurinol, 5-OH-tryptophan, carbidopa, dental extraction, lithotripsy, stone removal, hydration, ?deep brain stimulation?	Allopurinol, lithotripsy, stone removal, hydration	Allopurinol, hearing aids	Anticonvulsants and behavior therapies	Low purine diet, allopurinol, hydration, lithotripsy	Enzyme replacement, bone marrow transplantation; gene replacement
Prognosis	Some amelioration with treatment	Amelioration with treatment is good to excellent	Amelioration good	Prolonged stable impairment	Varies from assymptomatic to renal failure	

Abbreviations: HPRT, hypoxanthine: guanine phosphoribosyl transferase.

severe combined immune deficiency, which can present as late neonatal infections, rash, or growth failure. Dihydropyrimidine dehydrogenase deficiency causes urinary excretion of uracil, thymine, and 5-hydroxymethyluracil, and is associated with microcephaly, hypotonia, seizures, delayed myelination, and mental retardation. Replacement of underproduced β alanine has been proposed as a therapy; results are uncertain.

Nutrient defects

Deficiencies or excesses of vitamins, trace minerals, and micronutrients, or specific amino acids, are listed here for convenience (two of which can be considered amino acid disorders) (Box 12).

Cerebral folate deficiency can cause any combination of movement disorder, seizures, developmental delay or regression, anxiety, and sometimes, basal ganglion calcifications. This disease is caused by one of three mechanisms: a deficiency of folate intake, a defective cerebral folate receptor/transporter system, or antibodies to the cerebral folate receptor/transporter system. If the blood folate level is normal, the transporter defect is diagnosed by finding a deficiency of CSF 3-methyltetrahydrofolate. It is treated effectively with folinic acid, which does not require a transporter to enter the CSF. This treatment can cause worsening of seizures, paradoxically, if given to a person who does not have cerebral folate deficiency, or if not accompanied by simultaneous vitamin B12 therapy.

Box 12. Disorders of vitamins, minerals, and micronutrients

AVED (Ataxia from vitamin E deficiency)
Zinc deficiency (associated with dermatitis enteropathica; alopecia, moniliasis)
Copper deficiency and X-linked kinky hair disease (Xq12)
Copper removal deficiency (Wilson hepatolenticular degeneration)
Taurine deficiency (myopathy)
Selenium deficiency (painful myopathy, cardiomyopathy, blond hair roots)
Selenium toxicity (neuropathy)
Carnitine deficiency (myopathy, hepatopathy)
Hartnup disease (tryptophan transport and renal reabsorption defect; ataxia)
Cerebral folate deficiency (movement disorder, seizures, neurologic delay)
Neurodegeneration with brain iron deposition (formerly Hallervorden Spatz)
Pyridoxine (B6) deficiency, dependency, or responsivity

Box 13. Causes of hypoglycemia

Endocrine

Hyperinsulinism
    Transient neonatal
        Infant of diabetic mother
        Erythroblastosis fetalis
        Beckwith-Wiedemann syndrome
    Persistent
        Islet cell dysplasia
        Focal/diffuse adenomatosis
        Nessidioblastosis/insulinoma
    Drug-induced
        Insulin
        Oral hypoglycemic agents
    Other endocrine disorders
        Growth hormone deficiency[a]
        Corticotropin or cortisol deficiency[a]
        Glucagon deficiency[b]
        Somatostatin deficiency
        Thyroid hormone deficiency

Insufficient substrate

Postoperative hypoglycemia
Ketotic hypoglycemia[a]
Underlying liver disease
Sepsis
Hepatitis
Starvation and small-for-gestational-age infants
Cyanotic congenital heart disease

Inborn errors of metabolism

Carbohydrate
    Glycogen storage and synthesis diseases
    Galactosemia
    Fructosemia
Amino acidurias, (eg, tyrosinemia)
Organic acidurias
    Mitochondrial disorders
    Disorders of fatty acid oxidation and ketogenesis

Carnitine deficiency
Other causes of Reye-like syndrome (eg, urea cycle disorders)

TOXINS

Alcohol
Salicylates

[a] Hyperketotic syndromes: excess ketogenesis
[b] Hypoketotic syndromes: suppressed or defective ketogenesis

---

Toxins

Toxins cause their symptoms by blocking the function of an enzyme, receptor, or structural protein. When they impair the function of an enzyme of intermediary metabolism, they mimic metabolic disease or nutritional/vitamin deficiencies. An example is found in the way that acetaldehyde (a metabolite of ethanol) impairs pyruvate dehydrogenase, which is part of a thiamine-dependent enzyme complex. In neonates, toxins usually come by way of the mother's circulation, and include drugs of abuse, and rarely, lead or methyl mercury. Neonatal symptoms are not specific, and usually include hypotonia or hypertonia, and seizures during drug withdrawal. Iatrogenic toxicity is another source of toxins.

Diseases that cause hypoglycemia

It is convenient, educationally, to take this moment to summarize small molecule diseases and anticipate our discussion of large molecule storage diseases by listing the differential diagnosis where both classes of diseases can present with a common symptom (ie, hypoglycemia). Many diseases of small molecules cause hypoglycemia, because the body stores of glycogen or lipids are depleted during a fast. Glycogen storage disease is a class of storage disease that presents with hypoglycemia commonly. Causes of hypoglycemia are listed in Box 13, and many present during the neonatal period.

Large molecule diseases

The hallmark of large molecule disease is the storage of large molecules in tissues or body fluids [6–8]. They tend to cause dementia, epilepsy, movement disorders, gradual blindness, and spasticity, in the case of leukodystrophies. What constitutes "large molecules" is arbitrary; however, in general, the dysfunctional molecules have a structural, membrane, receptor, or other function in cells, but usually are not involved directly in intermediary energy metabolism and removal of acid or nitrogen. Because the disorders produce their symptoms in tandem with gradual accumulation of stored material, there are only a few of these disorders that present in the neonatal period.

Subclassification of large molecule diseases

Clues that are derived from phenotype have been incorporated in Table 1. Biochemically, once again, we can start from the perspective of "the food groups" to prompt our memory as to which tests to obtain. If a patient manifests no strong clues of a storage disease on history or physical examination, it may be economical to reserve testing for these disorders until after more common disorders and the small molecule diseases have been excluded. Emergency newborn diagnosis is helpful for some glycogen storage diseases, especially neonatal acid maltase disease (Pompe disease), for which there is now enzyme replacement therapy and which can be fatal in the newborn period. Nevertheless, early diagnosis is helpful to the patient and family, and it is beneficial to start enzyme replacement whenever possible. Box 14 contains an organization scheme of large molecule diseases, listed for educational purposes.

Diseases that are characterized by storage of sugars, glycoproteins, or glycolipids

Glycogen storage diseases [6] is a collection of disorders that is characterized by abnormal synthesis or degradation of glycogen, which results in lysosomal or cytoplasmic storage of unmetabolized glycogen in most forms of these diseases. Most are myopathic, hepatopathic, or both; however, blood, kidney, and brain can be affected. Cerebral glycogenosis may be a form of myophosphorylase deficiency. Fasting ketotic hypoglycemia is common to many of the glycogen storage diseases, and this may cause seizures. Myopathic forms often cause muscle cramps and may cause rhabdomyolysis. When liver is involved, hepatomegaly can be massive. Diagnosis usually requires enzyme analysis from blood, muscle, or liver. Enzyme replacement is available for Pompe disease (type II, neonatal acid maltase disease). All are autosomal recessive, except one form of phosphoglycerate kinase deficiency and two forms of phosphorylase b kinase, which are X-linked, whereas two other forms of phosphorylase b kinase are autosomal recessive. This depends on which subunit of the enzyme is affected. Aldolase deficiency is a newly described disorder of developmental delay, myopathy, rhabdomyolysis, hemolysis during febrile illness, and no glycogen found in muscle. Another syndrome has been described—mental retardation, cardiomyopathy, and autophagic vacuolar myopathy—but the enzyme defect is still under investigation. Lafora polyglucosan body disease occurs in adolescents and adults; it causes dementia, myoclonus, and epilepsy, and muscle biopsy reveals nonlysosomal, round, periodic acid–Schiff-positive inclusions in the perikarya of liver, muscle, skin, and neurons. When glycogen storage diseases present in neonates, they do so usually as hypoglycemia, with or without seizures, some-

---

Box 14. Organization scheme of large molecule diseases

Diseases that are characterized by storage of sugars, glycoproteins, or glycolipids

   Glycogen storage diseases
   Mucopolysaccharidoses
   N-acetyl galactosaminidase deficiency (Schindler) (discussed
      under lipidoses)
   Oligosaccharidoses (discussed under lipidoses)
   Congenital disorders of glycoprotein synthesis
      (Golgi apparatus disorders)

Diseases that are characterized by accumulation of cholesterol and complex lipids

   Peroxisomal disorders of long-chain fatty acid metabolism
   Intracellular cholesteroloses
   Sphingolipidoses
   Mucolipidoses
   Oligosaccharidoses (glycoproteinoses)
   Neuronal ceroid lipofuscinoses

Miscellaneous storage diseases

   Glutamyl ribose-5-phosphate storage disease (ADP-ribosyl
      protein lyase deficiency)
   N-acetylaspartate excess (aspartoacylase deficiency =
      Canavan disease)
   Alexander disease

---

times with hypotonia, cardiomyopathy, and variable hepatomegaly. Pompe disease manifests a characteristic short PR interval, low voltage on ECG, and neonatal heart failure (Table 11).

Mucopolysaccharidoses [5–8] are characterized by dysmorphic features, visceromegaly, bony dysostosis that often leads to short stature, sometimes primary cerebral dysfunction, and sometimes compressive neuropathies and myelopathies, depending on the specific disorder. All store mucopolysaccharides (glycosaminoglycans), and most excrete these in the urine. They follow an autosomal recessive inheritance, generally. Some of the lipidoses also have chemical and clinical characteristics of the mucopolysaccharidoses (eg, multiple sulfatase deficiency and Sandhoff disease); they are discussed in the section on lipidoses. Presentation in the newborn is rare, but it may be recognized by hoarse cry, persistent stridor, short size, and rarely hypotonia, cataracts, or odontoid hypoplasia; usually coarse features are not present yet. Other features are listed in Table 12.

Oligosaccharidoses and N-acetyl galactosaminidase deficiency (Schindler) are discussed under lipidoses.

Glutamyl ribose-5-phosphate lysosomal storage disease is caused by ADP-ribosyl protein lyase deficiency, and is X-linked. The product is not excreted and diagnosis is made only by noting storage in renal or brain tissue. This disease causes infant-onset dementia, progressive neuronal loss, and renal failure. Neonates may have hypotonia and renal impairment.

Congenital disorders of glycoprotein synthesis (Golgi apparatus disorders) were first called carbohydrate-deficient glycoprotein syndromes [12,13]. The new name preserves the initials of the original title, but expresses the pathophysiology better. These disorders are characterized by defective glyco-sylation of proteins in the Golgi apparatus. This is, in a way, the reverse of the oligosaccharidoses. The proteins are normal, but they are glycosylated insuf-ficiently, so that their function, transport, and survival are impaired. The most common screening test is to identify hypoglycosylated transferrin isoforms ("carbohydrate-deficient transferrin") in plasma. Phosphomannomutase defi-ciency was the first form identified, and Dol-P-mannosidase deficiency was re-ported more recently. All tissues and organs can be affected. Common symptoms include microcephaly, seizures, apnea, hypotonia from combined neuropathy and myopathy, cerebellar hypoplasia and olivary gliosis in some forms, growth failure, diarrhea, mild hepatic and renal dysfunction, and mild coagulopathy from factor XI dysfunction. Fatal neonatal cases with apnea and infantile spasms have been noted. The diseases are autosomal recessive, and no treatment is successful, although addition of mannose to patients who have phosphomannomutase defi-ciency may diminish diarrhea and aid growth.

Miscellaneous storage diseases

Canavan disease (N-acetylaspartate excess from aspartoacylase deficiency) is characterized by megalencephaly, hypotonia, swallowing difficulties, optic atrophy, seizures, and developmental delay that cause fatal neurodegeneration [5,8]. Head MRI and CT scans reveal strikingly watery myelin. Pathology reveals spongy degenerative leukodystrophy. Head magnetic resonance spectroscopy and urine demonstrate increased N-acetylaspartate. The disorder is autosomal reces-sive, with a moderate predominance in the Jewish population, and occurs in congenital, infantile, and juvenile ataxia forms. The gene defect is mapped to chromosome 17p. Gene therapy in this disease is being investigated.

Alexander disease is an autosomal recessive leukodystrophy that is char-acterized by megalencephaly and Rosenthal fiber hypertrophied astrocytes adherent to blood vessels in the white matter [8]. This disease can present in the newborn or early infantile period. It causes megalencephaly, growth failure from feeding incapacity, spasticity, dementia, and fatal neurodegeneration. In

Table 11
Glycogen storage diseases

Disease type	Enzyme defect	Tissue affected	Chromosome	Distinctive feature
0	UDPG-Glycogen transferase	Liver, muscle		
Ia vonGierke	Glucose-6-phosphatase	Liver, kidney (gut, muscle)	17q23	Uric acid high. Gout. Anemia. Short stature. Prolonged bleeding time. Hyperlipidemia, xanthomas. Lactic acidemia.
Ib	Glucose-6-phosphate transport protein (translocase)	Liver, neutrophils (gut, kidney)		Neutropenia, anemia. Uric acid high; stones. Gout. Inflammatory bowel disease. Short stature. Hyperlipidemia. Lactic acidemia.
Ia sp	Stabilizing (regulatory) protein	Liver		
Ic	Microsomal phosphate transporter	Liver		
Id	Microsomal glucose transporter	Liver		

II Pompe	a-1,4-glucosidase (acid maltase)	Generalized cardiac	17	Short PR interval, cardiomegaly. Fatal neonatal heart failure, macroglossia, severe hypotonia. Milder adult form with respiratory muscle failure.
III	Amylo-1,6-glucosidase (debrancher)	Liver, muscle (red & white cell)	1	Amylopectinosis
IV Andersen	Amylo-(1,4-6)-transglucosidase (brancher)	Liver (muscle, red & white cell)	3	
V McArdle	Muscle phosphorylase (myophosphorylase)	Muscle	10; 11 14;	Cramps, easy fatigue
VI	Liver phosphorylase	Liver (white cell)	10; 11 14;	
VII	Muscle phosphofructokinase	Muscle, red cells	1; 10; 21	Hemolytic anemia
VIII/IX Tarui	Phosphohexosisomerase (inhibitor) Phosphoglycerate kinase Phosphorylase b kinase	Liver (white cell)	X; 16q12; 7p12	The kinase form is X-linked
X	Phosphoglycerate kinase Phosphorylase kinase	Muscle	16q12; 7p12	
XI	Lactate dehydrogenase Phosphoglucomaltase	Liver, muscle	11; 12	
XII	Cyclic AMP-dependent kinase	Liver		

Abbreviation: UDPG, uridine diphosphate glucose.

Table 12
Mucopolysaccharidoses

Disease	MPS I (Hurler) (Scheie milder)	MPS II (Hunter)	MPS III (Sanfilippo A-D)	MPS IV (Morquio)	MPS V (formerly Scheie)	MPS VI (Maroteaux-Lamy)	MPS VII (Sly)
Enzyme defect	Iduronidase	Iduronate sulfatase	Heparan N-sulfatase	Galactose 6-sulfatase	Obsolete	Aryl sulfatase B	β-glucuronidase
Clinical features	Corneal clouding. Coarsening. Skeletal dysostosis. Visceromegaly. Heart disease. delay and dementia. Seizures	Cornea normal, coarsening, skeletal dysostosis, joint restriction, visceromegaly, short stature. delay, dementia and seizures late.	Cornea normal. No coarsening. Mild visceromegaly. Delays and hyperactivity.	Corneal clouding slight. Coarsening mild. Skeletal dysostosis is distinctive. Odontoid hypoplasia. Short stature. Visceromegaly. Normal mentation, compression neuropathies, and myelopathy.	Obsolete	Corneal clouding slight. Coarsening mild. Skeletal dysostosis is distinctive. Short stature. Visceromegaly, normal mentation. Compression neuropathies and myelopathy.	Corneal clouding slight. Skeletal dysostosis is distinctive. Short stature. Visceromegaly. Wide range of mental function.
Hallmark laboratory findings	Dermatan sulfate, Heparan sulfate	Dermatan sulfate, Heparan sulfate.	Heparan sulfate	Keratan sulfate, Chondroitin 6-sulfate	Obsolete	Dermatan sulfate	Dermatan sulfate, heparan sulfate, chondroitin 4-sulfate
Genetics	Autosomal recessive	X-linked recessive	Autosomal recessive	Autosomal recessive	Obsolete	Autosomal recessive	Autosomal recessive
Treatment	Enzyme replacement. Supportive	Enzyme replacement. Supportive	Supportive	Supportive	Obsolete	Supportive	Supportive

Abbreviation: MPS, mucopolysaccharidoses.

older presentations, it can resemble multiple sclerosis with megalencephaly. The most common forms are infantile, but juvenile- and adult-onset forms can occur. There is no treatment.

Diseases that are characterized by storage of fats

Peroxisomal diseases are characterized by dysfunction of the peroxisome (Box 15) [6]. They bridge the categories of small molecule diseases and large molecule diseases. They cause fluid accumulation of unmetabolized long-chain fatty acids in the plasma, but these are not "stored" in fixed intracellular collections, as occurs in other large molecule diseases. The known roles of the peroxisome include generation of hydrogen peroxide for biochemical reactions; synthesis of plasmalogens (eg, phosphatidylethanolamine); β-oxidation of very long–chain and long-chain fatty acids; oxidation of phytanic acid and pipecolic acid; some steps of bile acid formation; and some steps of dicarboxylic acid metabolism. Defects of the peroxisome lead to disruption of one or more of these steps. Therefore, the clinician's most efficient diagnostic screening test for peroxisomal disease is to measure the excessive relative accumulation of very long–chain and long-chain fatty acids in the blood. After that has been established, the

---

Box 15. Some inherited disorders of the peroxisome

Disorders of peroxisomal assembly (neonatal presentations)

   Zellweger cerebrohepatorenal syndrome
   Neonatal adrenoleukodystrophy
   Infantile Refsum disease
   Hyperpipecolic acidemia
   Rhizomelic chondrodysplasia punctata

Single peroxisomal enzyme deficiency

   X-linked adrenoleukodystrophy/adrenomyeloneuropathy
   Acyl-CoA oxidase deficiency
   Bifunctional enzyme deficiency
   Peroxisomal thiolase deficiency
   Dihydroxyacetone phosphate deficiency
   Alkyl dihydroxyacetone phosphate deficiency
   Glutaric aciduria type III
   Refsum disease
   Hyperoxaluria type I
   Acatalasemia

metabolist can confirm a specific subtype of peroxisomal disease through analysis of enzymes in skin fibroblasts, or through gene tests. Inheritance usually is autosomal recessive, with the notable exception of X-linked adrenoleukodystrophy.

Peroxisomal diseases tend to present with signs of central with or without peripheral myelin dysfunction (leukodystrophy with or without demyelinating polyneuropathy), sometimes with liver or other organ dysfunction. In cases of newborn and infantile presentations, skeletal or other organ dysplasia is common. The most severe forms are neonatal. These newborn diseases include Zellweger cerebrohepatorenal syndrome and neonatal adrenoleukodystrophy, which are multisystem malformation syndromes of cortical dysplasia and hypomyelination, sometimes with renal microcysts and hepatic dysplasia (Zellweger), and chondrodysplasia with neonatal peripatellar calcifications (neonatal adrenoleukodystrophy). In these two diseases, optic pallor is often present, and seizures can be severe and intractable. Refsum disease is primarily a peripheral neuropathy that presents in early adulthood and is characterized by accumulation of phytanic acid. Neonatal Refsum disease is severe, and does not have the same metabolic defect or treatment as does the adult form, but does presently similarly with polyneuropathy and elevated phytanic acid levels.

Treatment is symptomatic, coupled with genetic counseling. A therapeutic diet contains the lipids glyceryl trioleate and glyceryl trierucate (variants of "Lorenzo's oil"). This diet bypasses the defective pathways and has been shown to delay demyelination in asymptomatic patients with the X-linked adrenoleukodystrophy genotype. Adrenal hormone replacement is indicated if adrenal dysfunction is present. In Zellweger disease or neonatal adrenoleukodystrophy, supplementation with cholic, deoxycholic, and docosahexanoic acids may be helpful. Supplementation with vitamin K is indicated if there is severe liver dysfunction. A diet that is low in phytanic acid, sometimes augmented with plasmapheresis, treats Refsum disease. It is noteworthy that some peroxisomal disorders are accompanied by secondary pyruvate dehydrogenase dysfunction. Bone marrow transplantation is being studied in X-linked adrenoleukodystrophy.

Intracellular cholesteroloses

For educational convenience, some diseases of cholesterol metabolism can be grouped among small molecule diseases, and some can be grouped with the large molecule diseases, based on clinical presentation [5]. Cholesterol metabolites may collect outside cells in familial hypercholesterolemias, mevalonic aciduria, and cerebrotendinous xanthomatosis; those are listed in the small molecule disorders because the abnormal location of the lipid is predominantly extracellular. In contrast, diseases of intracellular storage of cholesterol metabolites (called "intracellular cholesteroloses" in this article) are listed here, under large molecule diseases. This is done because the lipid is stored as large inclusions within cells and the defective enzymes are lysosomal; although the stored metabolite is a small molecule, the clinical features are so similar to lipidoses that they must be evaluated, considered, and excluded along with lipidases. The intra-

Table 13
Intracellular cholesteroloses and Niemann-Pick

Disease	Wolman disease	Cholesterol ester storage	Niemann-Pick C	Niemann-Pick A	Niemann-Pick B
Enzyme defect	Lysosomal lipase	Lysosomal lipase	Lysosomal cholesterol esterification	Lysosomal sphingomyelinase	Lysosomal sphingomyelinase
Clinical features	Vomiting, diarrhea, growth failure, hepatosplenomegaly, developmental delay	Milder than Wolman	Infant hepatosplenomegaly, dementia, upgare paralysis, cataplexy, narcolepsy, rare seizures, dystonia, ataxia	Infant liver > splenomegaly, hydrops fetalis, growth failure, cherry red/black macula with halo, xanthomas, neurodegeneration	Infant to adult. Same as type A, but milder.
Hallmark laboratory findings	Adrenal calcifications, foamy lymphocytes and marrow histiocytes; stored cholesterol esters. Blood cholesterol and triglycerides may be normal.	Same as Wolman, but no adrenal calcifications.	Foamy histiocytes. Stored cholesterol. Poor fibroblast lysosomal cholesterol esterification, filipin stain +.	Foamy histiocytes. Stored cholesterol and sphingomyelin all cells and placenta. High transaminases, microcytic anemia, pancytopenia, pulmonary disease.	Like Type A. Lung > liver > > brain disease, but "Lewis variant" has sea blue histiocytes in spleen more than liver.
Genetics	Chromosome 10 recessive	Chromosome 10 recessive	18q11 recessive	11p15 recessive Ashkenazi	11p15 recessive Ashkenazi
Treatment	None; ? liver & marrow transplant	None; ? HMG- CoA reductase inhibitors; liver and marrow transplant	Research studies. Anticonvulsants, protryptilene and clomipramine for cataplexy. Anticholinergics for dystonia.	None	None
Prognosis	Poor	Poor	Poor	Guarded	Good

Table 14
Sphingolipidoses

	Enzyme defect	Accumulated substances	Visceromegaly	Cherry red macula	Special feature	Enzyme replacement
Niemann-Pick A, B	Sphingomyelinase	Sphingomyelin and cholesterol	3+	Red/black with halo	Organomegaly, lung disease	0
Niemann-Pick C	Cholesterol esterification	Cholesterol	1–2+	0	Upgaze paresis Cataplexy Dystonia	0
Gaucher	β-Glucosidase (glucocerebrosidase)	Glycosylceramide (glucocerebroside)	1–3+ Spleen infarcts.	0	Trismus and strabismus and retrocolis in type 2. Loss of voluntary lateral gaze in type 3.	+
Fabry	α Galactosidase A	Ceromide trihexoside	0	0	Lancinating pain Angiokeratoma Renal failure Strokes	+
Farber lipogranulomatosis	Ceramidase	Ceramide	+/–	+/–	Hoarse voice Lipid nodules	0
Gm1 gangliosidosis	β galactosidase	Gm1 ganglioside Galactosyl oligosaccharides Keratan sulfate	+/–	+ red/black	Morquio-like dysostosis Organomegaly	0

Disease	Enzyme		Substrate		Clinical	
Gm2 gangliosidosis Tay-Sachs	Hexosaminidase α	0	Gm2 ganglioside	+	Startle Blindness	0
Gm2 gangliosidosis Sandhoff	Hexosaminidase A & B B subunit	+/−	Gm2 ganglioside Oligosaccharides Glycosaminoglycans	+	Startle Blindness	0
Gm2 activator deficiency	Gm2 activator	0	Gm2 ganglioside	+	Equal to Tay-Sachs	0
Schindler	α Galactosidase B N-acetyl galactose-aminidase	0	N-acetyl-galactosaminyl oligosaccharides and glycopeptides	0	Neuroaxonal dystrophy	0
MLD	Arylsulfatase A; sulfatide activator (saposin B)	0	Galactosylsulfatide Lactosylsulfatide	+/−	Leukodystrophy Neuropathy later	0
Krabbe globoid leukodystrophy	Galactocerebroside (= β galactosidase) (= galactocylceramide β galactosidase)	0	Galactosylceramide	0	Leuko-dystrophy, very irritable infants, high CSF protein	0
Multiple sulfatase deficiency	Arylsulfatase A, B, C; other sulfatases	3+	Galactosylsulfatide Lactosylsulfatide Oligosaccharides Mucopolysaccharides	+	Like MLD and dysmorphic, osteodystrophy with spinal cord compression	0

Abbreviations: CSF, cerebrospinal fluid; MLD, metachromatic leukodystrophy; 0, not present; +/−, sometimes present; +, present.

cellular cholesteroloses include Niemann-Pick C disease, and cholesterol ester storage disease and its severe variant, Wolman disease. The intracellular cholesteroloses tend to cause dysfunction of gray matter, which produces dementia, seizures, and movement disorders, and also cause organomegaly. Niemann-Pick A and B are listed here for educational purposes, because their presentation is similar to Niemann-Pick C, but sphingomyelin, rather than cholesterol, is the primary stored material in types A and B disease. Niemann-Pick D is no longer considered a separate entity, but is type C in a Canadian population. Table 13 compares cholesteroloses, and highlights a few unique features. Presentation in the newborn period is extremely rare.

Sphingolipidoses and "glycolipidoses" are defects of lysosomal metabolism of sphingolipids that cause more intralysosomal than intracytoplasmic accumulation of complex sphingolipids, "glycolipids," and glycopeptides [5–7]. (Glycolipid is a term that can be used to designate composites of oligosaccharides and lipid derivatives. Glycopeptide is a term that can be used to designate composites of oligosaccharides and peptide derivatives.) If the accumulation is in oligodendrocytes or Schwann cells, the predominant features are those of a leukodystrophy (demyelinating dementia, spasticity, ataxia, and later demyelinating neuropathy). If the accumulation is in gray matter neurons or astrocytes, the predominant features are those of a "poliodystrophy" (dementia, seizures, retinal dysfunction, movement disorder, axonal neuropathy). The substance accumulated in the cells may be different from that which is excreted in urine. Cell death is usually slow, and is caused by the accumulation itself or by toxic or deficiency effects of metabolites in the affected pathways of normal sphingomyelin formation. Presentations occur as infantile, late childhood, and adult forms. They generally follow autosomal recessive inheritance, except for Fabry disease, which is X-linked. Treatment is usually supportive, and all defects are fatal, except for Gaucher's and Fabry disease, which are responsive to enzyme replacement. All Niemann-Pick disorders have features that are similar to Gaucher's disease, except the liver usually is more involved than the spleen in Niemann-Pick, whereas the spleen is usually larger than the liver in Gaucher's disease. Niemann-Pick and Gaucher's diseases produce histologically similar vacuoles and sea blue foamy histiocytes as a histologic hallmark, but the accumulated stained lipid substance is different in each disease. There are three forms of Gaucher's disease. Type 1 presents in childhood or teen years, and sometimes progresses to parkinsonian rigidity in early middle age; type 2 is a fatal neonatal and infantile form that presents with the tetrad of trismus, strabismus, and retrocolis along with hepatosplenomegaly; and type 3 causes massive splenomegaly with loss of voluntary lateral gaze. In the case of oligosaccharidoses and mucopolysaccharidoses, abnormal oligosaccharides and glycosaminoglycans (mucopolysaccharides) can be detected in urine; enzyme testing confirms a diagnosis. Sandhoff disease and multiple sulfatase deficiency combine features of oligosaccharidosis, mucopolysaccharidosis, and sphingolipidosis. The lipidoses that are most likely to present in the newborn period are Gaucher's disease type 2, Krabbe globoid cell leukodystrophy, Tay-Sachs Gm2

Table 15
Mucolipidoses

	Enzyme defect	Accumulated substances excreted in urine
Mucolipidosis I (sialidosis)	α-Neuraminidase	Sialylyoligosaccharides Sialylglycopeptides
Mucolipidosis II (I-cell disease)	UDP-N-acetylglucosamine: lysosomal enzyme, N-acetylglucosamine-1-phosphotransferase	Sialylyoligosaccharides, Glycoproteins, Glycolipids
Mucolipidosis III (pseudo-Hurler polydystrophy)	Same phosphotransferase as mucolipidosis I	Sialylyoligosaccharides, Glycoproteins, Glycolipids
Mucolipidosis IV (sialolipidosis)	Gangliosialidase	Gangliosides Phospholipids Mucopolysaccharides

Abbreviation: UDP, uridine diphosphate.

gangliosidosis, Gm1 gangliosidosis, and multiple sulfatase deficiency. Krabbe disease presents as a hypertonic infant who has a high CSF protein and is irritable; the old mnemonic is "Krabbe kids are crabby" (Table 14).

Mucolipidoses are characterized by lysosomal storage and urinary excretion of mucolipid sialyloligosaccharides, sialylglycopeptides, glycolipids, and sometimes mucopolysaccharides [3,7]. Clinical features include variable coarsening of features, visceromegaly, cloudy cornea, neural degeneration, and retinal degeneration. Diagnosis is made by combining clinical features, urinary screening, and enzyme assay in fibroblasts or leukocytes. All are autosomal recessive, all can present in the newborn, and the only treatments are symptomatic management and genetic counseling (Table 15).

Oligosaccharidoses (glycoproteinoses) are diseases that are caused by the inability to disassemble glycoproteins [3,7]. For educational simplicity, this can be considered the reverse of congenital disorders of glycoprotein synthesis, although the impaired degradation does not occur in the Golgi apparatus. They also are called oligosaccharidoses because they are characterized often by lysosomal storage of products that are bound to oligosaccharides. Their symp-

Table 16
Oligosaccharidoses (Glycoproteinoses)

Disease	Enzyme defect	Accumulated substances excreted in urine
α-Mannosidosis	α-Mannosidase	α-Mannosyl-oligosaccharides
β-Mannosidosis	β-Mannosidase	β-Mannosyl-oligosaccharides
Fucosidosis	Fucosidase	Fucosyl-oligosaccharides Fucosyl-glycosphingolipids
Aspartylglucosaminuria	Aspartylglucosaminidase	Aspartylglucosamine
Galactosialidosis	Protective protein for α-Neuraminidase and β galactosidase	Sialyloligosaccharides Galactosyloligosaccharides
Sialic acid storage disease	Sialic acid transport	Free sialic acid

Table 17
Neuronal ceroid lipofuscinoses

	Enzyme defect	Inclusions
Infantile (Haltia- Santavuori)	Palmitoyl-protein thioesterase	Granular osmiophilic deposits
Late infantile (Jansky-Bielschowsky)	Tripeptidyl peptidase I	Curvilinear bodies; subunit C of mitochondrial ATP synthase
Juvenile (Spielmeyer-Vogt-Batten)	438 amino acid membrane protein	Curvilinear and laminated (fingerprint) bodies; Subunit C of mitochondrial ATP synthase
Adult (Kufs)	Not Known	Mixed osmiophilic and laminar inclusions

toms include varying degrees of dysmorphic features, visceromegaly, dementia, seizures, global neurodegeneration with seizures, myoclonus, movement disorder, ataxia, progressive cerebral atrophy that can be severe, and storage in skin, endothelia, and all affected organs. All are autosomal recessive, all can present in the newborn, all are rare, and the only proven treatments are symptomatic management and genetic counseling (Table 16).

Neuronal ceroid lipofuscinoses cause dementia, intractable epilepsy, movement disorder, retinal blindness, global neurodegeneration, and death [3,7]. EEGs often show a photoconvulsive response, and the electroretinogram is nearly always abnormal. Their pathologic hallmark is accumulation of complex osmiophilic inclusions, which, by light microscopy, originally were called lipofuscin. Patients can suffer icthyosis, especially in the adult form. Strictly speaking, these are not lysosomal storage diseases. They were considered lipidoses in the past, because of the accumulation of membranous structures that contain sphingolipids. Usually there is only slight organomegaly or coarse features, or none at all. They occur in four age presentations. There is no reliable diagnostic urinary product; the obsolete assay for urinary dolichols is not sufficiently predictive. The infantile form can present in the newborn as hypotonia, seizures, and little visual interest (Table 17).

Other neurogenetic disorders

Other neurogenetic disorders include chromosomal disorders (eg, trisomy 21), subtelomeric disorders, nucleotide repeat disorders (eg, myotonic dystrophy), other genetic mutations and deletions (eg, Angelmann or Prader-Willi syndromes), and heritable disorders of unknown cause.

Leukodystrophies

Leukodystrophies are disorders that are characterized by disruption of myelin formation or by destruction of normal myelin (Box 16). This class of disease can

Box 16. Diagnostic algorithm for infantile storage diseases and leukodystrophies

Dysmorphic +/− mild organomegaly, +/− neurologic symptoms?
Mucopolysaccharidoses (Urine Berry spot positive)
    Mental retardation
        Hurler
        Hunter
        Hunter-Scheie
        Sanfilippo
        β Glucuronidase deficiency
        Mucosulfatidosis
        Multiple sulfatase deficiency
    No mental retardation
        Scheie
        Morquio
        Maroteaux-Lamy
Oligosaccharidoses (Urine Berry spot negative)
    Urine sialic acid increased
        Mucolipidosis I
        Mucolipidosis II
        Mucolipidosis III
    Urine sialic acid not present:
        Fucosidosis
        Mannosidosis
        Aspartylglucosaminuria
        Mucolipidosis IV
Peroxisomal diseases
Chromosomal diseases
Visceromegaly without dysmorphic features?
Disordered sugar metabolism
    Galactosemia
    Fructosemia
    Glycogen storage diseases
    Childhood mucopolysaccharidoses
Disordered fat metabolism without acidosis
    Wolman
    Cholesterol ester storage disease
    Niemann-Pick A-C
    Farber disease
    Tangier disease
    Sandhoff (some)
    Childhood mucolipidoses
    Urea cycle defects

Disordered fat metabolism with acidosis
  Sometimes in organic and amino acidurias
  Mevalonic aciduria
  Sometimes in disorders of fatty acid oxidation
Metabolic diseases with heart failure
Neurologic diseases without dysmorphic features
  or visceromegaly
Predominantly gray matter disease
  Tay-Sachs
  Sandhoff
  Gm1 gangliosidosis
  Alexander disease
  Neuroaxonal dystrophy
  Neuronal ceroid lipofuscinosis
  Many mitochondrial diseases
  Some organic and amino acidopathies and urea
    cycle defects
Predominantly white matter disease
  Canavan spongy degeneration
  Adrenoleukodystrophy
  Krabbe globoid-cell leukodystrophy
  Metachromatic leukodystrophy
  Pelizaeus-Merzbacher proteolipid protein mutation diseases

Data from Lyon L, Adams RD, Kolodny EH. Neurology of hereditary metabolic diseases of children. 2nd edition. New York: McGraw-Hill; 1996.

be subdivided into three groups: dysmyelination, myelinolysis, and demyelination. Dysmyelination signifies inherited disorders of myelin chemistry, which cause biochemical instability in myelin or defective myelin formation. Myelinolysis signifies disorders where there is normal myelin genotype chemistry, but assembly and water content is disrupted by toxic or metabolic factors that cause formation of vacuoles in myelin sheaths to produce a "spongy myelinopathy." Demyelination signifies disorders where the original myelin was normal, but was damaged by inflammatory processes (infectious, immune, or other etiologies). It is clear from this organization that leukodystrophies can be caused by disorders that originate from the full panoply of etiologies (eg, small molecule or large molecule diseases). In some cases, such as in adrenoleukodystrophy or after trauma, as leukodystrophy progresses, demyelination may be added to dysmyelination or myelinolysis. This topic has been addressed well elsewhere [6,7,14–16] and is not discussed in detail here, other than to state that Krabbe disease (globoid cell leukodystrophy), neonatal adrenoleukodystrophy, and Pelizaeus-Merzbacher disease (proteo-lipid protein gene defect) are the most likely leukodystrophies to present in the neonatal period, and are caused by dysmyelination. Neonatal leukodystrophy that was caused by hexachlorophene soaks in the 1970s is an example of myelinolysis, which also can be caused by organic acidemias, aminoacidurias, urea cycle defects, and nearly any metabolic disturbance. In the neonatal period, demyelination can occur from infection, but is rare because of the minimal amount of myelin that is present in the newborn.

Hereditary ataxias

The hereditary ataxias are disorders with the common salient symptom of ataxia. Although some of these disorders can present with a variety of symptoms, by definition, they usually present as difficulty with gait. As such, their characteristic presentation does not occur in the newborn period. The disorders that also can present in a way other than ataxia have been discussed in other sections of this article. This category has been mentioned here for educational completeness only.

Summary, misconceptions, and hazardous pearls

Over the years, "clinical pearls" were taught to help simplify the diagnosis of neurometabolic disease. These did increase the efficiency of finding some of these rare diseases. The last 2 decades' progress of biochemical neurogenetics has shown some of these pearls to be unreliable, or potentially misleading. Some of the pearls can lead a clinician to exclude diseases prematurely. The following are a discussion of some of these hazards of differential diagnosis.

It was once taught that malformations imply large chromosomal defects, by virtue of the belief that the large portion of DNA that is disrupted by the large chromosomal defect affects many enzymes and structural proteins. It is true that large chromosomal defects often cause congenital malformations; however, it also is true that small molecule diseases can cause dysmorphic features. This is the concept that is known as "metabolic dysplasia," whereby the presence in the fetus of a toxic metabolite, or the absence of a useful metabolite, can cause abnormality of organogenesis. Three examples are instructive, each of which was presented above. The first example is that pyruvate dehydrogenase deficiency can cause the same facial features as can fetal alcohol syndrome. This is probably because the primary toxic agent in fetal alcohol syndrome is acetaldehyde, which is toxic to the pyruvate dehydrogenase. Another example is that of Smith-Lemli-Opitz syndrome, which is a multisystem dysplastic syndrome that is manifested by characteristic facial features, hypotonia, hypospadias, 2-3 syndactyly, mental impairment, and a panoply of neurologic symptoms. It is caused by a deficiency of 7-dehydrocholesterol reductase. This causes an excess of 7-dehydrocholesterol and a deficiency of cholesterol, which disrupts organogenesis and neural and myelin formation. Symptoms are improved by treatment with large doses of cholesterol. The third example is that of Zellweger cerebrohepatorenal syndrome. It is caused by defective peroxisomal function and was described above. The lesson of all of these examples is that when one is called to diagnose the cause of a malformation syndrome, it is prudent to check chromosomes and subtelomeric studies; however, other disorders cannot be excluded yet by presumption. It is also useful to look for the hallmarks of small and large molecule diseases, such as metabolic acidosis or organomegaly, and to screen for these disorders. In short, malformations can be caused by small molecule diseases, large molecule diseases, or chromosomal defects.

It is generally advised to obtain a newborn screen (blood spot) test for metabolic disease after the child has been fed. This is prudent because some diseases, such as phenylketonuria and branched-chain amino acidopathy ("maple syrup urine disease"), exhibit increased urinary excretion of their unmetabolized intermediates after the patient is given a protein load from milk. It has crept into the thoughts of clinicians that a protein load is the only way to find metabolic disease, and, by extension, that a newborn who has not yet fed will not display the neurologic effects of an organic acidemia or aminoacidemia. In fact, a fasting state can be the best stressor to make some diseases manifest, such as is found with the hypoketotic hypoglycemia of fatty acid β-oxidation disorders. The lesson is that it may be necessary to obtain urine amino acids and organic acids during the fasting and the protein-loaded state if the diagnosis of a suspected metabolic disorder remains elusive. In short, some organic and amino acidopathies can be diagnosed on newborn screen during the fasting state.

It was once taught to pediatricians to not test for neurometabolic disease unless the patient had loss of milestones. The truth is that neurodegenerative disease often is neurometabolic, but neurometabolic disease is not always degenerative. Often, the patient fails to develop well, and may have no loss of milestones ever, or perhaps only after a febrile illness or the onset of seizures many years later; thereafter, an affected patient may stay at a diminished, but steady, state. This is exemplified by glutaric aciduria type I, which is caused by glutaryl CoA dehydrogenase deficiency. These children may be born macrocephalic, but are otherwise normal. At some time, usually during a viral syndrome, they develop an acute "encephalitic-like crisis." This crisis is characterized by acute necrosis of the caudate and putamen, sometimes also with frontotemporal atrophy, and are left with severe dystonia, choreoathetosis, dyskinesia, seizures, and spasticity. If, however, a person who has glutaryl CoA dehydrogenase deficiency is treated with the proper diet and passes through the age of 7 years without this encephalitic-like crisis, the child will have no deterioration and will be functionally normal. Similar phenomena are found in other diseases. The lesson is that if one waits to test for neurometabolic disease only in patients who have neuro-degeneration, some patients will develop severe disease, and neurometabolic diseases will be missed. Instead, refer to the indications to test for neurometabolic disease (see Box 1), in addition to signs of neurodegeneration. In short, neurometabolic diseases do not always present as neurodegeneration.

It is taught commonly to medical students that it is best to follow the rule of parsimony: look for a single cause of disease that accounts for all symptoms. In the case of neurometabolic disease, there usually is a nexus of causality that involves a "model" of disease [17]. In this model, three factors are required to bring on illness: a host factor (in this case, a genetic disorder of metabolism); a developmental proclivity (eg, pre-7-year-old risk period for glutaric aciduria type I); and a trigger (eg, viral syndrome, birth, trauma, dehydration, or even menses), that causes a shift toward catabolism or dependence on the dysfunctional metabolic pathway that, in turn, leads to a deterioration of neural function. That deterioration can be sudden (eg, Reye-like syndrome, encephalitic-like syndrome) or intermittent ataxia. Alternately, that deterioration can be slow or subacute, and lead to gradual neurodegeneration, or intermittent minor declines. With this triple-risk factor model in mind, the lesson is that if a patient has a severe form of a common viral illness, it may be prudent, when possible, to perform a few screening tests for metabolic disease (eg, testing for unexplained or persistent acidosis). There is a corollary to this. Each neurometabolic disease can present with a variety of severities in different patients, depending on the severity of the underlying gene defect, social or other circumstances during the particular critical biochemical developmental period of presentation, or the severity of the trigger (viral or otherwise). Therefore, a laboratory or clinical test for a neurometabolic disease may be normal when the patient is not acutely ill, or when the child is young, as in the case of late childhood– or adult-onset disorders. The triple-risk factor model of disease does not dispel the principle of parsimony, because the patient's neurometabolic disease still remains the fundamental cause of symptoms; however, the triple-risk model modifies the principle of parsimony, and puts it into the broader context of developmental physiology, common exogenous triggers, and biopsychosocial complexities. Some investigators will be uncomfortable with this idea of modifying the principle of parsimony, which also has been called "Occam's razor" or the "KISS" principle ("keep it simple, stupid"); however, Occam himself described the principle as follows: "Entities should not be multiplied more than necessary." There are many situations, however, where the simplest solution is not accurate and not sufficient, and it is necessary to modify the simple solution. (As if to symbolize that modifications of his principle are often necessary, even the name "Occam" has been spelled in several official varieties, including "Occum" and "Ockham".) In short, the principle of parsimony can lead to missing the diagnosis of neurometabolic disease, if it is not coupled with an awareness of the triple-risk factor model of disease.

The final note concerns the problem of missing one of these diagnoses. Each disease is rare. Most are complex. Most of them present nonspecifically or mimic more common diseases. They may be missed because they first become manifest during a simultaneous febrile illness or other stress, which obscures the coexistent neurometabolic disease. At the time when many of the readers of this article were in training, some of these diseases had not been discovered, their diagnosis was not provable without autopsy, or the disorders were not taught in our training institutions or textbooks. Progress has moved so rapidly in genomics and biochemistry that some of what is written in this article may be outdated by the time it is published. The reader never will encounter most of these diseases, or will be asked to assist with management only once or twice in a career. The barriers to sharing management over great distances are daunting, and we cannot expect that all such patients can be sent away to large academic centers for care. Moreover, we all feel loyalty to the people of our geographic region, and feel a strong obligation to provide as much service as we can to our fellow community members. Before a diagnosis is made, the patient's care is impeded severely without the guidance that is derived from a confirmed diagnosis. It is always disturbing that it can take months before a diagnosis is known. This delay can occur even if the clinicians have a high suspicion that some neurometabolic disease is present, and even with expert and ardent diagnostic effort. All of this occurs under constant urgent pressure to provide simultaneous care for the sick patient as well as all of the other patients who are under our care. Patients may benefit from us explaining to them how long it may take to make a full diagnosis; they need courage to continue the diagnostic process. Rarely is there a situation where the title of "patient" is more appropriate, because rarely does a patient and family require more patience than in the evaluation of a potential neurometabolic disease. Their stress from the disease is magnified by uncertainty. The effort is enough to make clinician, patient, and family lament. With such burdens, it is unreasonable to expect that we would never miss one of these diagnoses, or miss an aspect of management. It is more unfortunate for our communities if anxiety over the risks that are associated with diagnosing and managing these diseases were to block us from engaging as active participants. Instead, it can be a goal of a compassionate, concerned, and competent clinical environment to keep these diagnoses in the differential diagnosis, to use newborn screens whenever they are available, to encourage the expansion of reliable newborn screening, and to share the load of diagnosis and management with colleagues. Despite our efforts, perfection is not possible. It is this article's intent, however, to help you to provide babies and their families with your scientific acts of caring.

References

[1] Leslie ND. Principles of metabolism. In: Osborn LM, DeWitt T, First L, et al, editors. Pediatrics. Philadelphia: Elsevier; 2005. p. 110–21.
[2] Enns GM, Steiner RD. Diagnosis and treatment of children with suspected metabolic disease. In: Osborn LM, DeWitt T, First L, et al, editors. Pediatrics. Philadelphia: Elsevier; 2005. p. 1866–75.
[3] Victor M, Ropper AH. Principles of neurology. 7th edition. New York: McGraw-Hill; 2001.
[4] Wilson G, Cooley WC. Preventive management of children with congenital anomalies and syndromes. Cambridge (UK): Cambridge University Press; 2000.
[5] Nyhan WL, Ozand PT. Atlas of metabolic diseases. London: Chapman & Hall Medical; 1998.

[6] Rosenberg RN, Prusiner SB, DiMauro S, et al. The molecular and genetic basis of neurological disease. 2nd edition. Boston: Butterworth-Heinemann; 1997.

[7] Lyon L, Adams RD, Kolodny EH. Neurology of hereditary metabolic diseases of children. 2nd edition. New York: McGraw-Hill; 1996.

[8] Thoene JG, Coker NP. Physicians' guide to rare diseases. 2nd edition. Montvale (NJ): Dowden; 1995.

[9] Lockman LA. Coma. In: Swaiman K, editor. The practice of pediatric neurology. St. Louis (MO): Mosby; 1982. p. 150.

[10] Filiano JJ, Goldenthal MJ, Rhodes CH, et al. Mitochondrial dysfunction in patients with hypotonia, epilepsy, autism, and developmental delay: HEADD syndrome. J Child Neurol 2001; 17(6):435–9.

[11] Kuban KK, Filiano JJ. Neonatal seizures. In: Cloherty JP, Stark AR, editors. Manual of neonatal care. 3rd edition. Boston: Little Brown; 1991. p. 367–81.

[12] Kim S, Westphal V, Srikrishna G, et al. Dolichol phosphate mannose synthase (DPM1) mutations define congenital disorder of glycosylation Ie (CDG-Ie). J Clin Invest 2000;105(2):191–8.

[13] Jones KL. Smith's recognizable patterns of human malformation. 5th edition. Philadelphia: Saunders; 1997.

[14] Cooley WC. Down syndrome. In: Osborn LM, DeWitt T, First L, et al, editors. Pediatrics. Philadelphia: Elsevier; 2005. p. 1060–4.

[15] United States National Institutes of Health. Available at: http://genetests.com.

[16] United States National Library of Medicine. Online Mendelian inheritance in man. Available at http://www.Pubmed.gov/OMIM.

[17] Filiano JJ, Kinney HC. A perspective on neuropathologic findings in victims of the sudden infant death syndrome: the triple risk model. Biol Neonate 1994;65:194–7.

ELSEVIER
SAUNDERS

CLINICS IN
PERINATOLOGY

Clin Perinatol 33 (2006) 481–501

Cerebral Palsy due to Chromosomal Anomalies and Continuous Gene Syndromes

John H. Menkes, MD[a,b,*], Laura Flores-Sarnat, MD[c]

[a]Division of Pediatric Neurology, University of California, Los Angeles, CA, USA
[b]Department of Pediatric Neurology, Cedars-Sinai Medical Center, 8700 Beverly Boulevard,
Los Angeles, CA 90048, USA
[c]Division of Pediatric Neurology, Alberta Children's Hospital, 1820 Richmond Road SW,
Calgary, Alberta T2T 6E6, Canada

When cerebral palsy is defined as a disorder of movement and posture that is due to nonprogressive disturbances that occur in the developing fetal and infant brain, a significant proportion—up to 10%—is the consequence of chromosomal anomalies and continuous gene syndromes. Abnormalities of chromosomes are constitutional or acquired. Acquired chromosomal abnormalities develop post-natally, affect only one clone of cells, and are implicated in the evolution of neoplasia. Constitutional abnormalities develop during gametogenesis or early embryogenesis and affect a significant portion of the subject's cells. When cerebral palsy is defined as a disorder of movement and posture that is due to non-progressive disturbances that occur in the developing fetal and infant brain, a significant proportion—up to 10%—is the consequence of chromosomal anomalies and continuous gene syndromes. Abnormalities of chromosomes are constitutional or acquired. Acquired chromosomal abnormalities develop post-natally, affect only one clone of cells, and are implicated in the evolution of neoplasia. Constitutional abnormalities develop during gametogenesis or early embryogenesis and affect a significant portion of the subject's cells. The intro-duction of chromosomal banding techniques with increasing degrees of reso-lution, the widespread use of fluorescence in situ hybridization (FISH), and supplemental molecular analyses have refined cytogenetic analysis and have permitted detection of uniparental disomies (UPDs) and innumerable subtle,

* Corresponding author. Department of Pediatric Neurology, Cedars-Sinai Medical Center, 8700 Beverly Boulevard, Los Angeles, CA 90048.
 E-mail address: jhansmenk@aol.com (J.H. Menkes).

0095-5108/06/$ – see front matter © 2006 Elsevier Inc. All rights reserved.
doi:10.1016/j.clp.2006.03.001

often submicroscopic (cryptogenic), deletions, duplications, or translocations. These techniques have removed any clear dividing line between changes that are considered to be chromosomal abnormalities and those that are considered to be molecular defects [1]. Because more than 30,000 genes are expressed in the human brain, it comes as no surprise that impaired brain function is the most common symptom of chromosomal anomalies.

The incidence of chromosomal anomalies in unselected, apparently normal newborns is significant. Using banding techniques, Jacobs and colleagues [2] found a 0.92% prevalence of structural chromosomal abnormalities in unselected newborns; however, the cost of a systematic surveillance of the newborn population using high-resolution chromosomal banding, DNA polymorphisms, and subtelomeric FISH panels remains prohibitive. The limitations of prenatal and neonatal surveillance programs are discussed more fully by Hook and colleagues [3]. Major duplications or deficiencies in autosomes tend to be lethal [4], with death occurring in utero or in the immediate postnatal period [5]. Few of the autosomal trisomies are compatible with survival. Thus, the most common trisomy, chromosome 16, accounts for 7.5% of all spontaneous abortions, but is not compatible with live birth, and only 2.8% of cases of trisomy 13, 5.4% of cases of trisomy 18, and 23.8% of cases of trisomy 21 are live born [3].

Diagnosis during the neonatal period

Chromosomal disorders and contiguous gene syndromes should be considered in any neonate that presents with any of the following conditions:

The syndrome of muscular hypotonia with brisk deep tendon reflexes (atonic cerebral palsy) in the absence of a history of perinatal asphyxia or trauma.

Whenever neonatal hypotonia is accompanied by two or more major congenital anomalies, particularly when these involve the mesodermal or endodermal germ layers.

In the presence of minor congenital anomalies, particularly when these involve the face, hands, feet, or ears. Abnormalities of the palmar creases and abnormalities in the scalp hair whorl pattern are important pointers to the presence of chromosomal disorders. Because skin creases form at 11 to 12 weeks' gestation, these abnormalities indicate an insult in early intrauterine life.

The authors also obtain a cytogenetic survey in children who have congenital microcephaly.

In such subjects a cytogenetic examination is an essential part of the evaluation, and the yield of 10% contrasts with a yield of 1% for routine metabolic screening [6].

In most laboratories, phytohemagglutinin-stimulated lymphocytes serve for the analysis. Chromosomal banding is always indicated; the most popular banding technique in North America is Giemsa-trypsin banding (G banding). When an anomaly is identified, more than one technique might be needed to delineate its location and the size of any deletion or extra chromosomal fragment. When the location for the abnormality is suspected (eg, chromosome 15q for Prader-Willi syndrome), molecular cytogenetic analyses that use FISH techniques or high-resolution studies that focus on that site are indicated. FISH probes are available for most of the known microdeletion syndromes (Table 1) [7]. Chromosome-specific subtelomeric probes are available commercially, and if financially feasible, should form part of the evaluation.

DNA studies are routine in the evaluation of the fragile X syndrome. When these study results are negative, and the phenotype is highly suggestive of the fragile X syndrome, mutation analysis for the FMR-1 gene should be performed. Subtle chromosomal deletions or other anomalies are detected best by examining cells in late prophase or early metaphase using high-resolution analysis; this technique is more laborious and expensive than standard analysis. A newer alternative is the use of comparative genomic hybridization (CGH) [7]. CGH and array CGH not only detect subtelomeric deletions, but also deletions and duplications along the lengths of the chromosomes, assuming that the deletion or duplication is not so small as to be spaced between two adjacent probes in the set [8].

Current cytogenetic techniques are so sensitive that they have uncovered minor chromosomal anomalies in unselected newborn populations. It is unclear how many of the less common chromosomal variations are consistently responsible for neurologic symptoms, and how many are the consequences of the

Table 1
Microdeletion syndromes with prominent neurologic symptoms

Chromosome	Syndrome	FISH probe	Reference
4p16	Wolf-Hirschhorn	+	See text
5p16	Cri du chat	+	See text
7p13	Cephalopolysyndactyly	+	[75]
7q11.23	Williams	+	See text
7q34	Holoprosencephaly	−	[76]
8q24	Langer-Giedion	+	[77]
11p15 [a]	Beckwith-Wiedemann	+	[78]
11q13	Wilms tumor, aniridia, mental retardation, genitourinary anomalies hemihypertrophy (WAGR syndrome)	+	[79]
15q12	Prader-Willi/Angelman	+	See text
16p13.3	α-Thalassemia, mental retardation	+	[80]
16p13.3	Rubinstein-Taybi	+	[62]
17p11.2	Smith-Magenis	+	[81]
17p13	Miller-Dieker	+	See text
22q11.2	Velocardiofacial; Di George	+	See text
Xq21.1	Choroideremia, mental retardation	+	[82]

Abbreviation: +, can be detected.
[a] Developmental dysregulation rather than deletion of a cluster of imprinted genes.

same environmental event (eg, exposure to virus, drugs, irradiation) that induced the abnormal offspring. The coming availability of multicolor FISH and array CGH to screen children who have nonspecific mental retardation for cryptic subtelomeric deletions could result in detection of abnormalities in an additional 6% of mentally retarded children [2,9].

Autosomal abnormalities

Down syndrome (trisomy 21)

Down syndrome (trisomy 21) is the most common autosomal anomaly in live births. The most recent figures in the United States (1997) indicate a prevalence of 9.9 per 10,000 live births, and 43% occur in births to women aged 35 years and older [10]. This is significantly less than the prevalence of 1 in 500 that was recorded in 1950, and reflects the effectiveness of prenatal screening programs [11].

Down syndrome is associated with an extra chromosome 21 or an effective trisomy for chromosome 21 by its translocation to another chromosome, usually chromosome 14, or, less often, to another acrocentric chromosome, especially chromosome 21 or 22.

On a clinical basis, it is impossible to distinguish between patients who have Down syndrome that is caused by ordinary trisomy 21 or by translocation. The frequency of trisomy 21 increases with maternal age, and reaches a prevalence of 1 in 54 births in mothers aged 45 years or older. In contrast to ordinary trisomy, the incidence of translocation Down syndrome is independent of maternal age. Most translocations that produce Down syndrome arise de novo in the affected child and are not associated with familial Down syndrome.

By the use of polymorphic DNA markers, several studies concluded that the extra chromosome is derived maternally, and mainly is the consequence of errors in the first meiotic division in more than 90% of cases [12]. The mean maternal age associated with errors in meiosis is approximately 33 years, significantly higher than the mean reproductive age in the United States. In 4.3% of cases, there were errors in paternal meiosis. In these cases, and in the remainder that are caused by errors in mitosis, maternal age is not increased [13].

To understand the molecular pathogenesis of Down syndrome, two questions must be answered: (1) How does the presence of a small acrocentric chromosome in triplicate and the increased expression of genes on this chromosome produce the anatomic and functional abnormalities of the Down syndrome phenotype? and (2) Are we able to identify specific regions of chromosome 21 whose duplication is responsible for each of the phenotypic features of Down syndrome? These questions are addressed by Roizen and Patterson [14].

Principally, malformations affect the heart and the great vessels. Approximately 20% to 60% of subjects who have Down syndrome have congenital heart disease. Defects in the atrioventricular septum were the most common abnormalities that were encountered by Rowe and Uchida [15] in 36% of their patients, most of whom were younger than 2 years of age. Among the other malformations, gastrointestinal anomalies are the most common. These include duodenal stenosis or atresia, anal atresia, megacolon, and Hirschsprung's disease. Malformations of the spine, particularly of the upper cervical region, occasionally can produce neurologic symptoms.

Grossly, the brain is small and spherical, and the frontal lobes, brainstem, and cerebellum are smaller than normal. Generally, the number of secondary sulci is reduced; the tuber flocculi persist. Traditionally, the superior temporal gyrus is described as poorly developed. This appearance is the result of a superior temporal sulcus that is deeper than and "buries" the superior temporal gyrus (unpublished data). In other parts of the cerebral and cerebellar cortices neuronal density is reduced, cortical interneurons are lost, there is an accumulation of undifferentiated fetal cells in the cerebellum, and a reduction in the number of spines along the apical dendrites of pyramidal neurons, which are believed to indicate a reduction in the number of synaptic contacts [16].

The most intriguing neuropathologic observation is the premature development of changes within the brain that are compatible with a morphologic diagnosis of Alzheimer's disease. These changes are found in 15% of subjects who have Down syndrome who are aged 11 to 20 years, in 36% of subjects who are aged 21 to 30 years, and in all subjects who die at age 31 years or older [17].

Underlying the evolution of Alzheimer's disease in children who have Down syndrome is an excessive buildup of amyloid β-protein (AβP). This buildup is believed to be the consequence of an overexpression of the gene for amyloid β precursor protein, mapped to chromosome 21q21. This observation has been the topic of intense recent investigation that was reviewed by Lott and Head [18] and by Mrak and Griffin [19].

The clinical picture of Down syndrome is protean and consists of an unusual combination of anomalies, rather than a combination of unusual anomalies.

The birth weight of infants who have Down syndrome is less than normal, and 20% weigh 2.5 kg or less [20]. Neonatal complications are more common than normal and are a consequence of fetal hypotonia and a high incidence of breech presentations. Physical growth is delayed consistently, and the adult who has Down syndrome has a significantly short stature. The mental age that is achieved varies considerably. It is related, in part, to environmental factors, including the age at institutionalization for nonhome-reared individuals, the degree of intellectual stimulation, and the evolution of presenile dementia even before puberty.

Mosaicism can be found in approximately 2% to 3% of patients who have Down syndrome. In these instances, the subject exhibits a mixture of trisomic and normal cell lines. As a group, these individuals tend to achieve higher intellectual development than do nonmosaic subjects, and, in particular, they possess better verbal and visual-perceptual skills [21].

Aside from mental retardation, specific neurologic signs are rare and are limited to generalized muscular hypotonia and hyperextensibility of the joints.

This is particularly evident during infancy. Numerous case reports and series have associated atlantoaxial instability and dislocation with Down syndrome. The instability, seen in some 15% to 40% of patients, results from laxity of the transverse ligaments that hold the odontoid process close to the anterior arch of the atlas [22]. Usually, the instability is asymptomatic, but neck pain, hyperreflexia, progressive impairment of gait, urinary retention, and an acute traumatic dislocation has been encountered.

In addition to these neurologic abnormalities, patients who have Down syndrome exhibit several dysmorphic features. None of these is present invariably, nor are any consistently absent in the healthy population, but their conjunction contributes to the characteristic appearance of the subject. These are summarized in Box 1.

Currently (2002), the median age at death is 58 years for subjects who have Down syndrome [23]. Leukemia, notably treatment-related deaths; respiratory illnesses; congenital anomalies; and cardiovascular diseases account for most of the excess mortality [24,25].

Other abnormalities of autosomes

Aside from trisomy 21, trisomies that involve the other, larger chromosomes are associated with multiple severe malformations of brain and viscera, and affected children usually do not survive infancy. Trisomies of chromosomes 13 and 18 are the two entities that are encountered most commonly. The incidence of these and other chromosomal abnormalities are presented in Table 2 [26].

Trisomy 13 (Patau syndrome)

This condition occurs in fewer than 1 in 5000 births [27]. The clinical picture is characterized by feeding difficulties, apneic spells during early infancy, and striking developmental retardation. Subjects have varying degrees of median facial anomalies, including cleft lip or palate, premaxillary agenesis, and micrognathia. The ears are low set and malformed, and many infants are deaf. Polydactyly, flexion deformities of the fingers, and a horizontal palmar crease are common. Cardiovascular anomalies are present in 80% of patients, most commonly in the form of a patent ductus arteriosus or a ventricular septal defect. Approximately 33% of patients have polycystic kidneys. Also, there is an increased frequency of omphalocele, neural tube defects, microcephaly, and microphthalmus.

The major neuropathologic abnormality is holoprosencephaly (arrhinencephaly), a complex group of malformations that have in common absence of the olfactory bulbs and tracts and other cerebral anomalies, notably only one ventricle and absence of the interhemispheric fissure. On autopsy, several microscopic malformations are observed, including heterotopic nerve cells in the cerebellum and in the subcortical white matter. The prognosis for children who have chromosome 13 trisomy is poor and only a small percentage survives into the second year.

Box 1. Dysmorphic features in Down syndrome

Eyes

Oblique (upslanting) palpebral fissures
Persistence of a complete median epicanthal fold
Brushfield spots (slightly elevated light spots encircling the
    periphery of the iris)
Blepharitis, conjunctivitis
Lenticular opacifications, keratoconus

Ears

Small, low-set external ear with simple helix and hypoplastic tragus
Narrow diameter of the external auditory meatus
Congenital malformations of the bones of the middle ear
Permanent fixation of the stapes, shortening of cochlear spiral
Recurrent acute and chronic otitis
Hearing loss

Mouth

Radial furrows of lips
Protruding and fissured tongue
Neck short, with roll of fat and redundant skin in nape of neck
Low hairline

Extremities

Short
Incurved fifth digit, hypoplastic middle phalanx
Simian line (single transverse palmar crease)
Diastasis between first and second toes (sandal gap)

Skin

Xeroderma, hyperkeratotic lichenification

Autoimmune disorders

Juvenile rheumatoid arthritis-like progressive polyarthritis
Diabetes mellitus type I
Elevated antithyroid antibody
Gonadal deficiency and infertility

Table 2
Prevalence of chromosomal anomalies among 3658 newborns in a Danish population between 1980 and 1982

Chromosomal anomalies	Total	Rate per 1000
Autosomal chromosomes		
+ 13	0	–
+ 18	1	0.27
+ 21	5	1.37
+ 8	1	0.27
+ ring	2	0.55
13/14 translocation	2	0.55
14/21 translocation	1	0.27
Reciprocal translocations	7	1.91
Inversion chromosome 2 and 6	2	0.55
Inversion chromosome 9[a]	35	9.57
Duplications	2	0.55
Others	1	0.27
Total autosomal anomalies	59	16.13
Sex chromosome Anomalies		
47,XXY	3	1.60
47,XYY	2	1.07
47,XXX	3	1.68
45,XO (including mosaics)	4	2.24
Others	3	1.63
Total sex chromosome anomalies	15	4.10
Total chromosome anomalies	74	20.23

[a] No physical abnormalities accompany balanced translocations or inversion of chromosome 9.
Data from Nielson J, Wohlert M, Faaborg-Anderson J, et al. Incidence of chromosome abnormalities in newborn children. Comparison between incidences in 1969–1974 and 1980–1982 in the same area. Hum Genet 1982;61:98–101.

Trisomy 18 (Edwards syndrome)

The incidence of this condition seems to be on the increase; the most recently recorded prevalence (1999) in Hawaii was 4.7 cases per 10,000 [27]. The anomaly is seen much more frequently in female subjects; the most recent male:female ratio was 0.65 [28]. This suggests that a high proportion of affected male fetuses succumb during gestation. Like other autosomal trisomies, trisomy 18 results from an error in maternal meiosis.

The clinical picture is highlighted by a long narrow skull with prominent occiput, characteristic facies, low-set malformed ears, a mildly webbed neck, and marked physical and mental retardation. A typical picture of camptodactyly (flexion contractures of the fingers) and abnormal palmar flexion creases occurs. Many other inconstant anomalies of the extremities also occur; most are due to agenesis of particular muscles [29]. As in trisomy 13, omphalocele, polycystic kidneys, and congenital heart disease are common. A striking dermatoglyphic pattern—less common in other autosomal anomalies—is the presence of simple arches on all fingers.

No consistent central nervous system malformation is associated with the trisomy 18 syndrome. The most common anomaly is agenesis of the corpus callosum, which is associated occasionally with pontocerebellar hypoplasia, dysplasia of the inferior olivary and dentate nuclei of the cerebellar system, hypoplasia and dysplasia of the hippocampus, and nerve cell heterotopia of the cerebellum or white matter.

The prognosis for children who have trisomy 18 is poor, and 90% die by 1 year of age. The mean survival time is 10 months for girls, and 23 months for boys [30]. The natural history of trisomy 18 and trisomy 13 in long-term survivors has been well characterized [30].

Chromosome trisomy 9

A rare trisomy, the associated central nervous system malformations are a dilated fourth ventricle and malformed cerebellum that resembles the Dandy-Walker malformation. Additional features that distinguish it from simple posterior fossa malformations are agenesis of the corpus callosum, cerebral cortical migratory disturbances, mild ventriculomegaly, abnormally formed hippocampi, poorly convoluted inferior olivary nuclei, and syringomyelia [31].

Mosaic trisomy syndromes have been recognized for chromosomes 8, 9, 16, and 20. Mosaicisms for other autosomal trisomies have been reported rarely. Their clinical appearance was reviewed by Schinzel [32].

Structural autosomal anomalies

Several cytogenetically visible structural anomalies of the autosomal chromosomes have been reported and have been accompanied by neurologic defects, notably mental retardation and microcephaly. The most common of these entities is a deletion of the short arm of chromosome 5 (5p−), which causes the cri du chat syndrome, and the deletion of the short arm of chromosome 4 (4p−; Wolf-Hirschhorn) syndromes.

Cri du chat syndrome

Through the combined phenotypic and molecular analysis of affected individuals, the genes that are responsible for this condition have been mapped to 5p15.2 and 5p15.3. As a rule, mental retardation depends on the 5p deletion size and location, but in many instances there also are aberrations in copy number [33].

Cri du chat syndrome is seen in 1 in 20,000 to 50,000 births. A low birth weight and failure in physical growth are associated with a characteristic cry that is likened to that of a meowing kitten. Infants have microcephaly, large corneas, moon-shaped facies, ocular hypertelorism, epicanthal folds, transverse palmar (simian) creases, and generalized muscular hypotonia. The brain, although small, is grossly and microscopically normal, which represents a rare example of true microcephaly.

Wolf-Hirschhorn syndrome

The Wolf-Hirschhorn syndrome is caused by partial monosomy of the short arm of chromosome 4; one of the regions that is critical for the development of this disorder is 4p16.3. The syndrome is characterized by a facies that has been likened to that of a helmet of a Greek warrior. Frontal bossing; a high frontal hairline; a broad, beaked nose; prominent glabella; and ocular hypertelorism are seen. Major malformations occur commonly, especially cleft lip and palate, and mental retardation is usually severe. Epilepsy is a common feature, and is characterized by the presence of alternative hemiconvulsions, focal clonic seizures, and frequent status epilepticus [34].

Deletions in the region that are responsible for Wolf-Hirschhorn syndrome overlap those that are seen in Pitt-Rogers-Danks syndrome. The latter entity has a different phenotype and mental retardation is less severe than is seen in the Wolf-Hirschhorn syndrome. Wright and coworkers [35] proposed that the two conditions result from the absence of similar, if not identical genetic segments, and that the clinical differences between the two syndromes result from allelic variation in the remaining homolog.

Wolf-Hirschhorn syndrome can be diagnosed prenatally on the basis of the chromosomal abnormalities, or by the presence of characteristic facial dysmorphism [36].

Partial deletions and partial trisomies have been described for almost every chromosome, but few of these entities are sufficiently characteristic to allow the practitioner to suspect the diagnosis without cytogenetic analysis. In particular, the phenotypic expressions of ring chromosomes overlap those of partial deletions, and show so much variability that one cannot arrive at any conclusions with respect to their clinical pictures. Furthermore, certain features, especially microcephaly, are common to many of the chromosomal anomalies, and they also are encountered in the absence of any discernible chromosomal defect.

Subtelomeric abnormalities

Deletions, duplications, and cryptic imbalance rearrangements of the telomeres—the terminal segments of chromosomes—have received an increasing amount of attention in the past few years. It has become apparent that abnormalities in these regions are responsible for at least 5% to 10% of nonsyndromic mental retardation, as well as for cases of mental retardation that are associated with multiple congenital anomalies. Several techniques have been used to screen for these abnormalities. FISH is being replaced by CGH in which an abnormal and a control genome are compared for DNA copy differences. The latter technique is being adapted for rapid and sensitive automation [37].

Sex chromosome abnormalities

Sex chromosome abnormalities consist of various aneuploidies that involve the sex chromosomes. As determined by most surveys of the newborn population or of cells that are obtained at amniocentesis [38], the prevalence of sex chromosome abnormalities is approximately 2.5 in 1000 phenotypic male subjects and 1.4 in 1000 phenotypic female subjects (see Table 2). Although considerable geographic variation occurs, the two most common abnormalities in phenotypic male subjects are the XYY and the XXY (Klinefelter's) syndromes. Because monosomy X (45,X) is highly lethal, a significantly lower incidence of sex chromosome abnormalities is found in newborns than is found at amniocentesis. In a large proportion of subjects who have sex chromosome abnormalities, particularly phenotypic male subjects, the condition remains undiagnosed throughout life [38]. Most (75%) abnormalities in female subjects involve the XXX syndrome, with less than 25% being monosomy X (Turner syndrome) or variants thereof.

Klinefelter's syndrome

The condition occurs in 1 in 500 to 1000 male births [39], with a 40 times greater prevalence of the condition in karyotyped first-trimester miscarriages [40]. Although affected persons are tall with an eunuchoid habitus, the diagnosis usually is not made until adult life, and hormone assays are normal before the onset of puberty. Neurologic examination shows decreased muscle tone and some dysmetria or tremor; the major deficits in unselected subjects are cognitive disorders with a mild reduction in IQ, delayed auditory sequential memory, and a variety of learning disorders [41].

XYY karyotype

The XYY karyotype is encountered with a frequency as high as 4 in 1000 male newborns [42]. In the past, the XYY karyotype was believed to be associated with unusually tall stature, a predisposition to criminality, and dull normal intelligence. Controlled studies have shown a small, statistically significant deficit in verbal and full-scale IQs, but none in the performance scores [43]. Boys who have XYY syndrome can exhibit minor neurologic abnormalities, including intention tremor, mild motor incoordination, and limitation of motion at the elbows secondary to radioulnar synostoses. Careful behavioral studies confirmed that patients who have XYY syndrome tend to have a higher incidence of temper tantrums and exhibit other forms of overt impulsive behavior, poor long-term planning, and an inability to handle aggression in a socially acceptable manner [43]. In addition there is an increased incidence of criminal convictions during adolescence and adulthood [44].

Other sex chromosomal polysomies

In a phenotypically male subject, the greater the number of X chromosomes, the more severe is the mental retardation. XYYY subjects are only mildly retarded, whereas XXXYY male subjects have major intellectual deficits. Subjects who have the XXXY syndrome have severe mental retardation, small testes, microcephaly, and a variety of minor deformities. The XXXXY chromosomal anomaly is characterized by mental retardation, hypotonia, and a facial appearance that is reminiscent of Down syndrome [45]. In the phenotypic female subject, the presence of more than two X chromosomes also is associated with mental retardation. The most common of these disorders is the XXX syndrome, which is seen in 1 in 1000 newborn girls [46]. Although no specific clinical pattern exists for female subjects who have the XXX sex chromosome complement and there is considerable variability in their cognitive abilities, most have an IQ that is less than that of their siblings and are at risk for language problems, learning disabilities, and impaired social adaptation. Female subjects who demonstrate tetrasomy and pentasomy X usually are mentally retarded, with the observed degree of retardation increasing with the number of supernumerary X chromosomes.

Turner syndrome (Ullrich-Turner syndrome)

When cytogenetic techniques are combined with DNA analysis, most subjects who have this condition are 45,X mosaics who have a normal XX cell line, another abnormal cell line, or both. A significant proportion has some Y chromosome material [47]. As a rule, the apparent absence of the X chromosome is not associated with a gross intellectual deficit, however most patients have right-left disorientation and a defect in perceptual organization (space-form blindness). This is particularly true for those subjects who have an apparent 45,X karyotype and is less marked in children who have obvious mosaicism [48]. The defects in perceptual organization correlate with an MRI that indicates a reduced volume of cerebral hemisphere and parieto-occipital brain matter, which is more marked on the right [49].

Chromosomal anomalies in various dysmorphic syndromes (contiguous gene syndromes, microdeletion syndromes)

In addition to deletions that are detected readily cytogenetically, combined molecular and cytogenetic analysis has led to the identification of small deletions in several clinically well-defined syndromes (see Table 1). The term "contiguous gene syndrome," which was coined by Schmickel [50], refers to the patterns of phenotypic expression that result from the inactivation or overexpression as a result of deletion, duplication, or other means, of a set of adjacent genes in a specific chromosome region.

These conditions are distinct from the various syndromes that result from gross chromosomal deletion or duplication in that they are not readily demonstrable by classic cytogenetic techniques [51]. The number of recognizable syndromes has continued to multiply over the last few decades, and their clinical diagnosis has become increasingly difficult. Books, like the one by Jones [52], are invaluable assistants for that task, but even with their aid, diagnosis often is in dispute. An on-line database for the diagnosis of genetic and dysmorphic syndromes has been prepared by McKusick and his group [53] and is updated continuously by the National Center for Biotechnology Information. It can be accessed at.

Prader-Willi and Angelman syndromes

These two disorders with a marked difference in clinical expression are associated with interstitial deletions of chromosome 15q11-q13. The observation that the clinical picture of deletion 15q11-q13 depended on whether the deleted chromosome is derived from mother or father, provided the first clear example of genomic imprinting in the human. Certain regions of the human genome normally exhibit gene expression from only one of the two inherited genes. This monoallelic expression of biallelic genes is regulated by a variety of mechanism. The decision about which of the two alleles is expressed can be on a random basis, or it can be according to the parent of origin. The term "genomic imprinting" refers to the differential expression of genetic material depending on whether it is inherited from the male or female parent. The absence of biparental contributions to the genome, which cannot be detected by routine cytogenetic examination, may be responsible for a large proportion of syndromes for which no chromosomal anomaly has been demonstrated. Hall [54] also suggested that the phenotypic differences in any given chromosomal syndrome may reflect the parental origin of the affected chromosome. Some children with a cytogenetically normal karyotype have UPD, rather than biparental inheritance of a specific chromosome pair. In some instances UPD has no effect on the phenotype; in other instances it exerts a profound effect. A more extensive discussion of imprinting in Prader-Willi and Angelman syndromes is provided by Davies and coworkers [55].

Prader-Willi syndrome is marked by obesity, small stature, hyperphagia, and mental retardation. Its prevalence has been estimated at 1 in 10,000 to 25,000 births. When chromosomes are examined by FISH analysis, approximately 70% of patients who have Prader-Willi syndrome demonstrate a deletion of the proximal part of the long arm of chromosome 15 (15q11-q13). These deletions, which are visible occasionally by high-resolution banding techniques, occur exclusively on the paternally derived chromosome. Some of the remaining subjects who have Prader-Willi syndrome have other abnormalities in the same region of chromosome 15. In about 20% of subjects karyotype appears normal, but restriction fragment length polymorphism analyses show the presence of two maternally derived chromosomes 15, and no paternal chromosome 15, which is consistent with maternal UPD for chromosome 15. Thus, in at least 95% of patients, partial or complete absence of the paternal chromosome 15 occurs. In the remainder of the patients, the condition results from mutations in the imprinting center.

The clinical picture is mostly uniform [56]. Breech presentation is common. Characteristically, the face is long, the forehead is narrow, and the eyes are almond shaped. Symptoms of hypothermia, hypotonia, and feeding difficulties become evident in infancy. Occasionally, hypotonia is so striking that infants are evaluated for muscle disorders. Small hands and feet are noted in early childhood. Over the years, hyperphagia and excessive weight gain develop. Overeating is believed to reflect reduced satiation, rather than increased hunger. Hypotonia tends to improve, but short stature, hypogonadism, and mild to moderately severe mental retardation become evident [52,56]. Most patients have hypersomnolence; daytime hypoventilation also has been observed.

Anatomic examinations of the brain have not been helpful in providing insight into the cause of the mental retardation and hypotonia, but MRI has suggested abnormalities in cortical development [57].

The diagnosis of Prader-Willi syndrome is prompted by historic and clinical features and is confirmed by methylation polymerase chain reaction analysis of the promoter region of the gene for small nuclear ribonucleoprotein polypeptide N, which is part of the imprinted gene cluster at 15q11-q13 [58]. Although healthy subjects have biparental and always different methylation patterns, subjects who have Prader-Willi or Angelman syndromes that are caused by deletions or UPD show a uniform methylation pattern, which reflects the absence of the one of the parental alleles [58].

A deletion of the maternally derived chromosome 15q11-q13 is seen in approximately 75% of children who have the Angelman ("happy puppet") syndrome. The remainder has paternal UPD, a defect in the imprinting center, a defect in a gene that is involved in the ubiquitin-mediated protein degradation pathway [59], or an as yet unexplained defect.

The prevalence of Angelman syndrome is less than 1 in 10,000. The clinical picture is marked by severe mental retardation, microcephaly, and puppet-like, jerky, but not truly ataxic, movements. Frequent paroxysms of unprovoked laughter lend the syndrome its name. Seizures are common and the interictal EEG shows bifrontally dominant rhythmic runs of notched slow waves, or slow and sharp waves, especially during sleep when they can become continuous [60]. Examination of the brain shows mild cerebral atrophy, but normal gyral development. Marked cerebellar atrophy is seen, with loss of Purkinje and granule cells, and a marked decrease in dendritic arborizations [61].

Diagnosis may be made by FISH analysis in the case of deletions of 15q, but methylation studies detect a higher proportion of cases.

Other conditions with uniparental disomy have now been recognized. They are summarized in Table 3.

Table 3
Symptomatic uniparental disomies

Chromosome	Clinical manifestations	Reference
pUPD6	Transient neonatal diabetes mellitus	[83]
mUPD7	Russell-Silver syndrome	
pUPD11	Beckwith-Wiedemann syndrome	[70]
mUPD14	Prader-Willi–like appearance, short stature, mental retardation	[84]
pUPD14	Skeletal anomalies, unusual facies, mental retardation	[85]
mUPD15	Prader-Willi syndrome	See text
pUPD15	Angelman syndrome	See text

Uniparental disomies of the other chromosomes have no apparent phenotypic effect [82].

Miller-Dieker syndrome

Miller-Dieker syndrome is characterized by lissencephaly—one of the most severe cerebral malformations—which is characterized by microcephaly; severe to profound mental retardation; and an unusual facies that is marked by a high forehead, vertical soft tissue furrowing, and a small, anteverted nose [52]. More than 90% of subjects have visible or submicroscopic deletions of 17p13.3 [51]. The Miller-Dieker syndrome is a major cause for lissencephaly, and about one third of patients who have isolated lissencephaly have deletions or point mutations of the LIS-1 gene in 17p13.3. Prenatal diagnosis can be established after the 24th week of gestation by ultrasound and is confirmed by fetal MRI.

Rubinstein-Taybi syndrome

This syndrome is marked by microcephaly; a hypoplastic maxilla with a narrow palate; a prominent, beaked nose; the presence of broad thumbs and great toes; a moderate degree of mental retardation; and in rare instances, the Dandy-Walker malformation. Postnatal growth retardation occurs, and other facial abnormalities are common. These include downward-slanting palpebral fissures; low-set ears; heavy, highly arched eyebrows; and long eyelashes [62]. Many patients who have the Rubinstein-Taybi syndrome have breakpoints or deletions of chromosome 16p13.3, and mutations in a gene for a nuclear protein that is involved in cyclic AMP–regulated gene expression. Alternatively, a gene that codes for a histone acetyltransferase that regulates transcription by way of chromatin remodeling could be responsible for the clinical manifestations of the syndrome [63].

Cornelia de Lange syndrome (Brachmann–de Lange syndrome)

Cornelia de Lange syndrome (Brachmann–de Lange syndrome) is characterized by marked growth retardation; severe mental retardation; a low-pitched, growling cry; bushy eyebrows; hirsutism; and various malformations of the hands and feet [52]. The condition is believed to result from mutations of a gene, mapped to chromosome 5p13.1 and involved in the regulation of cell proliferation and neuronal plasticity [64].

Williams syndrome

This disorder is caused by a heterozygous deletion in chromosome 7q11.23 and is marked by an unusual elfinlike facies, supravalvular aortic stenosis, hypercalcemia, and significant physical and mental retardation.

Usually, mental retardation is not severe, and language ability may be good, with some children having an extraordinary talent for music. Hypersociability ("everybody in the world is my friend") is a striking characteristic and is evident in young children. This contrasts with severe deficits in several nonverbal tasks, notably spatial cognition, planning, and problem solving. By contrast, a patient with a severe delay in expressive speech showed duplication of the Williams syndrome locus [65].

MRI shows cerebral hypoplasia and alterations in the relative size of paleocerebellar to neocerebellar portions of the vermis. There is a significant reduction in white matter in the posterior half of the brain, and the size of the posterior portion of the corpus callosum is reduced [66].

Velocardiofacial syndrome and Di George syndrome (catch-22 syndrome)

Velocardiofacial syndrome is the most frequent microdeletion syndrome with a prevalence that approximates 2 in 10,000. It is characterized by an overt or submucous cleft palate, velopharyngeal insufficiency that results in a distinctive hypernasal speech, cardiac malformations that often are conotruncal defects, and parathyroid deficiency with hypocalcemia. The face is marked by a prominent, bulbous nose; ocular hypertelorism; a squared nasal root; and micrognathia. Most children have learning disabilities or suffer from mild mental retardation [67]. Approximately 25% of subjects develop a variety of psychiatric disorders in late adolescence or adult life, and there seems to be an increased susceptibility to schizophrenia.

Cytogenetic analysis using FISH probes has shown deletions within 22q11.21. At least 30 genes have been mapped to this area, but deletions or mutations of TBX1, a gene that has been mapped to 22q11.2, have been found in nearly all patients who have this syndrome.

Numerous other malformation syndromes are encountered frequently in the practice of child neurology. Most are characterized by mental retardation and small stature. Some of these conditions have been reviewed by one of us [68]. In due time and with a better understanding of molecular pathogenesis all of these entities will be found to represent contiguous gene syndromes or single gene defects.

Fragile X syndrome

The fragile X gene (FMR-1) contains a trinucleotide sequence (CGG), which is repeated from 6 to 55 times in the normal genome. In persons who have the fragile X syndrome, this repeat is expanded (amplified) to several hundred copies (full mutation), whereas asymptomatic carriers for fragile X carry between 50 and 230 copies (premutation). The premutation tends to remain stable during spermatogenesis, but frequently expands to a full mutation during oogenesis. All male subjects with a full mutation, but only 53% of female subjects with a full mutation, are mentally impaired. The marked expansion of the CGG repeat sequence is accompanied by inactivation through methylation of a sequence that is adjacent to, but outside of, the *FMR-1* gene, which is believed to represent the promoter region for gene transcription. As a consequence, the *FMR-1* gene is not expressed in most patients who have fragile X syndrome; its gene product, the fragile X mental retardation protein (FMRP), is reduced or completely absent. FMRP is believed to act as a translational repression and regulates translation of dendritic RNAs and normal maturation of synaptic connections [69].

To date, no specific neuropathology has been recognized. On gross examination, the posterior vermis is reduced in size, with a compensatory increase in the size of the fourth ventricle. Ultramicroscopy shows abnormal synapses, which suggests defective neuronal maturation or arborization.

The condition is common, and is second only to Down syndrome as a genetic cause for mental retardation. Fragile X is a clinically subtle dysmorphic syndrome. The male patient has a long face; prominent brow; square chin; large, floppy ears; and macro-orchidism without any obvious evidence of endocrine dysfunction [70]. Approximately 10% of subjects have a head circumference that is greater than the 97th percentile.

The neurologic picture is highlighted by retarded language development and hyperactivity. Most male subjects are moderately to severely retarded, and there is a considerable prevalence of autistic symptoms [71]. Delayed motor development is seen in some 20% of male subjects, and seizures have been experienced by 25% to 40% of male subjects. A neurologic syndrome that is marked by ataxia, progressive dementia, peripheral neuropathy, and mild Parkinsonian features is seen in some premutation carriers [72,73].

Diagnosis of the fragile X syndrome in affected individuals and carriers can be made readily by means of molecular DNA techniques. Four other fragile sites have been found cytogenetically on the long arm of chromosome X. The most common of these is FRAXE, which is located on band Xq28. It often is associated with a mild form of mental retardation [74].

References

[1] Strachan T, Read AP. Human molecular genetics. 3rd edition. London: Garland Science; 2004.
[2] Jacobs PA, Browne C, Gregson N, et al. Estimates of the frequency of chromosome abnormalities detectable in unselected newborns using moderate levels of banding. J Med Genet 1992; 29:103–8.
[3] Hook EB, Healy N, Willey A. How much difference does chromosome banding make? Ann Hum Genet 1989;54:237–42.

[4] Griffin DK. The incidence, origin and etiology of aneuploidy. Int Rev Cytol 1996;167:263–96.
[5] Kuleshov NP. Chromosome anomalies of infants dying during the perinatal period and premature newborn. Hum Genet 1976;31:151–60.
[6] Shevell M, Ashwal S, Donley D, et al. Practice parameter: evaluation of the child with global developmental delay: report of the Quality Standards Subcommittee of the American Academy of Neurology and the Practice Committee of the Child Neurology Society. Neurology 2003;60:367–80.
[7] Ferguson-Smith M, Smith K. Cytogenetic analysis. In: Rimoin DL, Connor JM, Pyeritz RE, et al, editors. Principles and practice of medical genetics. 4th edition. New York: Churchill Livingstone; 2002. p. 690–722.
[8] Carvalho B, Ouwerkerk E, Meijer GA, et al. High resolution microarray comparative genomic hybridization analysis using spotted oligonucleotides. J Clin Pathol 2004;57:644–6.
[9] Bendavid C, Haddad BR, Griffin A, et al. Multicolor FISH and quantitative PCR can detect submicroscopic deletions in holoprosencephaly patients with a normal karyotype. J Med Genet 2006 [Epub].
[10] Olsen CL, Cross PK, Gensburg IJ. Down syndrome: interaction between culture, demography, and biology in determining the prevalence of a genetic trait. Hum Biol 2003;75:503–20.
[11] Böök JA, Reed SC. Empiric risk figures in mongolism. JAMA 1950;143:730–2.
[12] Hassold T, Sherman S. Down syndrome: genetic recombination and the origin of the extra chromosome 21. Clin Genet 2000;57:95–100.
[13] Antonarakis SE. Human chromosome 21: genome mapping and exploration, circa 1993. Trends Genet 1993;9:142–8.
[14] Roizen NJ, Patterson D. Down's syndrome. Lancet 2003;361:1281–9.
[15] Rowe DR, Uchida IA. Cardiac malformation in mongolism. A prospective study of 184 mongoloid children. Am J Med 1961;31:726–35.
[16] Suetsugu M, Mehraein P. Spine distribution along the apical dendrites of the pyramidal neurons in Down's syndrome. Acta Neuropathol 1980;50:207–10.
[17] Wisniewski KE, Wisniewski HM, Wen GY. Occurrence of neuropathological changes and dementia of Alzheimer's disease in Down's syndrome. Ann Neurol 1985;17:278–82.
[18] Lott IT, Head E. Alzheimber disease and Down syndrome: factors in pathogenesis. Neurobiol Aging 2005;26:383–9.
[19] Mrak RE, Griffin WS. Trisomy 21 and the brain. J Neuropathol Exp Neurol 2004;63:679–85.
[20] Levinson A, Friedman A, Stamps F. Variability of mongolism. Pediatrics 1955;16:43–54.
[21] Fishler K, Koch R. Mental development in Down syndrome mosaiciscm. Am J Ment Retard 1991;96:345–51.
[22] Pueschel SM, Scola FH. Atlantoaxial instability in individuals with Down syndrome: epidemiologic, radiographic, and clinical studies. Pediatrics 1987;80:555–60.
[23] Glasson EJ, Sullivan SG, Hussain R, et al. The changing profile of people with Down's syndrome: implication for genetic counselling. Clin Genet 2002;62:390–3.
[24] Day SM, Strauss DJ, Shavelle RM, et al. Mortality and causes of death in persons with Down syndrome in California. Dev Med Child Neurol 2005;47:171–6.
[25] Christensen MS, Heyman M, Mottonen M, et al. Treatment-related death in childhood acute lymphoblastic leukaemia in the Nordic countries: 1992–2001. Br J Haematol 2005;131:50–8.
[26] Nielsen J, Wohlert M, Faaborg-Andersen J, et al. Incidence of chromosome abnormalities in newborn children. Comparison between incidences in 1969–1974 and 1980–1982 in the same area. Hum Genet 1982;61:98–101.
[27] Forrester MB, Merz RD. Trisomies 13 and 18: prenatal diagnosis and epidemiologic studies in Hawaii, 1986–1997. Genet Test 1999;3:335–40.
[28] Carothers AD, Boyd E, Lowther G, et al. Trends in prenatal diagnosis of Down syndrome and othrautosomal trisomies in Scotland 1990 to 1994, with associated cytogenetic and epidemiological findings. Genet Epidemiol 1999;16:179–90.
[29] Ramirez-Castro JL, Bersu ET. Anatomical analysis of the developmental effects of aneuploidy in man – the 18-trisomy syndrome: II. Anomalies of the upper and lower limbs. Am J Med Genet 1978;2:285–306.

[30] Baty BJ, Blackburn BL, Carey JC. Natural history of trisomy 18 and trisomy 13: I. Growth, physical assessment, medical histories, survival, and recurrence risk. Am J Med Genet 1994; 49:175–88.

[31] Golden JA, Schoene WC. Central nervous system malformations in trisomy 9. J Neuropath Exp Neurol 1993;52:71–7.

[32] Schinzel A. Catalogue of unbalanced chromosome aberrations in man. 2nd edition. Berlin: Walter de Gruyter; 2001.

[33] Zhang X, Snijders A, Segraves R, et al. High-resolution mapping of genotype-phenotype relationships in cri du chat syndrome using array comparative genomic hybridization. Am J Hum Genet 2005;76:312–26.

[34] Battaglia A, Carey JC. Seizure and EEG patterns in Wolf-Hirschhorn (4p-) syndrome. Brain Dev 2005;27:362–4.

[35] Wright TJ, Clemens M, Quarrell O, et al. Wolf-Hirschhorn and Pitt-Rogers-Danks syndromes caused by overlapping 4p deletions. Am J Med Genet 1998;75:345–50.

[36] Sase M, Hasegawa K, Honda R, et al. Ultrasonographic findings of facial dysmorphism in Wolf-Hirschhorn syndrome. Am J Perinatol 2005;22:99–102.

[37] Koolen DA, Reardon W, Rosser EM, et al. Molecular characterisation of patients with subtelomeric 22q abnormalities using chromosome specific array-based comparative genomic hybridisation. Eur J Hum Genet 2005;13:1019–24.

[38] Ferguson-Smith MA, Yates JRW. Maternal age specific rates for chromosome aberration and factors influencing them: report of a collaborative study on 52,965 amniocenteses. Prenat Diagn 1984;4:5–44.

[39] Allanson JE, Graham GE. Sex chromosome abnormalities. In: Rimoin DL, Connor JM, Pyeritz RE, editors. Principles and practice of medical genetics, 4th edition. New York: Churchill Livingstone; 2002. p. 1184–201.

[40] Ljunger E, Cnattingius S, Lundin C, et al. Chromosomal anomalies in first-trimester miscarriages. Acta Obstet Gynecol Scand 2005;84:1103–7.

[41] Bender B, Fry E, Pennington B, et al. Speech and language development in 41 children with sex chromosome anomalies. Pediatrics 1983;71:262–7.

[42] Sergovich F, Valentine GH, Chen AT, et al. Chromosome aberrations in 2159 consecutive newborn babies. N Engl J Med 1969;280:851–5.

[43] Radcliffe SG, Butler GE, Jones M. Edinburgh study of growth and development of children with sex chromosome abnormalities. IV. Birth Defects Orig Artic Ser 1990;26:1–44.

[44] Gotz MJ, Johnstone EC, Ratcliffe SG. Criminality and antisocial behaviour in unselected men with sex chromosome abnormalities. Psychol Med 1999;29:953–62.

[45] Peet J, Weaver DD, Vance GB. 49,XXXXY: a distinct phenotype. Three new cases and review. J Med Genet 1998;35:420–4.

[46] Linden MG, Bender BG, Harmon RJ, et al. 47,XXX: what is the prognosis? Pediatrics 1988;82: 619–30.

[47] Alvarez-Nava F, Soto M, Sanchez MA, et al. Molecular analysis in Turner syndrome. J Pediatr 2003;142:336–40.

[48] Temple CM, Carney RA. Intellectual functioning of children with Turner syndrome: a comparison of behavioural phenotypes. Dev Med Child Neurol 1993;35:691–8.

[49] Murphy DGM, De Carli C, Daly E, et al. X-chromosome effects on female brain: a magnetic resonance imaging study of Turner's syndrome. Lancet 1993;342:1197–2000.

[50] Schmickel RD. Contiguous gene syndromes: a component of recognizable syndromes. J Pediatr 1986;109:231–41.

[51] Budarf ML, Emanuel BS. Progress in the autosomal segmental aneusomy syndromes (SASs): single or multi-locus disorders. Human Molec Genet 1997;6:1657–65.

[52] Jones KL. Smith's recognizable patterns of human malformation. 6th ed. Philadelphia: WB Saunders; 2005.

[53] OMIM-Online Mendelian Inheritance in Man. Available at: http://www.ncbi.nlm.nih.gov/entrez/query.fcgi?db=OMIM.

[54] Hall JG. Genomic imprinting: nature and clinical relevance. Ann Rev Med 1997;48:35–44.

[55] Davies W, Isles AR, Wilkinson LS. Imprinted gene expression in the brain. Neurosci Biobehav Rev 2005;29:421–30.

[56] Holm VA, Cassidy SB, Butler MG, et al. Prader-Willi syndrome: consensus diagnostic criteria. Pediatrics 1993;91:398–402.

[57] Yoshii A, Krishnamoorthy KS, Grant PE. Abnormal cortical development shown by 3D MRI in Prader-Willi syndrome. Neurology 2002;59:644–5.

[58] Klein O, Cotter P, Albertson D, et al. Prader-Willi syndrome resulting from an unbalanced translocation: characterization by array comparative genomic hybridization. Clin Genet 2004;65: 477–82.

[59] Lossie AC, Whitney MM, Amidon D, et al. Distinct phenotypes distinguish the molecular classes of Angelman syndrome. J Med Genet 2001;38:834–45.

[60] Valente KD, Koiffman CP, Fridman C, et al. Epilepsy in patients with Angelman syndrome caused by deletion of the chromosome 15q11–13. Arch Neurol 2006;63:122–8.

[61] Jay V, Becker LE, Chan FW, et al. Puppet-like syndrome of Angelman: a pathologic and neurochemical study. Neurology 1991;41:416–22.

[62] Hennekam RCM, Stevens CA, Van de Kamp JJP. Etiology and recurrence risk in Rubinstein-Taybi syndrome. Am J Med Genet Suppl 1990;6:56–64.

[63] Roelfsema JH, White SJ, Ariyurek Y, et al. Genetic heterogeneity in Rubinstein-Taybi syndrome: mutations in both the CBP and EP300 genes cause disease. Am J Hum Genet 2005;76:572–80.

[64] Krantz ID, McCallum J, DeScipio C, et al. Cornelia de Lange syndrome caused by mutations in NIPBL, the human homolog of Drosophila melanogaster Nipped-B. Nature Genet 2004;36: 631–5.

[65] Somerville MJ, Mervis CB, Young EJ, et al. Severe expressive-language delay related to duplication of the Williams-Beuren locus. N Eng J Med 2005;353:1694–701.

[66] Schmitt JE, Eliez S, Warsofsky IS, et al. Corpus callosum morphology of Williams syndrome: relation to genetics and behavior. Dev Med Child Neurol 2001;43:155–9.

[67] Goldberg R, Motzkin B, Marion R, et al. Velo-cardio-facial syndrome: a review of 120 patients. Am J Med Genet 1993;45:313–9.

[68] Menkes JH, Falk RE. Chromosomal anomalies and contiguous gene syndromes. In: Menkes JH, Sarnat HB, Maria BL, editors. Child neurology. 7th edition. Philadelphia: Lippincott, William and Wilkins; 2006. p. 227–57.

[69] Zalfa F, Bagni C. Molecular insights into mental retardation: multiple functions for the fragile X mental retardation protein? Curr Issues Mol Biol 2004;6:73–88.

[70] De Arce MA, Kearns A. The fragile X syndrome: the patients and their chromosomes. J Med Genet 1984;21:84–91.

[71] Hagerman RJ, Jackson AW, Levitas A, et al. An analysis of autism in 50 males with the fragile X syndrome. Am J Med Genet 1986;23:359–74.

[72] Berry-Kravis E, Potanos K, Weinberg D, et al. Fragile X-associated tremor/ataxia syndrome in sisters related to X-inactivation. Ann Neurol 2005;57:144–7.

[73] Louis E, Moskowitz C, Friez M, et al. Parkinsonism, dysautonomia, and intranuclear inclusions in a fragile X carrier: A clinical-pathological study. Mov Disord 2006;21:420–5.

[74] Gu Y, Shen Y, Gibbs RA, et al. Identification of FMR2, a novel gene associated with the FRAXE CCG repeat and CpG island. Nat Genet 1996;13:109–13.

[75] Debeer R, Peeters H, Driess S, et al. Variable phenotype in Greig cephalopolysyndactyly syndrome: clinical and radiological findings in 4 independent families and 3 sporadic cases with identified GLI3 mutations. Am J Med Genet 2003;120A:49–58.

[76] Frints SG, Schrander-Stumpel CT, Schoenmakers EF, et al. Strong variable clinical presentation in 3 patients with 7q terminal deletion. Genet Couns 1998;9:5–14.

[77] Langer LO, Krassikoff N, Laxova R, et al. The tricho-rhino-phalangeal syndrome with exostoses (Langer-Giedion syndrome): four additional patients without mental retardation and review of the literature. Am J Med 1984;19:81–111.

[78] Pettenati MJ, Haines JL, Higgins RR, et al. Wiedemann-Beckwith syndrome: presentation of clinical and cytogenetic data on 22 new cases and review of the literature. Hum Genet 1986;74: 143–54.

[79] Crolla JA, Cawdery JE, Oley CA, et al. A FISH approach to defining the extent and possible clinical significance of deletions at the WAGR locus. J Med Genet 1997;34:207–12.

[80] Borgione E, Sturnio M, Spalletta A, et al. Mutational analysis of the ATRX gene by DGGE: a powerful diagnostic approach for the ATRX syndrome. Hum Mutat 2003;21:529–34.

[81] Spadoni E, Colapietro P, Bozzola M, et al. Smith-Magenis syndrome and growth hormone deficiency. Eur J Pediatr 2004;163:353–8.

[82] Yatema HG, van den Helm B, Kissing J, et al. A novel ribosomal S6-kinase (RSK4; RPS6KA6) is commonly deleted in patients with complex X-linked mental retardation. Genomics 1999;62: 332–43.

[83] Eggermann T, Zerres K, Eggermann K, et al. Uniparental disomy: clinical indications for testing in growth retardation. Eur J Pediatr 2002;161:305–12.

[84] Cox H, Bullman H, Temple IKJ. Maternal UPD(14) in the patient with a normal karyotype: clinical report and a systemic search for cases in samples sent for testing for Prader-Willi syndrome. Am J Med Genet 2004;127A:21–5.

[85] Chu C, Schwartz S, McPherson E. Paternal uniparental isodisomy for chromosome 14 in a patient with a normal 46, XY karyotype. Am J Med Genet 2004;127A:167–71.

ELSEVIER
SAUNDERS

CLINICS IN
PERINATOLOGY

Clin Perinatol 33 (2006) 503–516

Placental Pathology and Cerebral Palsy

Raymond W. Redline, MD

*Department of Pathology, University Hospitals of Cleveland, 11100 Euclid Avenue,
Cleveland, OH 44106, USA*

Cerebral palsy describes a group of nonprogressive disorders of movement and posture often accompanied by sensorineural deficits and functional disability that occurs in approximately 2.5 per 1000 live births [1,2]. Approximately 50% of cases develop after full-term births (>36 weeks) following an apparently normal gestation. The remainder are divided between very low birth weight infants (<1.5 kg) and a heterogeneous group of low birth weight (1.5–2.5 kg) and near-term (32–36 week) infants, some of whom have structural abnormalities of the central nervous system (CNS) or significant fetal growth restriction in utero. Although the proportion of affected children in each category has shifted owing to the increased survival of very low birth weight infants, it is remarkable that despite dramatic changes in antenatal diagnosis and intrapartum monitoring, the overall incidence of cerebral palsy has not changed much over the past 50 years.

Cerebral palsy has classically been separated into spasticity primarily affecting the lower limbs (spastic diplegia), one side of the body (spastic hemiplegia), or all limbs (spastic quadriplegia) and cases primarily affecting extrapyramidal pathways influenced by the basal ganglia (chorioathetoid type). A recent proposal has suggested that this classification be simplified to cerebral palsy with unilateral or bilateral limb involvement, followed by a specific description of impairments of movement and posture affecting other body regions (ie, trunk, each limb, and oropharynx), the accompanying anatomic and radiologic findings, and some statement as to the causation and timing of the precipitating brain injury [3]. This last requirement is often difficult to address satisfactorily. Some children display other neurologic abnormalities, including mildly abnormal muscle tone, seizures, developmental delay, and sensorimotor abnormalities that overlap with, but may not be classified as, cerebral palsy.

E-mail address: raymond.redline@uhhs.com

Neonatal encephalopathy, formerly known as hypoxic ischemic encephalopathy, is a transient clinical state defined by a depressed sensorium and abnormal neurologic examination at birth that in some cases may be due to episodes of hypoxia or other physiologic derangements during the intrapartum period [4]. Neonatal encephalopathy primarily affects term infants. Approximately one third of infants with moderate-to-severe neonatal encephalopathy develop cerebral palsy, usually of the spastic quadriplegic or chorioathetoid varieties [5,6]. Most of these infants will also have other severe neurosensory deficits and developmental delay. About one of eight cases of cerebral palsy follows a diagnosis of moderate-to-severe neonatal encephalopathy.

The etiologies of cerebral palsy and neonatal encephalopathy have been the subject of controversy for over 100 years. In part, this reflects the fact that each entity may represent the final common outcome of disparate causal pathways. Attention has focused around two major theories [7]. The first theory, championed by the part-time neuroanatomist Sigmund Freud, is that these disorders are the result of underlying abnormalities in brain structure that predate labor and delivery. The second theory, usually attributed to the orthopedic surgeon James Little, is that most cases are the result of severe intrapartum asphyxia. Various obstetric, pediatric, and neurologic societies have recently issued consensus statements opining that a relatively small proportion of cerebral palsy and neonatal encephalopathy has an intrapartum etiology [6,8]. These conclusions are primarily based on the presence of antenatal risk factors and the absence of clearly delineated intrapartum events in most cases. Strict clinical criteria have been proposed to identify the rare cases of intrapartum asphyxia. These statements need to be tempered by the findings of recent neuroradiologic studies suggesting that, irrespective of the presence or absence of antenatal risk factors or identifiable intrapartum events, the actual brain injury in most cases seems to occur in the immediate antepartum period [1,9].

The continuing controversy over the timing and etiology of cerebral palsy and neonatal encephalopathy revolves in part around two problems. First, the so-called "antenatal risk factors" are poorly defined and incompletely understood [10]. Second, the tools used to identify fetal distress during labor are nonspecific and show poor interobserver reproducibility [11,12]. Theories of causation have thus far failed to take into account two major considerations. First, some infants may inherit a predisposition to sustain significant injury in the event of a normally sublethal insult [13]. The fact that many affected probands have relatives with cerebral palsy, epilepsy, mental retardation, and developmental delay is likely a hint of the many important underlying genetic factors that can affect susceptibility to injury. Unfortunately, despite recent progress in studying the genetic epidemiology of complex disease processes and the molecular pathogenesis of brain development, we are far from being able to identify which mothers are at increased risk.

The second underused tool for understanding cerebral palsy and neonatal encephalopathy and the focus of this article is placental pathology. The placenta is the sole supply line for the substrates needed for fetal well being in utero. It is also the main barrier protecting the fetus from outside influences such as microorganisms, teratogens, physical trauma, and harmful immune responses. The placenta has been described as a diary of intrauterine life. In a sense this is certainly true, although it is a highly abridged version containing many digressions that have little to do with the main story line. The key is to focus on placental processes that are increased in patients with adverse outcomes. Only during the past 10 to 15 years have pathologists begun to carry out the type of studies needed to identify these factors. Placental lesions can be separated into those affecting the maternal supply line (uteroplacental vasculature), the fetal supply line (fetoplacental vasculature), and the different types of placental inflammation. A summary of the lesions in each group that have been associated with adverse neurologic outcomes in previous studies is provided in Box 1.

One of the keys to understanding the role of placental pathology in adverse outcomes is the ability to distinguish four types of information that it can provide (Box 2). Most dramatic, but least common, are "sentinel lesions," each of which can cause hypoxia sufficient to result in brain injury. The three lesions in this category are total separation of the placenta from the uterine vascular bed, disruption of the fetal placental vasculature leading to major fetal blood loss, and complete obstruction of umbilical blood flow.

More common are a group of thromboinflammatory processes involving large fetal placental vessels, processes that can potentially affect other portions of the

---

Box 1. Placental lesions associated with CNS abnormalities in multiple studies

Maternal supply line

Maternal arteriopathy [26,45,46]
Massive perivillous fibrin [48,49]
Subacute/chronic abruption [28,46,49]

Fetal supply line

Fetal thrombotic vasculopathy [14,22,26,28,49]
Meconium-associated vascular necrosis [14,49]
Pathologic umbilical cord abnormalities [18,19,28]

Inflammatory processes

Acute chorioamnionitis/fetal inflammation [14,19,23,26,27,30]
Chronic villitis [14,47,49]

Multiple placental lesions [19,30,49,64]

Box 2. Subcategories of placental pathology relevant to cerebral palsy

Sudden catastrophic events occurring before or during labor ("sentinel lesions")

Uteroplacental separation
Fetal hemorrhage
Umbilical cord occlusion
Amniotic fluid embolism

Thromboinflammatory processes affecting the fetal circulation

Fetal thrombotic vasculopathy
Chronic villitis with obliterative fetal vasculopathy
Meconium-associated fetal vascular necrosis
Chorioamnionitis with severe fetal vasculitis

Decreased placental reserve

Chronic maternal underperfusion
Diffuse chronic villitis
Chronic abruption/peripheral separation
Chronic fetal vascular obstruction
Massive perivillous fibrin deposition

Adaptive responses identified in the placenta

Increased circulating nucleated red blood cells
Villous chorangiosis
Distal villous immaturity

---

same vascular bed in the fetus, including the CNS. The four common lesions in this group are fetal thrombotic vasculopathy with extensive avascular villi, obliterative fetal vasculopathy secondary to chronic villitis, severe chorionic vasculitis secondary to chorioamnionitis, and vascular necrosis secondary to prolonged meconium exposure [14].

The third category consists of chronic patterns of injury that decrease the functional reserve of the placenta, handicapping its capacity to compensate for the normal stresses of parturition. The five processes in this group are chronic maternal underperfusion, chronic villitis, chronic abruption, chronic fetal vascular obstruction, and massive perivillous fibrin deposition [15].

Some findings may not affect placental function but rather reflect abnormalities occurring in the mother or fetus. These findings include increased circulating nucleated red blood cells, villous chorangiosis, and distal villous immaturity.

Sudden catastrophic events interrupting placental function before or during labor

Although most sudden catastrophic events during gestation are associated with recognizable structural changes in the placenta, two other situations should always be considered. Mothers may sustain a traumatic injury, drug overdose, or cardiovascular compromise that can abruptly interrupt uterine perfusion and damage the fetus. Alternatively, fetuses may develop organ damage that spares the placenta through inborn errors of metabolism or the effects of bioactive compounds or microorganisms that cross the placenta without affecting its structure or function.

With these usually apparent exceptions, there are three mechanisms for sudden catastrophic injury: (1) the placenta can become prematurely separated from the underlying maternal uterine vascular supply, either through primary rupture of vessels (abruptio placenta) or disruption of their supporting tissues (uterine rupture); (2) fetal placental blood vessels, small or large, can rupture, leading to significant blood loss, hypovolemia, and circulatory collapse; or (3) umbilical venous blood flow can be interrupted for a sufficient time period sufficient to cause ischemic damage to dependent fetal organs.

Abruptio placenta and uterine rupture are usually not exclusively pathologic diagnoses, particularly if a cesarean section has provided the opportunity for direct visualization of the uterus and its lining. On occasion, blood clots embedded in the placental parenchyma or secondary changes in the placenta can uncover an occult placental separation occurring before arrival in the hospital. Placental findings supportive of an abruption or uterine rupture include an indentation or rupture through the maternal surface (basal plate), forceful spread of blood within the deciduas basalis or behind the membranes, and parenchymal changes including irregular intervillous thrombi, acute villous stromal hemorrhage, and recent villous infarction [16].

Fetal hemorrhages can be separated into two groups: (1) occult small vessel hemorrhages secondary to rupture of villous capillaries and bleeding into the maternal circulation and (2) large vessel hemorrhages caused by disruption of vessels in the umbilical cord or chorionic plate with adjacent uteroplacental hemorrhage. Small vessel hemorrhages are reliably diagnosed by maternal Kleihauer-Betke (or flow cytometric) testing, which can reveal significant numbers of fetal red blood cells in the maternal circulation. Unfortunately, this testing is often not ordered. It is not unreasonable to assume that an infant with a low hematocrit in the absence of other obvious causes of fetal anemia, such as isoimmunization, parvovirus infection, or hemolysis, has sustained a fetomaternal hemorrhage unless proven otherwise. Placental findings that support a diagnosis of massive fetomaternal hemorrhage include a profound increase in the number of circulating nucleated red blood cells in the villous circulation, the finding of a large intervillous hematoma, villous edema, fetal arterial constriction, and villous capillary-venous dilatation.

Large vessel hemorrhages generally affect vessels that are not protected by Wharton's jelly or the chorionic plate. These vessels include those associated with membranous or furcate insertion of the umbilical cord (premature separation of umbilical vessels from surrounding umbilical cord stroma) and the large chorionic vessels connecting accessory lobes to the main placental disk. On rare occasions, another common placental finding, fresh blood between the amnion and the chorionic plate, can be physiologically significant. These subamnionic hemorrhages represent traumatic rupture of chorionic vessels and are usually caused by excessive traction on the umbilical cord after delivery of the infant (third stage of labor). Occasionally, particularly if the umbilical cord is short or entangled, sufficient traction on these vessels may develop in the first or second stages of labor to cause rupture and significant fetal blood loss. It is essentially impossible to distinguish the common third stage hemorrhages from the rare first and second stage hemorrhages by pathologic examination alone.

Pathologic lesions associated with complete umbilical vessel occlusion include tight true umbilical cord knots, occlusive umbilical vein thrombi, and tightly twisted (hypercoiled) umbilical cords. Other umbilical cord processes, such as prolapse or tight entanglements around body parts, can also cause complete obstruction of fetal blood flow. When this occurs, there may be an abrupt change in umbilical cord color, shape, or diameter that suggests chronicity. Although clinical umbilical cord entanglements as a group are not associated with cerebral palsy, certain pathologic umbilical cord lesions, such as an excessively long cord length, lesser degrees of hypercoiling, abnormal cord insertion sites, and paucity of Wharton's jelly, are significantly more common in infants with cerebral palsy, suggesting that episodes of physiologically significant vascular occlusion may occur in some of these cases [17–19].

Fetoplacental thromboinflammatory processes with onset before labor

Reports associating fetal inflammatory responses, vasospasm, and thrombosis of large fetal vessels in the placenta with adverse neurologic outcome have been steadily accumulating in the literature since the early 1990s [20–27]. A large series correlating the neuropathology of stillborn fetuses and early neonatal deaths with placental pathology also identified similar lesions [28]. In 2005 I reported the results of a study comparing the placental pathology of 125 consecutive medicolegal cases involving term infants with neonatal encephalopathy, cerebral palsy, or other related forms of long-term neurologic impairment with that of 250 term placentas submitted for a variety of other clinical indications [14]. The surprising finding was that over half of the medicolegal cases had one or more of four severe fetal thromboinflammatory lesions involving large fetal vessels of the placenta compared with less than 10% of controls. This highly significant association also held true for each of the four individual lesions when considered separately. Interestingly, the prevalence of these four lesions was not significantly different among affected infants with normal umbilical cord pH and base deficit values, suggesting that profound intrapartum acidosis is not necessarily part of the causal pathway by which they can cause brain injury.

Two of the fetal vascular lesions, fetal thrombotic vasculopathy and chronic villitis with obliterative fetal vasculopathy [29], begin weeks before delivery but continue to evolve and progress until parturition. Fetal thrombotic vasculopathy is defined by degenerative changes in the fetal capillary vascular bed of large portions of the terminal villous tree. These changes develop as the result of thrombosis or prolonged occlusion of the large fetal placental vessels supplying these regions. Operationally, the threshold for making this diagnosis has been set at an average of 15 or more affected villi per histologic section; however, lesser degrees of involvement are also more frequent in the placentas of infants with adverse neurologic outcomes. Chronic villitis with obliterative fetal vasculopathy is also associated with upstream vascular occlusion. In this situation, obstruction is the result of an inflammmatory vasodestructive process that develops when maternal leukocytes inappropriately cross the trophoblastic barrier to enter fetal tissue. The resulting villitis is usually confined to the terminal villi but occasionally spreads to the stem villi where it targets large fetal vessels. Obliterative vasculopathy is most frequently seen with villitis of unknown etiology but may also complicate infectious villitis caused by another organism's cytomegalovirus.

The other two fetal vascular lesions, chorioamnionitis with a severe fetal inflammatory response (intense chorionic vasculitis) and meconium-associated necrosis of vascular smooth muscle cells, develop as a consequence of subacute processes beginning days before delivery [27,30–32]. Both lesions are exaggerated forms of relatively common intrapartum processes that are distinguished by virtue of their duration, severity, and destructive effects on the fetal vessel wall. Intense chorionic vasculitis is characterized by a confluent neutrophilic infiltrate involving the amniotic aspect of large chorionic (or, less frequently, umbilical) vessels. This confluent infiltrate may lead to attenuation and disarray of the vascular wall or the formation of nonocclusive mural thrombi in the lumen but is not associated with apoptosis of individual vascular smooth muscle cells. Lesser degrees of fetal vascular inflammation are seen with equal frequency in cerebral palsy and control placentas.

An increased time of exposure to meconium-stained amniotic fluid leads to a gradual progression of pigment through the amnion into the chorionic plate and eventually into contact with large fetal vessels. In some cases, the toxic effects of meconium constituents, such as bile acids, can lead to apoptotic cell death of vascular smooth muscle cells at the periphery of chorionic or umbilical vessels [33]. This easily recognized histologic lesion is highly associated with adverse outcomes including cerebral palsy. Abundant meconium in the chorionic plate and chorionic vessel walls in the absence of vascular necrosis is also common, but to a lesser degree, in patients who have cerebral palsy, and several reports have described vasospasm following exposure of these vessels to meconium in vitro [19,34,35].

I believe there are two important factors explaining why lesions at one particular site, the large fetal vessels of the placental circulation, are so prevalent and strongly associated with neurologic injury. The first factor is that these vessels have a pivotal role in placental physiology. The placenta receives 40% to 50% of the total fetal cardiac output. This cardiac output is distributed into eight to ten paired fetal arteries and veins, each of which supplies a large area of the placenta without anastomotic connections [36]. Decreased fetal arterial blood flow can lead to stenosis of these arteries (fibromuscular sclerosis) and loss of a significant fraction of the circulatory bed [37]. Impaired fetal venous return can result in pooling of oxygenated fetal blood in the placenta and consequent fetal hypoxemia. Because fetal cotyledonary perfusion is thought to be regulated by maternal, not fetal oxygen tension, this process can also lead to significant circulatory mismatching of maternal and fetal blood flow [38]. The second reason why thromboinflammatory lesions of large fetal vessels are important is that the affected circulatory bed is in direct continuity with the rest of the fetal circulation. Thromboemboli, activated platelets, alloreactive maternal lymphocytes, and inflammatory microparticles can all potentially flow through the ductus venosus and foramen ovale to gain free access to other fetal circulatory beds including the CNS. Thromboinflammatory mediators such as cytokines, reactive oxygen intermediates, activated complement components, and other "danger signals" released as a result of tissue ischemia can all contribute to a "fetal inflammatory response syndrome" leading to diffuse endothelial damage and coagulopathy in various portions of the fetal circulation [39–41]. In support of this hypothesis is the finding that fetal thrombotic vasculopathy has been associated with fetal thrombocytopenia [42]. In some circumstances, vasoactive mediators may directly cause damage to the developing CNS; in others, they may sensitize the local vasculature, decreasing the threshold for other comparatively trivial events to exert their effects.

Placental lesions indicative of decreased placental reserve

It has been estimated that the normal human placenta has an excess reserve capacity between 33% and 40%. However, the operative word is "normal." Placentas can be abnormally small and have a decreased total gas-exchanging surface area. Alternatively, they may have decreased efficiency owing to diffuse chronic injury. Particularly important are placentas that are small and affected by diffuse chronic injury. These latter placentas often operate at such borderline capacity that any additional stressful insult can have a devastating effect. Such placentas probably account, at least in part, for the well-documented association of fetal growth restriction with cerebral palsy [43].

Diffuse chronic processes generally require weeks or more to develop and are easily recognized by placental examination. The most common is severe maternal underperfusion resulting in diffuse villous changes such as terminal villous undergrowth, increased syncytial knotting, villous agglutination, and the development of villous infarcts [44]. Some evidence in very low birth weight infants suggests that maternal underperfusion can have a biphasic effect, with an increased risk of neurologic impairment in infants with severely affected placentas and a mild protective effect with less severe disease [30,45,46]. The proposed explanation for the protective effect is habituation to mild degrees of hypoxia. Less common causes of diffuse chronic placental dysfunction include diffuse chronic villitis, chronic abruption-oligohydramnios sequence, chronic fetal vascular obstruction owing to umbilical cord abnormalities, and massive perivillous fibrin deposition (maternal floor infarction) [15]. Placental studies have identified each of these lesions as a significant predictor of abnormal neurologic outcome [47–49]. Other rare lesions that may result in placental hypoplasia or villous maldevelopment, such as confined placental mosaicism and diffuse multifocal chorangiomatosis, are also potential causes of decreased reserve but have not been studied in relation to neurologic outcome [50,51].

Placental changes indicative of a stressful intrauterine environment

Other placental findings are markers for processes affecting either the mother or fetus. In some cases, they may represent attempts to ameliorate an adverse environment; in others, they may be maladaptive consequences of it. Perhaps the most controversial of these findings is a significant increase in the number of circulating nucleated red blood cells in the fetal placental capillary circulation [52,53]. The significance and time required to elicit this finding have engendered a wide difference of opinion among various experts. My own interpretation based on reviews of cases of cerebral palsy over a 13-year period is that a finding of three or more villous capillary nucleated red blood cells in most high-power (40X) microscopic fields correlates with an absolute nucleated red blood cell count of more than 2500/cm^3 [49]. Based on personal experience and some animal experiments, I believe that increases of this magnitude represent a fetal bone marrow response to hypoxia that takes 6 to 12 hours or more to mount [54]. I believe that, in selected cases, pre-existing hypoxia may lead to the development of a preformed pool of nucleated red blood cells in the bone marrow that are released more quickly; however, the magnitude and duration of these more rapid responses tends to be less than that of responses developing over a longer time period.

A second adaptive response is a generalized increase in the number of fetal capillaries per terminal villous cross-section. The finding of large numbers of villi with 10 to 15 capillaries per villous cross-section has been termed *chorangiosis* and has been associated with decreased oxygen availability (maternal anemia, smoking, delivery at high altitude), increased levels of placental growth factors (diabetes, Beckwith-Wiedemann syndrome), and increased placental venous pressure (fetal thrombosis, fetal cardiac failure) [51,55–58]. This pattern has been ascribed to an imbalance between branching and nonbranching angiogenesis and may reflect differences in the relative availability of placental growth factor and vascular endothelial growth factor [59]. Approximately 10% of all term placentas with or without later cerebral palsy will show this pattern [19]. Although the severity of the process and the frequency of other coexisting chronic placental lesions seem to be greater in the group with adverse neurologic outcomes, this has not been systematically studied.

Pregnancies in mothers with abnormal glucose tolerance, increased pregnancy weight gain, or underlying obesity may be complicated by hyperglycemia or other metabolic derangements that result in the release of excessive amounts of insulin and other placental growth factors [60–62]. These conditions can lead to an adverse pattern of placental overgrowth characterized by increased placental supporting stroma and an increase in the number of villous capillaries developing away from the interhemal membrane (decreased vasculosyncytial membranes). These changes increase demand for oxygen by increasing the volume of nonfunctioning placental connective tissue while decreasing the ability of the placenta to provide oxygen by increasing the maternal-fetal diffusion distance. When combined with concomitant fetal overgrowth, they may result in paradoxical uteroplacental insufficiency despite an overabundance of placental tissue. The finding of decreased placental vasculosyncytial membranes has been associated with intrauterine fetal death but has not been specifically studied in placentas from infants with neurologic impairment [63].

Multiple placental lesions

Most would agree that multiple risk factors, such as an underlying genetic susceptibility, unrecognized antenatal fetal compromise, and acutely stressful events at parturition, can potentially interact to cause brain injury. Whether combinations of placental lesions can also act synergistically or in sequence to augment the risk for cerebral palsy is less clear. A crucial distinction in addressing this question is to separate multiple findings that are part of the same pathophysiologic sequence from those that represent separate processes affecting different physiologic compartments. The best example of the former are the multiple placental findings that accompany maternal underperfusion, such as villous infarction, syncytial knotting, intervillous fibrin deposition, placental undergrowth, and decidual vasculopathy [44]. Although the overall extent of each of these changes may increase the risk of fetal compromise, there is little reason why the total number of related indicators of the same underlying process should have any additive or synergistic effect. On the other hand, multiple lesions affecting different physiologic compartments could have important combinatorial effects. Recent studies have shown that for every additional independent placental lesion among the groups discussed previously there is a significant increase in the odds ratio for later neurologic compromise [14,30,49,64]. Furthermore, lesions in the chronic category that decrease placental reserve when combined with subacute thromboinflammatory processes beginning 1 day or more before delivery have a dramatically higher odds ratio for adverse neurologic outcome than do combinations of lesions occurring at the same time [19,49]. Data from several studies indicate that placentas from infants with later cerebral palsy are far more likely than those from other high-risk pregnancies to have combinations of lesions affecting different placental compartments, particularly when these lesions occur at different times.

Summary

Although cerebral palsy, neonatal encephalopathy, and other related forms of neurologic impairment may in rare situations be the consequence of primary brain malformations, slowly progressive metabolic diseases, or destructive primary infections, it is difficult to escape the conclusion that most cases are attributable to relatively sudden changes in normal homeostasis that result in brain injury. Acknowledging this fact in no way suggests that these sudden changes necessarily have to occur during labor and delivery, or that the range of stresses normally associated with labor and delivery are not intolerable for some fetuses. The contribution of placental pathology is to assist in characterizing the antenatal environment. In rare cases, the precise nature of the sudden insult can be ascertained. More frequently, a process known to be associated with the elaboration of active mediators that can contribute to brain injury will be identified. Underlying placental reserve as reflected by the extent of various chronic patterns of placental injury can be assessed, and other developmental patterns reflecting an abnormal antenatal environment can be taken into account.

Placental findings must always be placed in the context of available clinical data. Antenatal factors that appear with high prevalence in the author's studies and in other case series of infants later diagnosed with cerebral palsy include a family history of adverse neurologic outcomes, maternal abnormalities such as thyroid disease, maternal obesity, underlying thrombophilia, poor reproductive history, antenatal vaginal bleeding, intrapartum fever, and evidence of restriction or asymmetry of fetal growth. Particularly important data from the peripartum period include the operative findings at cesarean section (eg, abruption, uterine rupture, thick meconium, and cord entanglements), the immediate status of the newborn as assessed by cord blood gases and Apgar scores, and the temporal pattern of changes in the neonatal physical examination, laboratory studies, and neuroradiologic scans over the first few days of life.

Careful multidisciplinary reviews that include an expert assessment of the placental pathology constitute a powerful tool for understanding the various scenarios commonly associated with cerebral palsy. This approach provides the best hope for realizing the goal of subclassifying individual cases by etiology and timing and could potentially provide clues for future research efforts to understand more precisely the underlying genetic and metabolic abnormalities that place some infants at increased risk for perinatal brain injury.

References

[1] Hagberg B, Hagberg G, Beckung E, et al. Changing panorama of cerebral palsy in Sweden. VIII. Prevalence and origin in the birth year period 1991–94. Acta Paediatr 2001;90(3):271–7.

[2] Volpe J. Neurology of the newborn. Philadelphia: WB Saunders; 2001.

[3] Bax M, Goldstein M, Rosenbaum P, et al. Proposed definition and classification of cerebral palsy, April 2005. Dev Med Child Neurol 2005;47(8):571–6.

[4] Adamson SJ, Alessandri LM, Badawi N, et al. Predictors of neonatal encephalopathy in full-term infants. BMJ 1995;311(7005):598–602.

[5] Gaffney G, Flavell V, Johnson A, et al. Cerebral palsy and neonatal encephalopathy. Arch Dis Child 1994;70:F195–200.

[6] Hankins GD, Speer M. Defining the pathogenesis and pathophysiology of neonatal encephalopathy and cerebral palsy. Obstet Gynecol Suppl 2003;102(3):628–36.

[7] Lamb B, Lang R. Aetiology of cerebral palsy. Br J Obstet Gynaecol 1992;99:176–8.

[8] MacLennan A. A template for defining a causal relation between acute intrapartum events and cerebral palsy: international consensus statement. BMJ 1999;319:1054–9.

[9] Cowan F, Rutherford M, Groenendaal F, et al. Origin and timing of brain lesions in term infants with neonatal encephalopathy. Lancet 2003;361(9359):736–42.

[10] Nelson KB, Ellenberg JH. Antecedents of cerebral palsy: multivariate analysis of risk. N Engl J Med 1986;315:81–6.

[11] Parer JT, King T. Fetal heart rate monitoring: is it salvageable? Am J Obstet Gynecol 2000; 182(4):982–7.

[12] Freeman R. Intrapartum fetal monitoring: a disappointing story. N Engl J Med 1990;322:624–6.

[13] Nelson KB, Dambrosia JM, Iovannisci DM, et al. Genetic polymorphisms and cerebral palsy in very preterm infants. Pediatr Res 2005;57(4):494–9.

[14] Redline RW. Severe fetal placental vascular lesions in term infants with neurologic impairment. Am J Obstet Gynecol 2005;192:452–7.

[15] Redline RW, Patterson P. Patterns of placental injury: correlations with gestational age, placental weight, and clinical diagnosis. Arch Pathol Lab Med 1994;118:698–701.

[16] Redline RW. Hemorrhagic and thrombotic lesions of the placenta. In: Bick RL, editor. Hematologic complications in obstetrics, pregnancy, and gynecology. Cambridge (UK): Cambridge University Press; 2005.

[17] Machin GA, Ackerman J, Gilbert-Barness E. Abnormal umbilical cord coiling is associated with adverse perinatal outcomes. Pediatr Dev Pathol 2000;3(5):462–71.

[18] Baergen RN, Malicki D, Behling C, et al. Morbidity, mortality, and placental pathology in excessively long umbilical cords: retrospective study. Pediatr Dev Pathol 2001;4(2):144–53.

[19] Redline RW. Placental lesions and neurological outcome. In: Steer P, Sibley C, editors. Placenta and neurodisability. London: MacKeith Press; 2006.

[20] Sander CH. Hemorrhagic endovasculitis and hemorrhagic villitis of the placenta. Arch Pathol Lab Med 1980;104:371–3.

[21] Shen-Schwarz S, MacPherson TA, Mueller-Heubach E. The clinical significance of hemorrhagic endovasculitis of the placenta. Am J Obstet Gynecol 1988;159:48–51.

[22] Sander CH, Kinnane L, Stevens NG. Hemorrhagic endovasculitis of the placenta: a clinicopathologic entity associated with adverse pregnancy outcome. Compr Ther 1985;11:66–74.

[23] Bejar R, Wozniak P, Allard M, et al. Antenatal origin of neurologic damage in newborn infants. I. Preterm infants. Am J Obstet Gynecol 1988;159(2):357–63.

[24] Redline RW, Pappin A. Fetal thrombotic vasculopathy: the clinical significance of extensive avascular villi. Hum Pathol 1995;26:80–5.

[25] Kraus FT, Acheen VI. Fetal thrombotic vasculopathy in the placenta: cerebral thrombi and infarcts, coagulopathies, and cerebral palsy. Hum Pathol 1999;30:759–69.

[26] McDonald DG, Kelehan P, McMenamin JB, et al. Placental fetal thrombotic vasculopathy is associated with neonatal encephalopathy. Hum Pathol 2004;35(7):875–80.

[27] Leviton A, Paneth N, Reuss ML, et al. Maternal infection, fetal inflammatory response, and brain

damage in very low birth weight infants: Developmental Epidemiology Network Investigators. Pediatr Res 1999;46(5):566–75.

[28] Grafe MR. The correlation of prenatal brain damage with placental pathology. Neuropathol Exp Neurol 1994;53:407–15.

[29] Redline RW, Ariel I, Baergen RN, et al. Fetal vascular obstructive lesions: nosology and reproducibility of placental reaction patterns. Pediatr Dev Pathol 2004;7:443–52.

[30] Redline RW, Wilson-Costello D, Borawski E, et al. Placental lesions associated with neurologic impairment and cerebral palsy in very low birth weight infants. Arch Pathol Lab Med 1998; 122:1091–8.

[31] Redline RW, Faye-Petersen O, Heller D, et al. Amniotic infection syndrome: nosology and reproducibility of placental reaction patterns. Pediatr Dev Pathol 2003;6:435–48.

[32] Altshuler G, Arizawa M, Molnar-Nadasdy G. Meconium-induced umbilical cord vascular necrosis and ulceration: a potential link between the placenta and poor pregnancy outcome. Obstet Gynecol 1992;79:760–6.

[33] King EL, Redline RW, Smith SD, et al. Myocytes of chorionic vessels from placentas with meconium associated vascular necrosis exhibit apoptotic markers. Hum Pathol 2004;35:412–7.

[34] Altshuler G, Hyde S. Meconium-induced vasocontraction: a potential cause of cerebral and other fetal hypoperfusion and of poor pregnancy outcome. J Child Neurol 1989;4:137–42.

[35] Holcberg G, Huleihel M, Katz M, et al. Vasoconstrictive activity of meconium stained amniotic fluid in the human placental vasculature. Eur J Obstet Gynecol Reprod Biol 1999;87(2):147–50.

[36] Boyd JD, Hamilton WJ. The human placenta. Cambridge (UK): W. Heffer and Sons; 1970.

[37] Fox H. Pathology of the placenta, Vol. 7. 2nd edition. London: Saunders; 1997.

[38] Talbert D, Sebire NJ. The dynamic placenta. I. Hypothetical model of a placental mechanism matching local fetal blood flow to local intervillus oxygen delivery. Med Hypotheses 2004;62(4): 511–9.

[39] Gomez B, Romero R, Ghezzi F, et al. The fetal inflammatory response syndrome. Am J Obstet Gynecol 1998;179:194–202.

[40] Matzinger P. The danger model: a renewed sense of self. Science 2002;296(5566):301–5.

[41] Pierce BT, Pierce LM, Wagner RK, et al. Hypoperfusion causes increased production of interleukin 6 and tumor necrosis factor alpha in the isolated, dually perfused placental cotyledon. Am J Obstet Gynecol 2000;183(4):863–7.

[42] Redline RW. Clinical and pathological umbilical cord abnormalities in fetal thrombotic vasculopathy. Hum Pathol 2004;35(12):1494–8.

[43] Jarvis S, Glinianaia SV, Torrioli MG, et al. Cerebral palsy and intrauterine growth in single births: European collaborative study. Lancet 2003;362(9390):1106–11.

[44] Redline RW, Boyd T, Campbell V, et al. Maternal vascular underperfusion: nosology and reproducibility of placental reaction patterns. Pediatr Dev Pathol 2004;7:237–49.

[45] Burke CJ, Tannenberg AE. Prenatal brain damage and placental infarction: an autopsy study. Dev Med Child Neurol 1995;37:555–62.

[46] Kumazaki K, Nakayama M, Sumida Y, et al. Placental features in preterm infants with periventricular leukomalacia. Pediatrics 2002;109(4):650–5.

[47] Scher MS, Trucco GS, Beggarly ME, et al. Neonates with electrically confirmed seizures and possible placental associations. Pediatr Neurol 1998;19:37–41.

[48] Adams-Chapman I, Vaucher YE, Bejar RF, et al. Maternal floor infarction of the placenta: association with central nervous system injury and adverse neurodevelopmental outcome. J Perinatol 2002;22(3):236–41.

[49] Redline RW, O'Riordan MA. Placental lesions associated with cerebral palsy and neurologic impairment following term birth. Arch Pathol Lab Med 2000;124(12):1785–91.

[50] Robinson WP, Barrett IJ, Bernard L, et al. Meiotic origin of trisomy in confined placental mosaicism is correlated with presence of fetal uniparental disomy, high levels of trisomy in trophoblast, and increased risk of fetal intrauterine growth restriction. Am J Hum Genet 1997; 60(4):917–27.

[51] Ogino S, Redline RW. Villous capillary lesions of the placenta: distinctions between chorangioma, chorangiomatosis, and chorangiosis. Hum Pathol 2000;31:945–54.

[52] Hermansen MC. Nucleated red blood cells in the fetus and newborn. Arch Dis Child Fetal Neonatal Ed 2001;84(3):F211–5.

[53] Naeye RL, Lin HM. Determination of the timing of fetal brain damage from hypoxemia-ischemia. Am J Obstet Gynecol 2001;184(2):217–24.

[54] Blackwell SC, Hallak M, Hotra JW, et al. Timing of fetal nucleated red blood cell count elevation in response to acute hypoxia. Biol Neonate 2004;85(4):217–20.

[55] Soma H, Watanabe Y, Hata T. Chorangiosis and chorangioma in three cohorts of placentas from Nepal, Tibet and Japan. Reprod Fertil Dev 1996;7:1533–8.

[56] Mutema G, Stanek J. Increased prevalence of chorangiosis in placentas from multiple gestation. Am J Clin Pathol 1997;108:341.

[57] Altshuler G. Chorangiosis: an important placental sign of neonatal morbidity and mortality. Arch Pathol Lab Med 1984;108:71–4.

[58] Stanek J. Numerical criteria for the diagnosis of placental chorangiosis using CD34 immuno-staining. Trophoblast Res 1999;13:443–52.

[59] Benirschke K, Kaufmann P. Pathology of the human placenta. 4th edition. New York: Springer; 2000.

[60] Driscoll SG. The pathology of pregnancy complicated by diabetes mellitus. Med Clin North Am 1965;49:1053–65.

[61] Singer DB. The placenta in pregnancies complicated by diabetes mellitus. Perspect Pediatr Pathol 1984;8:199–212.

[62] Evers IM, Nikkels PG, Sikkema JM, et al. Placental pathology in women with type 1 diabetes and in a control group with normal and large-for-gestational-age infants. Placenta 2003;24(8–9):819–25.

[63] Stallmach T, Hebisch G, Meier K, et al. Rescue by birth: defective placental maturation and late fetal mortality. Obstet Gynecol 2001;97(4):505–9.

[64] Viscardi RM, Sun CC. Placental lesion multiplicity: risk factor for IUGR and neonatal cranial ultrasound abnormalities. Early Hum Dev 2001;62(1):1–10.

ELSEVIER
SAUNDERS

CLINICS IN
PERINATOLOGY

Clin Perinatol 33 (2006) 517–544

Neuroimaging Evaluation of Cerebral Palsy

Robert A. Zimmerman, MD*, Larissa T. Bilaniuk, MD

*Department of Radiology, The Children's Hospital of Philadelphia, 34th Street and
Civic Center Boulevard, Philadelphia, PA 19104, USA*

Cerebral palsy has many different etiologies and can arise during the in utero period, the birth process, or the postnatal period [1–4]. This article focuses primarily on the contributions of MRI in the evaluation of the fetus, the neonate, and the infant who eventually are clinically diagnosed to have cerebral palsy [5,6]. It is not intended to diminish the role of CT or ultrasound, modalities about which much has been written. The goal herein is to focus on the more recently introduced MRI techniques and improvements, such as ultrafast imaging, high-field imaging (3 Tesla), and diffusion imaging, when applied to the clinical problem of cerebral palsy.

The clinical differential diagnosis of cerebral palsy includes a wide spectrum of abnormalities that can occur in utero and peri- or postnatally. These abnormalities consist of hypoxic ischemic brain injury, vascular occlusive events (embolic and thrombotic), bleeding from vascular malformations, bleeding from coagulopathy, traumatic injury, metabolic disorders, genetic disorders, developmental malformations of congenital etiology, and infectious and inflammatory diseases.

MRI of the brain

Fetal brain

In the past decade, MRI has become a practical means of evaluating the fetal brain primarily owing to the development of ultrafast imaging techniques that permit acquisition of images in a short time in which each image is independent

---

* Corresponding author.

E-mail address: zimmerman@email.chop.edu (R.A. Zimmerman).

0095-5108/06/$ – see front matter © 2006 Elsevier Inc. All rights reserved.
doi:10.1016/j.clp.2006.03.005

from others as to the effect of motion. Unlike in regular MRI in which patient motion affects all of the images of a given series, in the ultrafast imaging used for fetal evaluation, only the image during which motion occurs is affected [6]. Ultrafast imaging (half-Fourier acquisition single-shot turbo spin echo [HASTE]) produces a T2-weighted image in 0.5 second. The time for a sequence when images are obtained in an axial, coronal, or sagittal plane is approximately 20 to 30 seconds. The entire imaging study usually takes 30 minutes. No sedation is used for the mother or the fetus. T1-weighted images take longer, about 22 seconds for a series of gradient echo images, and are more likely to be marred

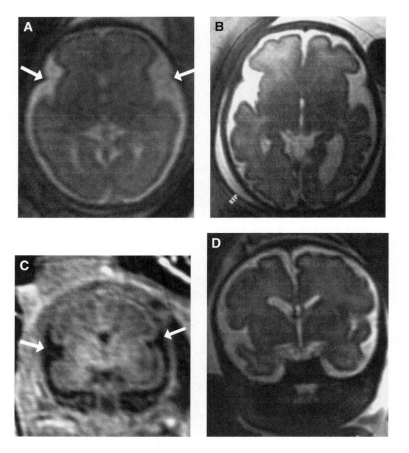

Fig. 1. Normal MRI of fetal brain. (*A*) Axial T2-weighted imaging at 23 weeks' gestation shows flat cortical surface to brain with shallow wide Sylvian fissures (*arrows*). (*B*) Axial T2-weighted imaging at 32 weeks' gestation. Gyral and sulcal development is evident. There continues to be underopercularization with wide Sylvian fissures. (*C*) Coronal T1-weighted imaging at 23 weeks' gestation shows lack of gyration and sulcation. Wide Sylvian fissures are apparent (*arrows*). (*D*) Coronal T2-weighted imaging at 32 weeks shows early gyral and sulcal development. (*E*) Sagittal T2-weighted imaging at 32 weeks' gestation shows aqueduct of Sylvius (*arrow*) and fourth ventricle.

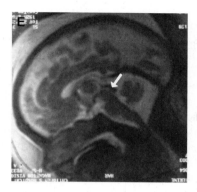

Fig. 1 (*continued*).

by patient motion. T1-weighted sequences are used when there is a question of hemorrhage or abnormal myelination. The third sequence that is used, echo planar imaging (EPI), results in hypointense bone and shows blood as a loss of signal owing to susceptibility effects arising from the blood products. EPI images can be obtained in 6 to 10 seconds.

For evaluation of the brain, all three cardinal planes, sagittal, coronal, and axial, are acquired with T2-weighted imaging (Fig. 1) and EPI. T1-weighted imaging is usually performed in one plane if indicated. The fetal MRI success rate is approximately 95%. Technical failures occur owing to too much fetal motion, maternal claustrophobia, or a large size of the patient (ie, overweight or advanced pregnancy), prohibiting her from fitting comfortably in the scanner. Indications for fetal MRI arise because of questions raised by screening fetal ultrasonography, such as ventricular enlargement, brain malformation, or brain injury. MRI is not performed during the first trimester because its usefulness and safety at this stage of development are not fully resolved. The authors perform MRI from 18 weeks' gestation and beyond.

Evaluation of the fetal brain by MRI

The literature and experience evaluating the fetal brain by MRI for etiologies resulting in cerebral palsy have been accrued at major centers in the United States, Europe, and Asia. In the authors' experience, the most common reason for performing fetal MRI of the central nervous system (CNS) has been ventriculomegaly. The etiology of ventriculomegaly has been threefold: hydrocephalus from obstruction (eg, aqueductal stenosis), malformation (eg, holoprosencephaly), or destruction of brain tissue (eg, periventricular leukomalacia, infarction).

Hydrocephalus diagnosed in utero does not have a known incidence. The incidence given for newborns is 0.3 to 2.5 cases per 1000 live births [7]. The normal value for the width of the lateral ventricle atrial region in the second trimester is 7 ± 1 mm [8]. A width up to 10 mm has been accepted as within normal limits in the second and third trimester, with 10 to 12 mm being borderline ventriculomegaly and 12 to 15 mm mild ventriculomegaly [9,10]. When hydrocephalus develops in a fetus, several factors must be taken into consideration. Because the brain is unmyelinated and soft, it has great compliance to accommodate ventricular dilatation; however, at the same time, there is intrauterine pressure on the head from the surrounding amniotic fluid. The two processes oppose each other. The ventricular pressure on the brain causes expansion of the ventricles and stretching of the overlying brain parenchyma while the amniotic pressure restrains expansion of the skull. As these processes progress and continue for a prolonged period, there is eventual axonal degeneration with neuronal loss and edema and gliosis within the brain tissue [11–13]. In addition, there may be a decrease in the number of synaptic connections and dendrites [4]. One important principle of fetal hydrocephalus is that the longer the hydrocephalus is present, the worse the prognosis [7].

Fifty percent of cases of isolated fetal hydrocephalus have as one of their etiologies the Chiari II malformation, aqueductal stenosis, or the Dandy-Walker malformation [7]. Mortality and morbidity are associated with fetal hydrocephalus [14]. The prognosis varies with different entities. With long-standing in utero hydrocephalus, a rupture of the cortex can occur owing to destruction of the cortical mantle. This event represents a further insult in addition to the injury produced by the increased pressure on the brain (Fig. 2).

Agenesis of the corpus callosum is the most frequent congenital anomaly associated with ventriculomegaly, usually without enlargement of the head and without obstruction of the ventricular system. The incidence of callosal agenesis is 0.3% to 0.7% in the general population and 2% to 3% in the developmentally disabled population [15,16]. Recognized etiologies include genetic and teratogenic factors, influenza, and the use of alcohol or cocaine [17,18]. Absence of

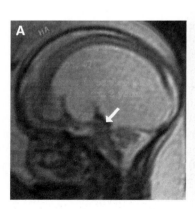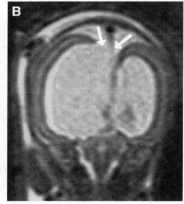

Fig. 2. Images from a 22-week-old fetus with hydrocephalus owing to obstruction at the level of the aqueduct of Sylvius. There is rupture of the cerebral cortical mantle. (*A*) Sagittal T2-weighted imaging shows a large head and huge lateral ventricle with the aqueduct occluded (*arrow*) at the level of the inferior colliculus. The fourth ventricle is of normal size. (*B*) Coronal T2-weighted imaging shows disruption of cortex of both cerebral hemispheres (*arrows*).

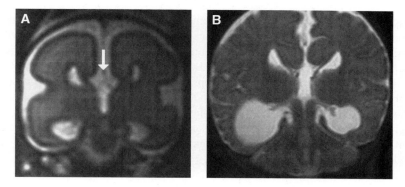

Fig. 3. Agenesis of the corpus callosum. (*A*) Coronal T2-weighted imaging in a 25-week-old fetus shows complete absence of corpus callosum (*arrow*). (*B*) Follow-up MRI with T2-weighted imaging at 2 months of age again shows a coronal absent corpus callosum and CSF separating the two cerebral hemispheres.

the corpus callosum is easily recognized on coronal and axial HASTE images (Fig. 3).

Holoprosencephaly has an incidence of 1 in 16,000 neonates but has a higher rate of occurrence in utero, with a reported incidence of 40 in 10,000 spontaneous abortions [19,20], indicating a high in utero failure rate owing to this malformation. In alobar and semilobar forms of holoprosencephaly, there is an incidence of up to 50% to 60% of abnormal chromosomes, with trisomy 13 being the most common [21,22]. In the most severe form, the alobar variety (Fig. 4), there is a monoventricle with no interhemispheric fissure and, often, significant facial maldevelopment. In semilobar holoprosencephaly, the occipital horns and

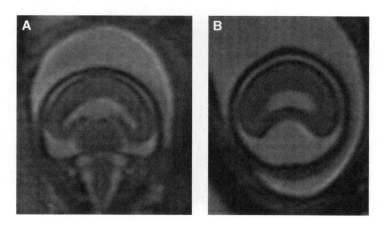

Fig. 4. Alobar holoprosencephaly in a 20 weeks' gestation fetus. (*A*) Coronal T2-weighted and (*B*) axial T2-weighted images show a single undivided cerebrum with a monoventricle and no interhemispheric fissure or falx.

temporal horns may have some development, but the thalami and basal ganglia are often fused, and the bodies of the lateral ventricles form a single cavity.

Hydranencephaly is caused by an in utero bilateral destruction of brain tissue within the vascular distribution of the internal carotid arteries and should not be mistaken for hydrocephalus or holoprosencephaly. There is a total absence of the cortical mantle in the anterior and middle cerebral artery vascular territories. Given the current resolution of fetal MRI, maximal hydrocephalus and hydranencephaly could be mistaken for each other if the hydranencephalic patient also had obstruction of cerebrospinal fluid (CSF) flow, a relatively rare occurrence in hydranencephaly.

Destructive in utero lesions producing ventriculomegaly

Anything that produces destruction and loss of tissue in the fetal brain can result in an enlarged ventricle (Fig. 5) [11,12]. In the evaluation of such cases, one should look for the presence or absence of cortex and adjacent white matter surrounding the ventricle. It is also important to look for the presence of blood products, best brought out by EPI. Hypoxic ischemic stresses in the fetus during the second trimester or in the markedly premature infant can cause rupture of the germinal matrix and bleeding, as well as infarction of the white matter, producing periventricular leukomalacia. The bleeding and infarction can occur in combination or individually. Periventricular leukomalacia is difficult to recognize in the fetus unless it is seen as cystic changes in the tissue surrounding the lateral

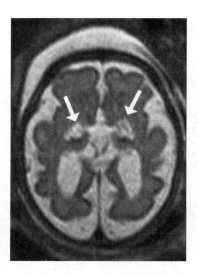

Fig. 5. Images from a 29-week-old fetus with profound asphyxia owing to maternal hypotension examined 7 weeks post insult. Axial T2-weighted imaging shows cystic cavitation of bilateral basal ganglia (*arrows*) and enlargement of occipital horns of lateral ventricles and third ventricle owing to volume loss.

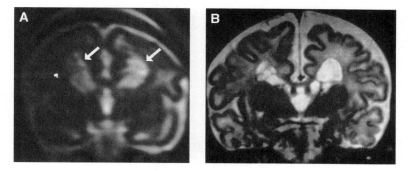

Fig. 6. Periventricular cystic leukomalacia. (*A*) Coronal T2-weighted images from a 32-week-old fetus show bilateral cystic changes (*arrows*) in the periventricular white matter above the lateral ventricles. (*B*) Follow-up coronal T2-weighted imaging at 6 weeks of age shows same findings.

ventricles or a loss of periventricular white matter, seen progressively over time, accompanied by ex vacuo enlargement of the ventricles (Fig. 6).

Second trimester in utero cerebral infarction results in porencephaly (Fig. 7). The etiologies include vascular occlusive disease, infection, trauma, an arterio-venous malformation with vascular steal, twin-twin transfusion, and fetal ma-ternal bleeding [6]. Fetal MRI shows a loss of cortex and adjacent white matter within the vascular territory with underlying expansion of the adjacent lateral ventricle (Fig. 7) [23,24]. The cases thus far detected in utero have been vi-sualized at the porencephalic stage, representing an old injury and not an acute stage. The use of diffusion imaging as part of fetal MRI offers the potential to visualize the acute infarction in utero as a restriction of the motion of water molecules at the site of cytotoxic edema.

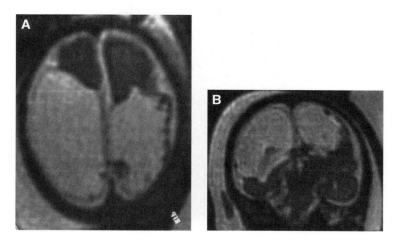

Fig. 7. Multiple old in utero infarctions in a 27-week-old fetus. (*A*) Axial T2-weighted and (*B*) coronal T2-weighted images show bilateral infarctions involving the cortex and white matter with massive atrophic enlargement of the lateral ventricles.

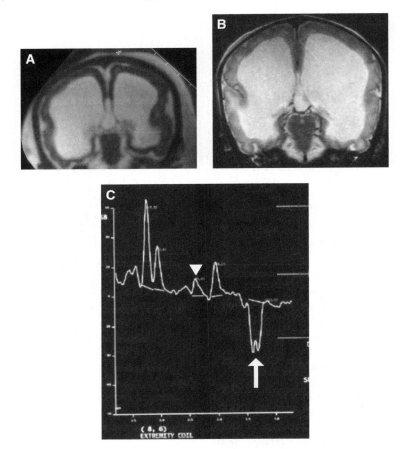

Fig. 8. Marked in utero white matter and basal ganglionic, thalamic gray matter loss with hydro-cephalus owing to inborn error of metabolism, pyruvate dehydrogenase deficiency. (*A*) Coronal T2-weighted images from a 38-week-old fetus show marked expansion of the lateral ventricles with tissue loss. (*B*) Follow-up coronal T2-weighted imaging at 2 days of age shows the same findings. (*C*) Proton spectroscopy performed at 2 days of age with TE of 135 msec shows large amount of lactate at 1.3 ppm (*arrow*) and elevated amounts of pyruvate at 2.4 ppm (*arrowhead*).

In utero insults of diverse etiologies, such as from inborn errors of metabolism and genetic abnormalities, can be demonstrated with fetal MRI (Fig. 8). Such insults may be confused with hypoxic ischemic injury if fetal imaging is not performed, if imaging is performed later in infancy, or if metabolic or genetic testing is not performed.

In utero hemorrhage

The etiologies for intracerebral hemorrhage in the fetus are manifold. Causes include alterations in maternal blood pressure such as those accompanying a vasovagal reaction, problems with placental circulation such as a partial abrup-

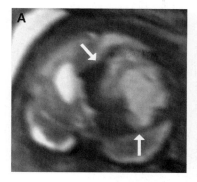
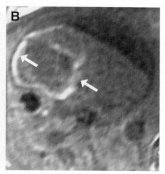

Fig. 9. Intracerebral hemorrhage in a 30-week-old fetus. (*A*) Coronal T2-weighted imaging shows large left frontal heterogeneous mass (*arrows*) representing intracerebral hemorrhage. (*B*) Sagittal T1-weighted imaging. Intracerebral hemorrhage has a hyperintense rim (*arrows*) representing the methemoglobin component of the hematoma.

tion, the presence of a bleeding disorder such as an alloimmune platelet disorder, and hypoxic ischemic episodes as a result of unrecognized cord entanglement and maternal abuse of drugs such as cocaine (Fig. 9). A 6% incidence of intraventricular hemorrhage was reported in an autopsy series of stillbirth infants [25]. Germinal matrix hemorrhage can be detected in the fetus using EPI sequences. The site of the germinal matrix hemorrhage is characteristic, as is the intraventricular and intraparenchymal extension (Fig. 10). Whenever there is an intraparenchymal hemorrhage in a fetus, one should look for abnormal flow voids that may indicate the presence of an arteriovenous malformation. In the authors'

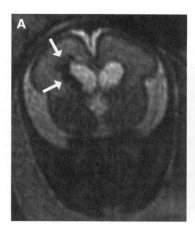
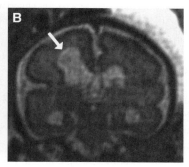

Fig. 10. Evolution of a germinal matrix hemorrhage in a fetus. (*A*) Coronal T2-weighted images from a 26-week-old fetus show a germinal matrix hemorrhage (*arrows*) around the right frontal horn. (*B*) Follow-up at 28 weeks' gestation shows excavation of brain at site of prior bleed with ex vacuo expansion of the lateral ventricle (*arrow*).

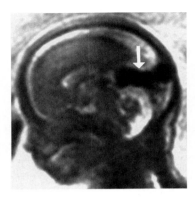

Fig. 11. Vein of Galen malformation in a 21-week-old fetus. Sagittal T2-weighted imaging shows marked enlargement of the vein of Galen and straight sinus (*arrow*).

experience, the most common malformation seen on fetal imaging has been the vein of Galen malformation. It is typically recognized by the enlarged flow void of the vein of Galen, straight and transverse sinuses (Fig. 11). Because of the vein of Galen malformation, there may be a steal of blood from the surrounding brain, resulting in loss of brain parenchyma owing to ischemia with compensatory enlargement of the ventricles. Sometimes the enlarged vein of Galen compresses the aqueduct of Sylvius, producing an obstructive hydrocephalus.

Neonatal brain

Technical considerations when performing MRI of the neonatal and infant brain are based on the corrected true age of the neonate taking into consideration the gestational age of the neonate at the time of birth, premature versus full term, relative to the time that imaging is performed. In very young infants, the use of special sequences helps to demonstrate abnormalities [26]. The choice of techniques and sequences is based to some extent on the acuteness of the imaging relative to the point in time when injury to the tissue has occurred. The newborn full-term infant has a brain that is extremely watery without much myelination. This anatomy affects the appearance of T1, T2, and fluid-attenuated inversion recovery (FLAIR) images. As the brain matures post 40 weeks' gestation, myelination takes place, resulting in less water in the brain; consequently, changes occur in signal intensity on T1- and T2-weighted images. T1-weighted images in a newborn infant benefit from a slightly longer repetition time (TR) and a short echo time (TE). For instance, a TR of 1500 msec with a TE of 11 msec will give a good image in a term infant. At 6 months, the TR is decreased to 1000 msec with the TE remaining constant. At 1 to 2 years, a TR of 750 msec will suffice. With the use of turbo spin echo (fast T2) images, the TR (6000–7000 msec) and the TE are kept long (99–120 msec) [27] for the term infant and the 1 year old. FLAIR images do not have a major role in evaluation of the neonate because myelination has not yet occurred. In the infant beyond 1 year of age, FLAIR images become useful by providing contrast among gliosis, increased water content in scar tissue, and myelinated brain, showing the injury processes [27]. To demonstrate blood products within the ventricles or brain parenchyma, gradient echo two-dimensional FLASH susceptibility scans are performed. These images show a loss of signal at the site of blood products because of dephasing of the proton spins by the iron in blood [27]. Postcontrast T1-weighted images are obtained only when there is a question of infection or tumor, and rarely when there is a need to demonstrate a disturbance of the blood brain barrier, such as can be seen with subacute infarcts. In the past decade, two additional techniques have become important in the evaluation of an infant suspected to have cerebral palsy. Diffusion-weighted imaging with the production of apparent diffusion coefficient maps (ADC) is extremely important when MRI is performed during the acute injury phase [28,29]. Because of cellular swelling, diffusion shows restriction of the motion of water as high signal intensity. The ADC map gives a numeric expression of the change in signal intensity owing to the restriction of the motion of water that can be compared with normal data or normal areas of the brain [26].

Proton spectroscopy performed with a TE of 135 to 144 msec has the capability of evaluating brain tissue for the presence of metabolites such as N-acetyl aspartate (neuronal marker), creatine (energy), and choline (cell membrane marker) [30]. In addition, when present, lactate can be demonstrated as an inverted doublet at 1.3 ppm [30]. This finding is valuable in the acutely injured brain occurring with hypoxic ischemia, infarction, and some metabolic diseases [31–33]. Proton spectroscopy performed with shorter TEs, such as 20 msec, can show multiple additional metabolites. These substances include myoinositol (a glial marker and osmolyte), taurine, sugars, acetone, and glutamate [30].

Physiology of injury at full term

Reduction of oxygenation to the fetus leads to bradycardia, which reduces the cerebral perfusion pressure as well as the oxygenation reaching the brain. The rapidity of the onset of this decrease in flow (ie, gradual or abrupt) influences the pattern of injury seen in the brain. In addition, maturity or lack of maturity of the developing brain increases or decreases the vulnerability of the tissues to the effects of the decrease in oxygenation and blood flow. Neurons that are mature and functional are more vulnerable to the lack of nutrients, whereas cortical areas of the brain that are immature and nonfunctional are accustomed to the in utero relatively hypoxic environment and are less vulnerable. With sudden decreases in blood flow and oxygen, there is little time for a redistribution of blood flow to protect the more mature neurons in the central gray matter of the basal ganglia, thalamus, and brainstem. With a more gradual onset of decreased flow and oxygen, there is time for a relative shift of flow to protect these more valuable and vulnerable structures. With a shift in blood flow to the brainstem and central gray matter, the burden of the injury falls on the supratentorial distal portions of the cortex and white matter in the so-called "watershed zones" located between the vascular territories, between the anterior and middle cerebral artery, and between the posterior and middle cerebral artery. The three major patterns of injury that emerge as a result of these physiologic and developmental responses to hypoxic ischemia have been described as profound asphyxia (near total asphyxia), partial prolonged asphyxia, and a mixed injury pattern, both profound and partial prolonged.

Profound asphyxia (near total asphyxia)

A sudden, marked, or catastrophic decrease in cerebral blood flow or oxygenation to the fetal brain or newborn infant produces a near total profound

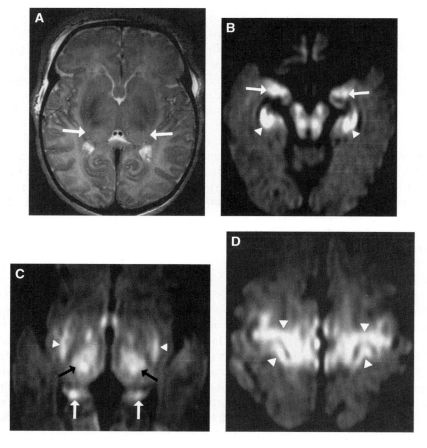

Fig. 12. Acute profound injury in a 3-day-old female infant demonstrated as increased signal on T2 imaging and as restricted diffusion owing to cytotoxic edema. (*A*) Axial T2-weighted imaging shows subtle increased signal in the thalami (*arrows*). (*B*) Axial diffusion-weighted imaging shows abnormal bilateral increased signal in the temporal lobes (*arrows*), hippocampi (*arrowheads*), and midbrain. (*C*) Axial diffusion-weighted imaging shows bilateral abnormal increased signal in the thalami (*black arrows*), putamina (*arrowheads*), and hippocampi (*white arrows*). (*D*) Axial diffusion-weighted imaging shows bilateral abnormal increased signal intensity in the pre- and postcentral gyri (rolandic cortex) (*arrowheads*). (*E*) On an axial (ADC) map, the abnormalities are depicted as areas of decreased signal intensity (*arrowheads*).

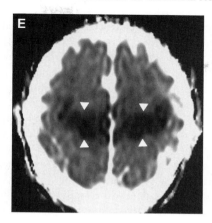

Fig. 12 (*continued*).

asphyxia [34]. The three most common causes for this decrease are placental abruption, cord prolapse, or uterine rupture [35]. Most profound asphyxias are terminal events occurring just immediately before delivery; however, the same injury pattern can occur when a newborn suffers a cardiac arrest post delivery, or when resuscitation is inadequate after a cardiovascular collapse. Profound asphyxia can occur in a fetus in utero before labor and delivery when the mother experiences a cardiac arrest or cardiovascular collapse as the result of a reaction to an anesthetic or other drugs, has a vasovagal reaction, or goes into shock secondary to trauma as in a motor vehicle accident. The same pattern of injury can also be seen in infants 1 to 2 months of age who sustain a cardiopulmonary arrest for a variety of reasons and are resuscitated.

Vulnerability to profound asphyxia in the term infant is manifested in mature neurons with high metabolic rates that are most sensitive to the deprivation of nutrients [27,29,36–41]. Such regions of vulnerability include the posterior putamina, the ventrolateral nucleus of the thalamus, the pre- and postcentral gyri (the rolandic cortex region that lies along the central sulcus), and the subrolandic white matter that is an area of active myelination at term [34,42]. In addition, the hippocampi, the superior vermis, and multiple small areas within the brainstem, primarily cranial nerve nuclei and internal capsules, are also highly sensitive to profound asphyxia (Fig. 12) [43]. More extensive areas of the basal ganglia can be involved, including other portions of the thalami, the full putamina, globus pallidus, and caudate nuclei. Extensive injuries to the basal ganglia are less common than injuries to the putamen.

Recognition of the acute injury process on neuroimaging is dependent on identification of edema at the site of cell death, that is, cytotoxic swelling. Of the three modalities commonly employed to examine the patient suspected to have an acute injury (ultrasound, CT, and MRI), MRI with the capability of diffusion imaging is the most sensitive (Fig. 12) [29,33,34,40,44]. With a sufficient accumulation of edema owing to cytotoxic swelling and vasogenic edema within the volume of the slice being imaged, a change occurs in the echogenicity with ultrasound, a decrease in density occurs with CT, and an increase in signal intensity occurs with T2-weighted imaging with MRI. Although blurring of the margins of the deep gray structures may be seen on CT in less than 24 hours (eg, 18 hours), full-blown hypodensity on CT depending on the size of the area of involvement usually requires 24 hours [27,35,36,45,46]. Ultrasound can demonstrate an extensive profound asphyxia in the central gray matter as increased echogenicity by 24 hours after the event. Nevertheless, when performing ultrasound and CT, if the area of involvement is not of sufficient size, studies performed 24 hours and even 48 hours after the event may be inadequate to demonstrate the presence or absence of the injury.

MRI with T2-weighted imaging will usually be positive by 24 hours after the event. Diffusion imaging is likely to be positive within the first 24 hours and will remain positive for at least 5 days post injury. Generally, in a newborn term infant with a large enough injury, edema becomes visible on ultrasound, CT, and T2-weighted imaging by 24 hours post event and increases to peak edema by 72 hours. The mass effect of the edema resolves by the end of the fifth day going into the sixth day. With sufficient edema in the central gray matter structures, the basal ganglia, and thalami, compression of the third ventricle occurs. In a more extensive injury with involvement of not only the basal ganglia and thalami but also other areas such as the rolandic cortex, there may be some degree of lateral ventricular compression as well. From 72 hours post event, the degree of ventricular compression may be seen to increase depending on the extent of the injury process [22,27,47]. As the disease process progresses past 72 hours out to the sixth day, the ventricular compression resolves, and the ventricles return to normal size. The echogenicity seen on ultrasound, the decreased density seen on CT, and the increased signal intensity seen on T2-weighted MRI may or may not change with the initial evolution of the injury.

As the edema resorbs, damaged tissue is left behind, which, on its own, can produce changes in echogenicity, density, and signal intensity. Subacutely, mineralization around dead neurons in the central gray matter can produce a relatively increased echogenicity. On CT, the subacute injury may or may not be visible until it becomes chronic and can be seen as increased density (Fig. 13E). Injury on T1-weighted imaging MRI may be seen subacutely as increased signal intensity owing to paramagnetic effects arising from calcifications at the site of injured neurons (Fig. 14) [27,37,47]. With further evolution of the injury process extending over the ensuing weeks to months, depending on the volume of tissue involved, reabsorption of tissue occurs, leading to encephalomalacia and scarring (gliosis), which results in atrophy of portions of the brain (Fig. 13). Gliosis is seen as areas of increased signal intensity on T2-weighted and FLAIR imaging because of the increased water content of the tissue relative to normal. This change is best shown on the T2-weighted images once myelination has occurred (ie, after 18 months), because the myelinated white matter is normally hypointense on T2-weighted and FLAIR images and contrasts well with the abnormal increased intensity of gliosis. Atrophy is seen as a decrease in the volume of tissue and an enlargement of the fluid-filled CSF spaces. Evidence of encephalomalacia within the brain often becomes more evident with time as tissue is reabsorbed (Fig. 13) [27,37,47]. As the child grows older, ultrasound loses its utility because of closure of the anterior fontanelle, and CT and MRI become the modalities for evaluation.

Partial prolonged asphyxia

As the fetus becomes full term, the watershed zones in the brain, the areas between vascular territories, shift from the periventricular region toward the

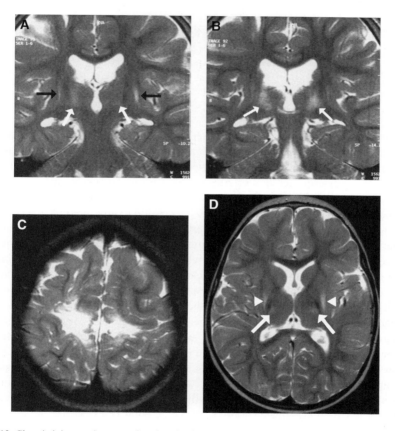

Fig. 13. Chronic injury owing to profound asphyxia. (*A,B*) Coronal T2-weighted imaging in a 7-year-old boy shows mild atrophic dilatation of the lateral and third ventricles. There is abnormal increased signal intensity in the posterior putamen (*black arrows*) and thalami (*white arrows*). (*C*) Axial T2-weighted imaging in a 4-year-old girl shows severe loss of tissue in the pre- and postrolandic gyri. (*D*) Axial T2-weighted imaging in a 3-year-old boy shows bilateral thalamic (*arrows*) and posterior putaminal (*arrowheads*) abnormal increased signal intensity. (*E*) Axial non–contrast enhanced CT imaging in an 18-month-old boy shows bilateral small calcified thalami (*arrows*) and relatively hypodense small basal ganglia (*arrowheads*). Lateral and third ventricles are enlarged owing to loss of brain volume.

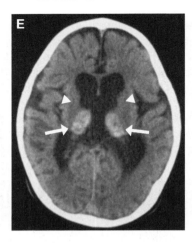

Fig. 13 (*continued*).

cortex and the subcortical white matter. The watershed regions lie anteriorly between the anterior and middle cerebral arteries, primarily in the parasagittal region of the anterior frontal and parietal lobes, and posteriorly between the middle and posterior cerebral arteries in the parasagittal region of the posterior parietal and occipital lobes. There is also an inferior watershed zone in the region of the posterior inferior temporal lobes [27]. Additionally, there is a watershed region between the branches of the vertebral and basilar arteries between the superior cerebellar, posterior inferior cerebellar, and anterior cerebellar arteries in the cerebellum, but this watershed is rarely found to be involved in a term infant with hypoxic ischemic brain injury. It can be involved in older infants, children, and adolescents [48]. Watershed territory injuries of the supratentorial brain occur in term fetuses and neonates when there is a reduction in blood flow and oxygenation. Such injuries most frequently are gradual in onset, leading to a progressive but significant reduction in blood flow and oxygenation to the tissue at the end of the vessels in the watershed zones. A series of such events occurring over 1 or more hours or even longer results in variable injury to either or both of the gray and white matter at the site of the watershed zone. Prolongation of the insult can produce involvement eventually extending beyond the usual watershed region and involving greater portions of the cerebral hemispheres. With further depletion of energy reserves and further diminishing of the fetal heart rate, a pattern of injury may develop that has elements of a partial prolonged asphyxia and profound asphyxia.

The partial prolonged asphyxic pattern of injury may occur silently in utero during the last weeks of gestation and become manifest following delivery or at a later point in time. More often it is recognized during the labor and delivery period, when it is associated with events such as cord compression with a nuchal cord, oligohydramnios producing cord compression, or placental insufficiency

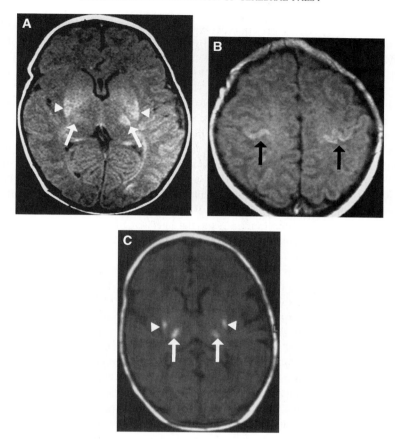

Fig. 14. Profound asphyxia in a 6-day-old male infant (*A*, *B*) and 6-week-old female infant (*C*) post profound asphyxia at birth. (*A*) Axial T1-weighted images show abnormal bilateral increased signal intensity in the putamina (*arrowheads*) and thalami (*arrows*). (*B*) Axial T1-weighted images show abnormal bilateral increased signal intensity in the perirolandic cortex (*arrows*). (*C*) Axial T1-weighted images show bilateral abnormal increased T1-signal intensity in the putamina (*arrowheads*) and thalami (*arrows*).

owing to abnormalities of placental growth and development. Partial prolonged asphyxia can occur in the postpartum perinatal period when there are difficulties in resuscitation of the infant. Neonates in the neonatal nursery can become hypoxic owing to pneumothorax or hypotensive events associated with episodes of apnea and bradycardia.

Ultrasound is of limited value in evaluating watershed injuries in the term infant unless the ultrasonographer focuses on the near field below the anterior fontanelle to demonstrate parasagittal areas of increased echogenicity, indicating an infarction in the watershed zone. Often, the area of injury is not appreciated because the performance of ultrasound concentrates on the periventricular white matter and central gray matter along with the third and lateral ventricles [49]. Ultrasound performed through the anterior fontanelle misses significant portions of the anterosuperior frontal lobes as well as the superior posterior parietal and occipital lobes, the most common sites for watershed infarction. In a large watershed injury, by 24 hours post injury, there is frequently enough edema such that increased echogenicity and a decrease in size of the interhemispheric fissure and portions of the lateral ventricles may be demonstrated, indicating the presence of the injury. Lesser injuries may not be visible on ultrasound. Small lateral ventricles seen on ultrasound in the 12 to 24 hours following birth are a frequent normal finding and not necessarily indicative of cerebral edema from brain injury [50]. As the edema resolves and necrosis occurs over the ensuing weeks, widening of the interhemispheric fissure occurs from loss of tissue (atrophy) with enlargement of the lateral ventricles. These changes are clues to the presence of brain injury and indicate the need for further evaluation with CT or MRI. CT is more sensitive than ultrasound because it shows the full extent of the brain and the brain tissue at risk for injury.

Watershed infarctions are seen 24 hours or more after injury as a loss of gray matter cortical density, with the cortex becoming hypodense with the development of edema, more the density of white matter (Fig. 15A) [27]. As a result, there is loss of the gray matter–white matter differentiation. This loss is most often seen in the parasagittal regions to the right and left of the midline, with frequent involvement of the frontal lobes and parietal occipital lobes together or separately (Fig. 15A) [51]. Watershed injuries may be predominately one sided and may be more anterior or posterior. Infrequently, the watershed injury may be solely unilateral and only anterior or posterior. The reasons for this asymmetry in a setting of a systemic global hypoxic ischemic injury are unknown. It is speculated that the pattern of injury may depend in part upon the anatomic variations in the circle of Willis and the relative availability of collateral blood flow. With a partial prolonged asphyxia that persists for a longer period, the area of injury can extend beyond the watershed zones into the adjacent cortices, producing massive cerebral edema in the supratentorial brain and leading to obliteration of most of the lateral ventricles. Significant brain swelling greater than at 24 hours post injury can be seen between 48 and 96 hours, with the swelling peaking at approximately 72 hours [27]. Intermediate degrees of brain swelling are seen at 36 hours and to some extent beyond 96 hours post injury. Resolution of edema on CT as end of mass effect is seen at 6 to 7 days [27]. Abnormal decreased density within the brain can persist beyond that time. As the edema resolves, the cortex seems to reappear on images obtained at 8 days and beyond. This observation is not a recovery of the cortex but the visualization of laminar cortical necrosis by CT imaging [27]. The injured cortex will atrophy with loss of tissue, enlargement of the subarachnoid space (sulci), and shrinkage of the involved portions of the hemispheres. In the chronic stages, some calcifications may be seen in the cortex, a dystrophic process. Subcortical cystic encephalomalacia is frequent, representing a complete replacement of portions of the white and even gray matter by fluid-filled cystic spaces within areas of

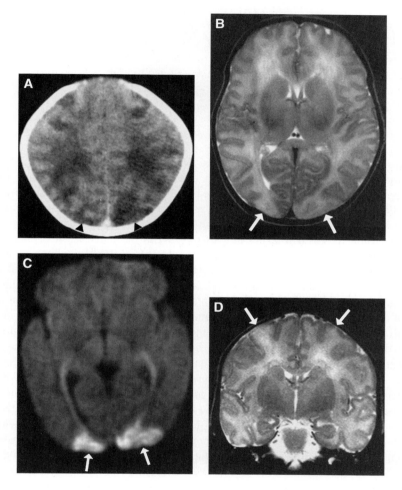

Fig. 15. Acute partial prolonged asphyxia resulting in acute watershed infarction. (*A*) Axial non–contrast enhanced CT in a 2-day-old female infant shows bilateral edema in the parietal and frontal watershed regions as a loss of gray matter density. (Note that in the normal regions a slightly higher density cortex can be seen adjacent to the inner table of the skull.) (*B–E*) Images taken at day 3 of life. (*B*) Axial T2-weighted images show bilateral watershed infarctions as a loss of cortical signal intensity (*arrows*) in the occipital lobes. As a result, the abnormal cortex has similar intensity to that of the white matter. (*C*) Axial diffusion-weighted imaging shows bilateral abnormal increased signal intensity, restricted diffusion, at sites of occipital infarctions (*arrows*). (*D*) Coronal T2-weighted imaging shows bilateral loss of cortical signal intensity at frontal sites of watershed infarction (*arrows*). (*E*) Coronal ADC map shows abnormal bilateral decreased signal, restricted diffusion, at sites of frontal watershed infarctions (*arrows*).

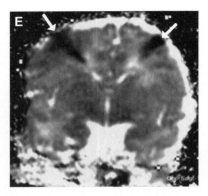

Fig. 15 (*continued*).

necrosis [52]. Ulegyria, a mushroomlike gyrus, may result secondary to atrophy of the under surface of the gyrus. This change represents a post-swelling phenomenon in which the vasculature to the base of the gyrus has been compromised by the swelling to a greater extent than at the apex, leading to more severe tissue loss within the gyrus at the depth of the sulcus [53].

Diffusion-weighted imaging as part of MRI is the most sensitive and successful technique for detection of the earliest changes of parasagittal injury owing to partial prolonged asphyxia [27,29]. The injury results in a restriction of the motion of water and is seen as high signal intensity on diffusion-weighted imaging at a field strength of B1000 and as an area of low signal on the ADC map, which can be measured and quantified relative to normal values (Fig. 15C,E). Twenty-four hours after injury, the cortex will lose its normal low signal intensity on T2-weighted images, becoming brighter because of edema and indistinguishable from the subadjacent bright unmyelinated white matter (Fig. 15B,D). Injury to the subcortical white matter, which is already of high water content in the newborn infant, may not be distinguished on T1 or T2 images by a change in signal intensity, because the addition of more water to watery tissue may not be seen as a difference in signal intensity. Nevertheless, edema in the white and gray matter increases their bulk and leads to compression of the lateral ventricles [27]. With resolution of edema and mass effect at 6 days and beyond, cortical laminar necrosis becomes evident as seen by an increase in signal intensity on T1-weighted images. This cortical high signal intensity will eventually disappear with time as the cortex is reabsorbed. T1- and T2-weighted images will eventually show volume loss possibly in the form of cystic encephalomalacia (Fig. 16A,B). Gliosis, which represents brain scar tissue, is seen on T2-weighted and FLAIR images as areas of increased signal intensity at sites of old damage [27]. It usually involves the cortex and subcortical white matter and may extend within the white matter toward the lateral ventricles.

Following injury, watershed infarctions may become reperfused by blood flow within arterioles. This relatively infrequent complication of watershed infarction can produce a different imaging appearance from that of a purely ischemic insult.

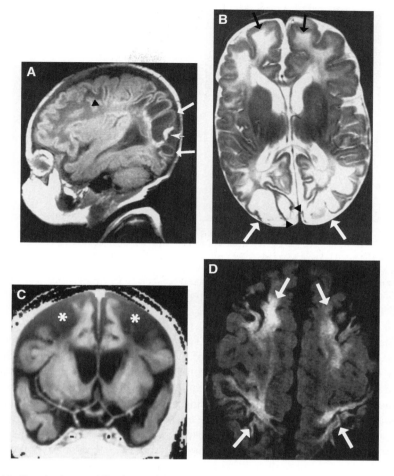

Fig. 16. Chronic changes following partial prolonged asphyxia. (*A,B*) Images from a 1-month-old female infant with birth-related asphyxia. (*A*) Sagittal T1-weighted imaging shows parieto-occipital cystic encephalomalacia (*thick arrows*) with a smaller area of frontal parasagittal involvement (*black arrowhead*). Foci of increased signal (*thin arrow*) are consistent with hemorrhage. (*B*) Axial T2-weighted imaging (same patient as in *A*) shows mild enlargement of lateral ventricles. Bilateral cystic encephalomalacia is present in the temporal occipital lobes (*white arrows*). Hemorrhagic cortex is present on the right (*arrowheads*). Bilateral frontal lobe white matter is abnormal (*black arrows*). (*C*) Coronal T1-weighted imaging in a 4-year-old boy shows loss of tissue in bilateral parasagittal watershed distribution (*asterisk*) with mild enlargement of lateral ventricles. (*D*) Axial FLAIR image in a 6-year-old girl shows bilateral increased signal intensity (*arrows*) and focal adjacent atrophic enlargement of sulci in frontal and parietal lobes in a parasagittal watershed distribution.

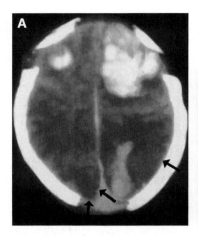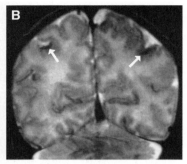

Fig. 17. Hemorrhage secondary to reperfusion of brain injured by partial prolonged asphyxia. (*A*) Non–contrast enhanced CT in a 1-day-old infant. Bilateral parasagittal bleeds are in watershed distribution. Note loss of gray/white matter differentiation at sites of bleeds as well as in parietal lobes at site of nonhemorrhagic infarction (*arrows*). (*B*) Post bilateral hemorrhagic watershed infarction in a 5-week-old infant. Coronal T2-weighted imaging shows residual hypointense blood products (*arrows*) at site of prior infarctions.

In the reperfusion situation, the blood vessels involved at the site of watershed damage are injured and are incapable of remaining intact when increased blood flow under pressure is resumed through them. As a result, rupture of the wall of the damaged arterioles occurs, leading to bleeding within the brain tissue located in the watershed zone [27]. This bleeding may occur focally in a small portion of the injured brain or may be extensive. Localization of the hemorrhagic process can help to characterize the disease process. Blood on ultrasound can be hyperechoic, but if a large hematoma is resolving, it becomes hypoechoic centrally. On CT, acute hemorrhage is hyperdense, but eventually the density decreases over the ensuing weeks (Fig. 17A). On MRI, blood has been characterized according to its chemical content. Deoxyhemoglobin is isointense on T1 images and hypointense on T2 images, intracellular methemoglobin is hyperintense on T1 images and hypointense on T2 images, extracellular methemoglobin is hyperintense on T1 and T2 images, and hemosiderin is hypointense on T2 and T1 images (Fig. 17B) [54]. Blood products are best demonstrated on MRI using a gradient echo T2* sequence for susceptibility [55]. Blood products appear on T2* imaging as a loss of signal intensity (blackness) because the iron in blood causes dephasing of the proton spins, resulting in loss of signal.

Severe partial prolonged asphyxia

In severe partial prolonged asphyxia, the period of reduced blood flow and oxygenation goes on for a sufficiently long time or to a sufficient degree of deprivation of nutrients that the area of cerebral cortical gray matter and subcortical white matter involvement extends beyond the typical watershed areas of the brain. This involvement produces a more homogeneous and extensive pattern of cortical and subcortical injury with edema and resultant mass effect that tends to involve large portions or all of the cerebral lobes bilaterally (Fig. 18A,B). Abnormalities on ultrasound (increased echogenicity), CT (decreased density), and T2-weighted MRI (increased intensity) are present by 24 hours post insult and on diffusion MRI even earlier. Maximal edema and resolution of edema

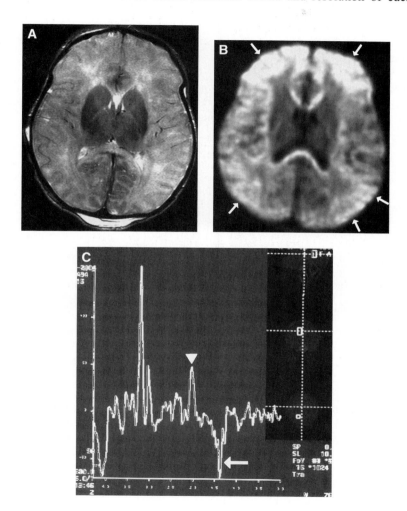

Fig. 18. Severe partial prolonged asphyxia in a 4-day-old male infant owing to a tight nuchal cord. (*A*) Axial T2-weighted imaging shows abnormal cortical and subcortical bilateral cerebral increased T2 signal intensity. Lateral ventricles are small. Basal ganglia and thalami are normal in signal intensity. (*B*) Axial diffusion-weighted imaging shows extensive gray and white matter injury (*arrows*) of both cerebral hemispheres with sparing of central gray matter. (*C*) Proton spectroscopy, single voxel, from right parietal lobe. TE of 135 msec shows decreased N acetylaspartate (Naa) (*arrowhead*) and markedly elevated lactate (*arrow*).

follow the same time course seen with lesser degrees of partial prolonged asphyxia. Frequently, during the subacute phase of injury, changes in the cortex consistent with cortical laminar necrosis are manifested on nonenhanced CT as abnormal increased density and on nonenhanced T1-weighted imaging as abnormal increased T1 signal intensity. Over time with further reabsorption of damaged tissue by macrophages, subcortical cystic encephalomalacia may occur in addition to the less impressive but still equally important finding of a global supratentorial cortical and subcortical atrophy. Enlargement of sulci and ventricles and the presence of chronic extra-axial fluid collections are frequent chronic findings.

Mixed partial prolonged asphyxia leading to terminal profound asphyxia

A mixed form of asphyxic injury occurs when energy substrates are depleted in a partial prolonged asphyxia, leading to a further insult in the form of a

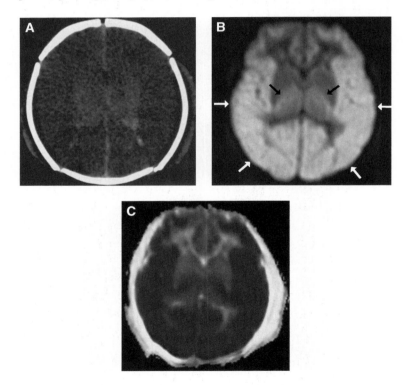

Fig. 19. Images from a 72-hour-old male infant post prolonged partial asphyxia resulting in mixed injury. (*A*) Axial CT, non–contrast enhanced imaging shows diffuse bilateral cerebral edema with loss of gray/white matter differentiation and collapse of the lateral ventricles. Thalami are also abnormally hypodense. (*B*) Axial diffusion-weighted imaging performed the same day as CT shows collapsed lateral ventricles and abnormal bilateral increased signal intensity involving the cortex (*white arrows*) and subcortical white matter as well as thalami (*black arrows*). Frontal lobes are less affected. (*C*) Axial ADC map shows affected brain as hypointense.

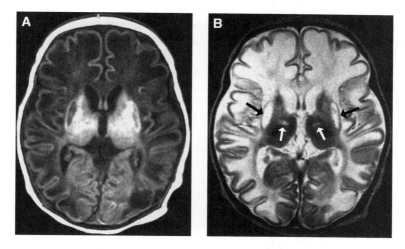

Fig. 20. Chronic mixed injury in a 21-day-old female infant. (*A*) Axial T1-weighted imaging shows atrophically enlarged lateral and third ventricles. The basal ganglia and thalami show abnormal increased signal intensity. The putamina centrally have less intensity owing to cavitation. Subcortical white matter is diffusely abnormally hypointense, while the cortex shows multiple regions of increased signal intensity consistent with laminar cortical necrosis. (*B*) Axial T2-weighted imaging shows diffuse abnormal increase in white matter signal intensity and cavitary changes in the putamina (*black arrows*) and thalami (*white arrows*).

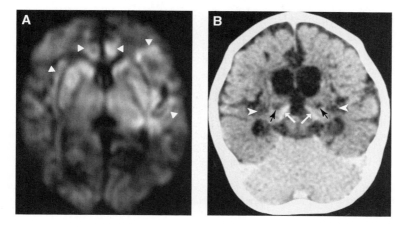

Fig. 21. Images from a 2-day-old female infant post placental abruption. (*A*) Axial diffusion-weighted imaging shows bilateral abnormal increased signal involving the thalami, putamina, and caudate nuclei. There are additional areas of cortical involvement (*arrowheads*). (*B*) Two-year follow-up axial CT shows atrophic enlargement of the lateral and third ventricles. There is abnormal decreased density in abnormally small basal ganglia (*white arrowheads*) and abnormal increased density (*white arrows*) and abnormal decreased density (*black arrows*) in very small thalami.

terminal near total collapse. This injury is seen clinically as a sudden bradycardic event superimposed on a prior more gradual abnormal decline in fetal heart rate. In addition to the damage from the partial prolonged asphyxia occurring in the watershed regions or (in more severe cases) beyond the watershed regions, the addition of the severe bradycardic events causes injury to the thalamus and putamina with the possibility of hippocampal, vermian, and brainstem injury as well (Fig. 19). The evolution of mixed injuries is similar to that previously described (Fig. 20).

Very severe near total (profound) asphyxia can show the classic profound pattern of injury but with a greater extent of cortical involvement that is not limited to the rolandic cortical region (Fig. 21). In such cases, the fetal bradycardia is particularly long (eg, 30 minutes) and in some instances longer if the fetus survives. The predominant pattern of injury is profound asphyxia with severe injury to the basal ganglia and thalamus predominating.

Summary

Injury to the fetal brain as a potential cause of cerebral palsy in the postnatal period can be demonstrated by performing fetal MRI. As experience increases and MRI techniques continue to improve, fetal MRI will have an increasing role in the evaluation of the fetal CNS and will contribute to the understanding of such injuries.

MRI is the modality of choice and provides definitive information in the postnatal evaluation of the term infant in whom hypoxic ischemic brain injury has occurred and in whom cerebral palsy will eventually be diagnosed.

References

[1] Nelson KB. The epidemiology of cerebral palsy in term infants. Ment Retard Dev Disabil Res Rev 2002;8:146–50.
[2] Kuban KCK, Leviton A. Cerebral palsy. N Engl J Med 1994;33:188–95.
[3] Cowan F, Rutherford M, Groenendaal F, et al. Origin and timing of brain lesions in term infants with neonatal encephalopathy. Lancet 2003;361:736–42.
[4] Ellis WG, Goetzman BW, Lindenberg JA. Neuropathologic documentation of prenatal brain damage. AJDC 142:858–66.
[5] Truwit CL, Barkovich AJ, Koch TK, et al. Cerebral palsy: MR findings in 40 patients. AJNR Am J Neuroradiol 1992;13:67–78.
[6] Zimmerman RA, Bilaniuk LT. Magnetic resonance evaluation of fetal ventriculomegaly-associated congenital malformations and lesions. Seminars in Fetal & Neonatal Medicine 2005; 10:429–43.
[7] Sutton LN, Sun P, Adzick NS. Fetal neurosurgery. Neurosurgery 2001;48:124–44.
[8] Cardoza JD, Goldstein RB, Filly RA. Exclusion of fetal ventriculomegaly with a single measurement: the width of the lateral ventricular atrium. Radiology 1988;169:711–4.
[9] Lipitz A, Yagel S, Malinger G, et al. Outcome of fetuses with isolated borderline unilateral ventriculomegaly diagnosed at mid gestation. Ultrasound Obstet Gynecol 1998;12:23–6.

[10] Bromley B, Frigoletto Jr FD, Benacerraf BR. Mild fetal lateral cerebral ventriculomegaly: clinical course and outcome. Am J Obstet Gynecol 1991;164:863–7.

[11] Del Bigio MR, Brunj JE, Fewer HD. Human neonatal hydrocephalus: an electron microscopic study of the periventricular tissue. J Neurosurg 1985;63:56–63.

[12] Rubin RC, Hochwald GM, Tiell M, et al. Hydrocephalus: II-cell number and size, and myelin content of the pre-shunted cerebral cortical mantle. Surg Neurol 1976;5:115–8.

[13] Weller RO, Shulman JK. Infantile hydrocephalus: clinical, histological, and ultrastructural study of brain damage. J Neurosurg 1972;36:255–67.

[14] McAllister II JP, Chovan P. Neonatal hydrocephalus: mechanisms and consequences. Neurosurg Clin N Am 1998;9:73–93.

[15] Grogono JL. Children with agenesis of the corpus callosum. Dev Med Child Neurol 1968;10: 613–6.

[16] Jeret JS, Serur D, Wisniewski K, et al. Frequency of agenesis of the corpus callosum in the developmentally disabled population as determined by computerized tomography. Pediatr Neurosci 1986;12:101–3.

[17] Dominguez R, Aquirre Vila Coro A, Slopis JM, et al. Brain and ocular abnormalities in infants with in utero exposure to cocaine and other street drugs. Am J Dis Child 1991;145:688–95.

[18] Conover PT, Roessmann U. Malformational complex in an infant with intrauterine influenza viral infection. Arch Pathol Lab Med 1990;114:535–8.

[19] DeMyer W. Holoprosencephaly. In: Vinken PJ, Bruyn GW, editors. Handbook of clinical neurology, vol. 30. Amsterdam: Elsevier; 1977. p. 431.

[20] Matsunaga E, Shiota K. Holoprosencephaly in human embryos: epidemiologic studies of 150 cases. Teratology 1977;16:261–72.

[21] Lehman CD, Nyberg DA, Winter 3rd TC, et al. Trisomy 13 syndrome: prenatal US findings in a review of 33 cases. Radiology 1995;194:217–22.

[22] Berry SM, Gosden C, Snijders RJ, et al. Fetal holoprosencephaly: associated malformations and chromosomal defects. Fetal Diagn Ther 1990;5:92–9.

[23] Kubik-Huch R, Huisman TAGM, Wisser J, et al. Ultrafast MR imaging of the fetus. AJR Am J Roentgenol 2000;174:1599–606.

[24] de Laveaucoupet J, Audibert F, Guis F, et al. Fetal magnetic resonance imaging (MRI) of ischemic brain injury. Prenat Diagn 1002;21:729–36.

[25] Vergani P, Strobelt N, Locatelli A, et al. Clinical significance of fetal intracranial hemorrhage. Am J Obstet Gynecol 1996;175:536–43.

[26] Zimmerman RA, Haselgrove JC, Wang Z, et al. Advances in pediatric neuroimaging. Brain Dev 1998;20:275–9.

[27] Zimmerman RA, Wong AM-C, Bilaniuk LT. Hypoxic and ischaemic brain insults in newborns and infants. In: Carty H, Brunelle F, Stringer DA, Kao SCS, editors. Imaging children. 2nd edition. Edinburgh: Elsevier Churchill Livingstone; 2005. p. 1807–62.

[28] Johnson AJ, Lee BC, Lin WL. Echoplanar diffusion-weighted imaging in neonates and infants with suspected hypoxic-ischaemic injury: correlation with patient outcome. AJR Am J Roentgenol 1999;172:219–26.

[29] Wolf RI, Zimmerman RA, Clancy R, et al. Quantitative ADC measurements in term neonates for early detection of hypoxic-ischemic brain injury: initial experience. Radiology 2001;218: 825–33.

[30] Wang Z, Zimmerman RA, Sauter R. Proton MR spectroscopy of the brain: clinically useful information obtained in assessing CNS diseases in children. AJR Am J Roentgenol 1996;167: 191–9.

[31] Barkovich AJ, Baranski K, Vigneron D. Proton MR spectroscopy for the evaluation of brain injury in asphyxiated, term neonates. AJNR Am J Neuroradiol 1999;20:1399–405.

[32] Ashwal S, Holshouser BA, Tomasi LG. Magnetic resonance spectroscopy determined cerebral lactate and poor neurological outcomes in children with central nervous system disease. Ann Neurol 1997;41:470–81.

[33] Groenendaal F, van der Grond J, Witkamp TD, et al. Proton magnetic resonance spectroscopic imaging in neonatal stroke. Neuropediatrics 1995;26:243–8.

[34] Menkes JH, Curran J. Clinical and MR correlates in children with extrapyramidal cerebral palsy. AJNR Am J Neuroradiol 1994;15:451–7.

[35] Leung AS, Leung EK, Paul RH. Uterine rupture after previous cesarean delivery: maternal and fetal consequences. Am J Obstet Gynecol 1993;169:945–50.

[36] Hill A. Current concepts of hypoxic-ischaemic cerebral injury in the term newborn. Pediatr Neurol 1991;7:317–25.

[37] Pasternak JF, Gorey MT. The syndrome of acute near-total intrauterine asphyxia in the term infant. Pediatr Neurol 1998;18:391–8.

[38] Roland EH, Poskitt K, Rodriguez E. Perinatal hypoxic-ischaemic thalamic injury: clinical features and neuroimaging. Ann Neurol 1998;44:161–6.

[39] Rosenbloom L. Dyskinetic cerebral palsy and birth asphyxia. Dev Med Child Neurol 1994;36: 285–9.

[40] Barkovich AJ. MR and CT evaluation of profound neonatal and infantile asphyxia. AJNR Am J Neuroradiol 1992;13:959–72.

[41] Roelants-van Rijn AM, Nikkels PGJ, Groenendaal F, et al. Neonatal diffusion-weighted MR imaging: relation with histopathology or follow-up MR examination. Neuropediatrics 2001;32: 286–94.

[42] Krageloh-Mann I, Helber A, Mader I, et al. Bilateral lesions of thalamus and basal ganglia: origin and outcome. Dev Med Child Neurol 2002;44:477–84.

[43] Rutherford MA, Pennock JM, Counsell SJ, et al. Abnormal magnetic resonance signal in the internal capsule predicts poor neurodevelopmental outcome in infants with hypoxic-ischemic encephalopathy. Pediatrics 1998;102:323–8.

[44] Barkovich AJ, Westmark KD, Bedi HS, et al. Proton spectroscopy and diffusion imaging on the first day of life after perinatal asphyxia: preliminary report. AJNR Am J Neuroradiol 2001;22: 1786–94.

[45] Winkler P, Zimmerman RA. Perinatal brain injury. In: Zimmerman RA, Gibby WA, Carmody RF, editors. Neuroimaging: clinical and physical principles. New York: Springer; 2000. p. 531–84.

[46] Lupton BA, Hill A, Roland EH, et al. Brain swelling in the asphyxiated term newborn: pathogenesis and outcome. Pediatrics 1988;82:139–46.

[47] Barkovich AJ. Brain and spine injuries in infancy and childhood. In: Pediatric neuroimaging. 4th edition. Philadelphia: Lippincott Williams & Wilkins; 2005. p. 190–290.

[48] Liu AY, Zimmerman RA, Haselgrove JC, et al. Diffusion-weighted imaging in the evaluation of watershed hypoxic-ischemic brain injury in pediatric patients. Neuroradiology 2001;43: 918–26.

[49] Rutherford M, Pennock JM, Dubowitz L. Cranial ultrasound and magnetic resonance imaging in hypoxic-ischaemic encephalopathy: a comparison with outcome. Dev Med Child Neurol 1994; 36:813–25.

[50] Nelson MD, Tavare CJ, Petrus L, et al. Changes in the size of the lateral ventricles in the normal-term newborn following vaginal delivery. Pediatr Radiol 2003;33:831–5.

[51] Pasternak JF. Parasagittal infarction in neonatal asphyxia. Ann Neurol 1987;21:202–4.

[52] Naidich TP, Chakera TMH. Multicystic encephalomalacia: CT appearance and pathological correlation. J Comput Assist Tomogr 1984;8:631–6.

[53] Villani F, D'Incerti L, Granata T, et al. Epileptic and imaging findings in perinatal hypoxic-ischemic encephalopathy with ulegyria. Epilepsy Res 2003;55:235–43.

[54] Gomori JM, Grossman RI, Goldberg HI, et al. Variable appearances of subacute intracranial hematomas on spin echo high-field MR. AJNR Am J Neuroradiol 1987;8:1019–26.

[55] Gomori JM, Grossman RI, Goldberg HI, et al. High-field MR imaging of ependymal siderosis secondary to neonatal intraventricular hemorrhage. Neuroadiology 1987;29:339–42.

ELSEVIER
SAUNDERS

Clin Perinatol 33 (2006) 545–555

CLINICS IN
PERINATOLOGY

Cerebral Palsy Life Expectancy

Jane L. Hutton, PhD, CStat

Department of Statistics, The University of Warwick, Coventry CV4 7AL, UK

Parents of children who have cerebral palsy (CP) of perinatal origin often wish to know how long their child is likely to live. Health and social care providers, whether state authorities, as in the United Kingdom (UK), or insurance companies in Europe or the United States of America (USA) need information on life expectancy to plan for the medical, educational, and social needs of these children and their families. Although the nature and timing of the causes of CP often are unclear [1,2], if liability is admitted, information on life expectancy is an essential component in deciding the quantum of a settlement. Despite these needs, reliable estimates of life expectancy have become available only in the last 16 years.

Early studies of life expectancy assessed only children who were in long-term institutional care [3,4]. Because children in institutional care are a special subset of all children who have CP and because institutional care might systematically improve or worsen survival [5], it is difficult to relate these estimates to the general population of people who have CP. Two studies that were based on small numbers and short follow-up were published in 1985 [6,7]. The first survival estimates that were based on a geographically defined cohort with rigorous follow-up were published in 1990, and demonstrated that most children would survive to adulthood [8]. The same year saw the first results from a large Californian service register [9] (see correction [10]). Reports on life expectancy in Australia [11], Canada [12], the UK [13–18], and the USA [19–22] have been published. The causes of death of people who had CP also have been reported [15,18,23–26].

E-mail address: j.l.hutton@warwick.ac.uk

0095-5108/06/$ – see front matter © 2006 Elsevier Inc. All rights reserved.
doi:10.1016/j.clp.2006.03.016

perinatology.theclinics.com

Life expectancy: aspects of estimation

To obtain a good estimate of the survival experience of a population of interest, such as people who have CP, we need to have a representative group of such people, with information on factors that affect life expectancy, and to know precisely when they died or how old they were when last known to be alive.

The most reliable source of information on survival is a cohort with the following characteristics:

Each person conforms to a specified definition of CP, and each person comes from a precisely defined geographic population

His/her date of birth is known

His/her sex, birth weight, gestational age, and severity of functional disability are recorded

Notification of death and date of death is guaranteed

Several definitions of CP have been proposed. The crucial components of all of the definitions are that the disability is of the brain; it produces disorders of movement or posture; it occurs pre- or perinatally and is nonprogressive; and although the disability is nonprogressive, the symptoms and signs may vary as the child matures. All syndromes that have progressive cerebral disability must be excluded from survival estimates, and early diagnoses should be verified as the child grows. A child who is diagnosed with severe CP in infancy may be shown not to have a disorder of movement or posture [27].

It is essential to assess the completeness of registers or databases that include people who receive treatment or services related to their syndrome [28]. If cases are collected from a service that focuses on provision of education for persons who have cognitive deficits, reliable information on people who have normal or good cognitive ability will not be available. A region with an excellent health service might attract people from other regions, so that the service disease register does not represent a geographic cohort.

In some countries, data on dates and causes of death or dates of emigration are available routinely through the official statistics systems; other countries do not release such data. To estimate the effects on survival of the severity of functional disability, each severity category must have a specific definition. The categories must be mutually exclusive.

Clinical experience alone is insufficient for reliable estimation of the probability of survival in CP [29]. Readers who require precise details of the methods that are used in life tables and other survival estimates should consult technical books [30–32] or use government statistics web sites (eg, [33]).

The definition of "life expectancy" is the arithmetic mean of all of the lifetimes of the relevant population. Care is needed in reading tables of life expectancy, because actuarial tables that are presented in government and actuarial publications usually give the "residual life expectancy for age x," which is the average additional number of years that a person aged x will live. For example, at birth (ie, age 0) a UK boy has life expectancy of 75.4 years and is expected to live to age 75.4, whereas at age 10 years, he has life expectancy of 66 years and is expected to live to age 76.0 years. The risks for death are high in the early years of life, so if he survives, his expected final age at death is higher than it was at birth.

Sometimes estimates of the median additional life are used. In the UK, civil courts wish to know the median, or the age at which 50 of a notional cohort of 100 people like the plaintiff will have died. If not all of a cohort of people who are being studied have died, it is not possible to estimate the mean lifetime directly; however, it is possible to estimate the pattern of survival to the age of the oldest person in the cohort. If more than half of the cohort has died, the median lifetime can be estimated. National life tables use information on persons who are currently alive to estimate life expectancy.

Disabilities and demographic factors

Although the usual slightly poorer survival of male subjects compared with female subjects is present, the sex effect is minimal relative to the effect of disability (Fig. 1). A combined estimate of UK CP survival shows that 85% of women live to age 30 years, compared with 83% of men (Table 1). Low birth weight ($\leq$ 2500 g; Fig. 2) and prematurity ($<$ 37 weeks' gestation; Fig. 3) also are associated strongly with survival, but not as might be expected; premature infants

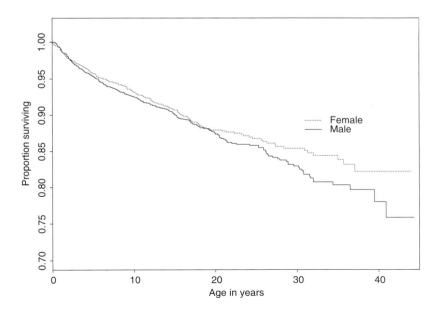

Fig. 1. Life expectancy by gender.

Table 1
United Kingdom 10-, 20-, and 30-year survival estimates

Characteristic		Percentage surviving to		
		10 y	20 y	30 y
Sex:	Female:	93	87	85
	Male:	92	87	83
Birth weight (g)	<1500	95	92	92
	1500–2499	95	90	86
	≥ 2500	91	85	81
Gestational age (wk)	< 32	95	93	92
	32–36	95	90	87
	≥ 37	91	85	81

have better survival than do term infants [13,15–17]. The UK CP 30-year survival is 92% for very low birth weight and premature infants, compared with 81% for term and normal weight births (Table 1). Part of this difference in survival arises from the higher proportions of severe disabilities among term or normal birth weight infants. For example, in one English cohort (Mersey), 36% of normal birth weight infants had severe mental disabilities, compared with 26% of those who weighed less than 1500 g at birth [16]. The clinical type of CP is associated with survival, in that quadriplegia is associated with a higher risk for death.

Reports from all of the recent studies of CP life expectancy agree that survival is significantly poorer in those who have severe disability [8,11–18,20,21]. In

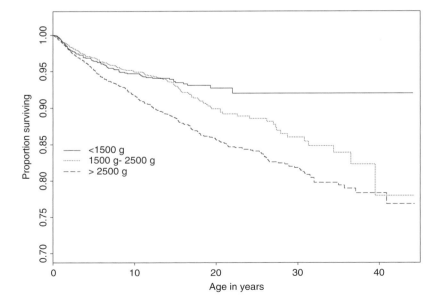

Fig. 2. Life expectancy by birth weight.

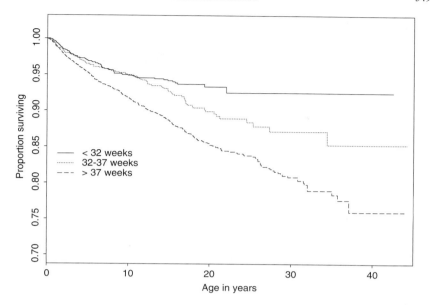

Fig. 3. Life expectancy by gestational age.

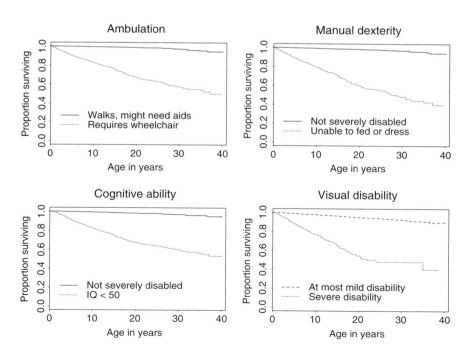

Fig. 4. Life expectancy by disabilities.

contrast, children who have mild disabilities have good life expectancy (Figs. 4 and 5). In the UK and Europe, common definitions of severe function abilities are used [8,14,17,34]. Severe manual disability is defined as the child being unable to feed or dress him/herself. A severe intellectual disability is defined as an intelligence quotient (IQ) of less than 50. Severe ambulatory disability indicates that the child is unable to walk, even with aids, and requires a wheelchair. A severe visual impairment is defined as vision in the better eye of less than 6/60. A severe hearing impairment is defined as a hearing loss in the better ear of more than 70 dB averaged across frequencies from 0.5 kHz to 4 kHz. Estimates for a general UK CP cohort—for each disability considered separately—show that 95% to 99% of children with no to moderate disability live to adulthood (age 20 years, Table 2). Of those who require a wheelchair or have severe intellectual disability, about 60% live to age 30 years. About half of those who have severe manual or visual disability live to age 30 years.

The Californian Mental Retardation Database records whether, when lying, people can lift their head or roll; whether epilepsy is present; and whether tube feeding (gastrostomy) is used [20,21]. The less mobility that a person has, the poorer is his/her life expectancy, and epilepsy and tube feeding are associated with increased risks for death.

The frequency and type of epileptic seizures and the level of control of seizures usually are not known, so the effect on survival cannot be assessed accu-

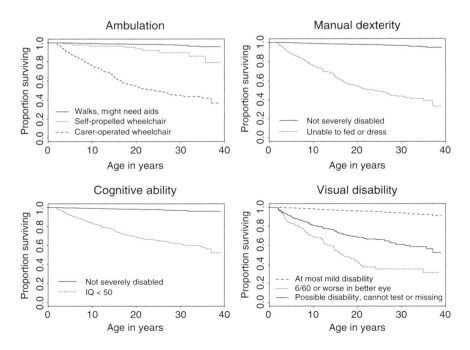

Fig. 5. Life expectancy by disabilities (Mersey only).

Table 2
United Kingdom 10-, 20-, and 30-year survival estimates

Disability	Percentage surviving to		
	10 y	20 y	30 y
Ambulation:			
Normal to moderate	99	99	98
Wheelchair required	82	67	58
Manual dexterity:			
Normal to moderate	99	98	97
Cannot feed or dress	79	59	49
Mental ability:			
Normal to moderate	99	98	97
IQ < 50	82	67	60
Vision:			
Normal to moderate	97	95	93
< 6/60 in better eye	76	54	47
Severe disabilities:			
None	99	99	99
One	99	96	95
Two	96	89	78
Three	84	65	59
Four	68	41	33
Missing[a]	81	75	69

[a] If any disability data are missing.

rately. Clinical assessment by the pediatrician and those who care for the child affect the decision to feed through a gastrostomy. Tube feeding is an indicator that the child has severe problems and is a poor prognosis for survival; however, gastrostomy is performed to improve prognosis and quality of life. Therefore, it is difficult to assess the impact of gastrostomy.

There is no evidence of much change in life expectancy over the last 40 years. The percentage of children in the Mersey [16] and North of England [15] geographic cohorts who survive to age 10 years has been 90% to 94% for births from 1960 to 1990. If deaths in the first 2 years of life are discounted by considering survival from age 2 to age 10, survival for five regions in the UK for births 1980 to 1997 vary from 93% to 98%. Some of this variation is associated with small differences in the severity of CP between regions. Comparison with a cohort of people that was born in the 1940s and 1950s does show some improvement in survival [18].

Combined effects of risk factors

Because children who have CP can have a wide range of levels of disabilities, it is sensible to consider the combined effects of multiple disabilities. Using statistical models that allow the joint effects of several variables to be assessed shows that severe cognitive, motor (manual and ambulatory), and visual disabilities all contribute information on the probability of survival. A summary of the joint impact can be made by considering the number of severe disabilities that a child has. Table 2 summaries a general UK CP population. Children who have only one severe disability are likely (95%) to live to age 30 years. In contrast, only one third of those who have four severe disabilities reach this age. Severe hearing disability does not add additional information when the other four functional disability categories are taken into account. The clinical type of CP also fails to add information after allowing for severity of disability.

In UK populations, low birth weight was associated with better survival after allowing for cognitive, motor, and manual disability [16]. A recent study of five UK geographic cohorts found that low birth weight was associated with better survival than was normal birth weight only in more affluent families [17].

In Mersey, the year of birth was associated with life expectancy only after allowing for disabilities and birth weight. Among children who were born weighing less than 2500 g, those who were born earlier had better survival than did those who were born later (see Fig. 1) [16]. The difference is small; the estimated percentage that survived from age two to age 20 was 97% for 1966 births and 91% for 1989 births. By 1989, the survival of low birth weight and normal birth weight infants was the same. This suggests that as neonatal intensive care improved, more frail infants survived to be diagnosed as having CP.

Variation in survival by region

There are some differences in the levels of disabilities between countries in the populations studied [11,15,17,18]. The Californian database has high levels of severe ambulatory impairments (73% in children, 35% in adults) compared with 26% to 36% in young people in the UK, Canada, and Australia, and 17% in a UK adult study. Canada and Australia record slightly lower rates of severe cognitive disability (16% and 24%, respectively) than do the other countries (21–44%). Manual disability is severe in 20% to 25% of subjects across these countries. Blindness is recorded in 6% to 11% of children. Although the prevalence of severe disabilities varied between the five UK regions, there were no difference in survival experience after disabilities were taken into account.

Two cohorts permit long-term follow-up of people who have CP [18,20,22]. In general, excess risks of death compared with the general population decreased with age [35]. An increase in the relative risk of death after age 50 years was found for the UK female cohort [18], but this was not reported for the Californian study. No such increase was observed for the UK men, who had a lower relative risk. A possible explanation is that men who have medical problems do better than women because female partners or parents act as caregivers. The Californian study reported a decline in ambulatory function over the age of 60 years, along with a poorer life expectancy for these individuals who had lost mobility [22].

Causes of death

CP is the most commonly recorded underlying cause of death in younger people, and is shown on about 30% of death certificates [15,23,24]. Deaths that are due to diseases of the respiratory system are much more prevalent than in the general population, especially for those who die before age 40 (20–30%) [15,18,23–26]. In an Australian cohort, 59% of the immediate causes of death were due to respiratory causes; 21% were related to inhalation of liquid or aspiration pneumonia. Other pneumonia or unattributed pneumonia accounted for 37% of deaths. Epilepsy (5–9%) and congenital malformations (7–8%) are common recorded causes of death.

In UK and USA adults older than 30 years, larger proportions of death are from cancers and diseases of the circulatory system. For those who are older than 40 years, digestive and nervous system causes of deaths are more prevalent than would be expected in the general population [18,25]. In the UK, deaths that are due to injuries and accidents occur much less often than would be expected [18], in contrast to the Californian experience [25]. Deaths are attributed less often to CP among older people—either as the underlying cause or as CP mentioned anywhere on the death certificate.

Summary

Many people who have CP live to be adults, particularly those without severe functional disabilities. These results provide broad indications of survival experience.

To estimate survival, the precise combination of different functional disabilities must be specified and consistent. It would be possible to reach a wide range of survival estimates by varying the combination and levels of disability. In any large clinical dataset, it is unusual for every variable to have a complete set of values. The reasons why some values are missing may bias a survival estimate severely. For example, when IQ is used as a measure of cognitive ability, a missing value for IQ could arise if the child had limited communication because of other severe impediments. Also, children who die young are more likely to have missing information. For the general UK CP cohort, the survival to 10 years for children who have at least one disability not recorded is as poor as that for those who have three disabilities. Subsequent survival is better than in those who have three disabilities.

Quality of life for a person who has CP is affected inevitably by quality of care. In settlement of quantum, the compensation that is awarded is aimed at optimizing the quality of life. Of course, only some people who have CP are recipients of such awards [36], the rest rely on state support. Quality of care and its possible effect on survival feature in legal cases. The recent finding of an inverse relationship between affluence and survival requires further analysis [17]. Unless the distinguishing criteria between favorable and unfavorable home environments are defined and applied to the database that is used to estimate survival, it is unwise to predict the effects of a "good" institution or home. In the UK, health and social care is coordinated for children; however, in general, adult care from different professionals is independent. Some UK pediatricians refer their young adult patients who have CP to geriatricians to ensure a coherent system of care.

A Lifestyle Assessment Score (LAS) has been developed to assess the impact of CP on children and their families using a range of 0 to 100 [37]. A questionnaire yields scores in six dimensions: physical dependency, clinical burden, mobility, schooling, economic burden, and social integration. The LAS combines these scores using weights that are derived from pediatricians, parents of children who have CP, and parents of children without disability. A typical child with an LAS of 30 completes most activities alone, poses little economic burden, and attends a mainstream school. A child with an LAS of 70 undertakes few self-help tasks, experiences severe economic difficulties, and is in a specialized educational setting. Although severe disabilities are associated with higher LAS scores, half of those who have severe disabilities have LAS scores of less than 70. Lifestyle is associated with quality of life but is not identical. Collaborative work is in progress that involves several CP registers in Europe to investigate the quality of life in children who have CP.

References

[1] MacLennan A for the International Cerebral Palsy Task Force. A template for defining a causal relation between acute intrapartum events and cerebral palsy: International Consensus Statement. BMJ 1999;319:1054–9.

[2] Bakketeig LS. Only a minor part of cerebral palsy cases begin in labour. BMJ 1999;319:1016–7.

[3] Dayton NA, Doering CR, Hilferty MM, et al. Mortality and expectation of life in mental deficiency in Massachusetts: analysis of the fourteen-year period 1917–1930. N Engl J Med 1932;205:555–70.

[4] Balakrishnan TR, Wolf LC. Life expectancy of mentally retarded persons in Canadian institutions. Am J Ment Defic 1976;80:650–62.

[5] Zaharia ES, O'Brien K. Mortality: an individual or aggregate variable? Am J Ment Retard 1996;101:424–9.

[6] Kudrjacev T, Schoenberg BS, Kurland LT, et al. Cerebral palsy: survival rates, associated handicaps and distribution by clinical subtype. Neuro 1985;35:900–3.

[7] Von Wendt L, Rantakolio P, Suakkonen A-L, et al. Cerebral palsy and additional handicaps in a 1-year birth cohort from northern Finland—a prospective follow-up study to the age of 14 years. Ann Clin Res 1985;17:156–61.

[8] Evans PM, Evans SJW, Alberman E. Cerebral palsy: why we must plan for survival. Arch Dis Child 1990;65:1329–33.

[9] Eyman RK, Grossman HJ, Chaney RH, et al. The life expectancy of profoundly handicapped people with mental retardation. N Engl J Med 1990;323:584–9.

[10] Grossman HJ, Eyman RK. Survival estimates of severely disabled children. Pediatr Neurol 1998;19(3):243–4.

[11] Blair E, Watson L, Badawi N, et al. Life expectancy among people with cerebral palsy in Western Australia. Dev Med Child Neurol 2001;43:508–15.

[12] Crichton JU, Mackinnon M, White CP. The life-expectancy of persons with cerebral palsy. Dev Med Child Neurol 1995;37:567–76.

[13] Hutton JL, Cooke T, Pharoah POD. Life expectancy in children with cerebral palsy. BMJ 1994; 309:431–5.

[14] Williams K, Hennessy E, Alberman E. Cerebral palsy: effects of twinning, birthweight and gestational age. Arch Dis Child 1996;75:F178–82.

[15] Hutton JL, Colver AF, Mackie PC. Effect of severity of disability on survival in north east England cerebral palsy cohort. Arch Dis Child 2000;83:468–74.

[16] Hutton JL, Pharoah POD. Effects of cognitive, sensory and motor impairment on the survival of people with cerebral palsy. Arch Dis Child 2002;86:84–9.

[17] Hemming K, Hutton JL, Colver A, et al. Regional variation in survival of people with cerebral palsy in the United Kingdom. Pediatrics 2005;116:1383–90.

[18] Hemming K, Hutton JL, Pharoah POD. Long term survival for a cohort of adults with cerebral palsy. Dev Med Child Neurol 2006;48:90–5.

[19] Eyman RK, Grossman HJ, Chaney RH, et al. Survival of profoundly disabled people with severe mental retardation. Am J Dis Child 1993;147:329–36.

[20] Strauss D, Shavelle RM. Life expectancy of adults with cerebral palsy. Dev Med Child Neurol 1998;40:369–75.

[21] Strauss D, Shavelle RM, Anderson TW. Life expectancy of children with cerebral palsy. Pediatr Neurol 1998;18:143–9.

[22] Strauss D, Ojdana K, Shavelle R, et al. Decline in function and life expectancy of older persons with cerebral palsy. NeuroRehabilitation 2004;19:69–78.

[23] Evans PM, Alberman E. Certified cause of death in children and young adults with cerebral palsy. Arch Dis Child 1990;65:325–9.

[24] Maudsley G, Hutton JL, Pharoah POD. Cause of death in cerebral palsy: a descriptive study. Arch Dis Child 1999;82:309–94.

[25] Strauss D, Cable W, Shavelle R. Causes of excess mortality in cerebral palsy. Dev Med Child Neurol 1991;41:580–5.

[26] Reddihough DS, Baike G, Walstab JE. Cerebral palsy in Victoria, Australia: mortality and causes of death. J Paediatr Child Health 2001;37:183–6.

[27] Nelson KB, Ellenberg JH. Children who "outgrew" cerebral palsy. Pediatrics 1982;69:529–36.

[28] Buehler JW. Surveillance. In: Rothman KJ, Greenland S, editors. Modern epidemiology. 2nd edition. Philadelphia: Lippincott-Raven; 1998. p. 435–57.

[29] Strauss D, Shavelle RM. Doctors are not experts on life expectancy. Expert Witness 1998;3: 11–3.

[30] Cox DR, Oakes D. Analysis of survival data. London: Chapman & Hall; 1984.

[31] Collett D. Modelling survival data in medical research. 2nd edition. London: Chapman & Hall; 2003.

[32] Armitage P, Berry G. Statistical methods in medical research. 2nd edition. Oxford (UK): Blackwell; 1987.

[33] Government Actuary's Department. Available at: http://www.gad.gov.uk. Accessed February 1, 2006.

[34] Surveillance of Cerebral Palsy in Europe (SCPE) Collaborative Group. Prevalence and characteristics of children with cerebral palsy in Europe. Dev Med Child Neurol 2002;44:633–40.

[35] Strauss D, Shavelle RM. Life expectancy of persons with chronic disabilities. J Insur Med 1998; 30:96–108.

[36] Greenwood C, Newman S, Impey L, et al. Cerebral palsy and clinical negligence litigation: a cohort study. Br J Obstet Gynaecol 2003;110:6–11.

[37] Mackie PC, Jessen EC, Jarvis SN. The lifestyle assessment questionnaire: an instrument to measure the impact of disability on the lives of children with cerebral palsy and their families. Child Care Health Dev 1998;24:473–86.

ELSEVIER
SAUNDERS

CLINICS IN
PERINATOLOGY

Clin Perinatol 33 (2006) 557

Erratum

Erratum to "Cardiovascular Drugs for the Newborn" [Clin Perinatol 32 (4) (2005) 979–997]

Robert M. Ward, MD[a],*, Ralph A. Lugo, PharmD[b]

[a]*University of Utah, Division of Neonatology, 50 North Medical Drive, Salt Lake City, UT 84132, USA*
[b]*College of Pharmacy, University of Utah, 30 South 2000 East, Room 267, Salt Lake City, UT 84112-5820, USA*

An error appeared in the article "Cardiovascular Drugs for the Newborn" by Drs. Robert M. Ward and Ralph A. Lugo in the December 2005 issue of the *Clinics in Perinatology*.

On page 992, the second sentence in the second paragraph should read: "A group of 70 infants born at 23 to 31 weeks' gestation who had hypoxic respiratory failure defined by arterial–alveolar oxygen gradient (aAO2) less than 0.22 were randomized to treatment with 5 ppm NO or no treatment, and pulmonary blood flow velocity was measured by Doppler."

In the last sentence in the same paragraph, "AaO2" should be "aAO2".

DOI of original article title 10.1016/j.clp.2005.09.013.

* Corresponding author.

ELSEVIER
SAUNDERS

CLINICS IN
PERINATOLOGY

Clin Perinatol 33 (2006) 559–572

Index

Note: Page numbers of article titles are in **boldface** type.

A

Abetalipoproteinemia, 449, 452–453

Abruptio placenta
asphyxia in, 529
cerebral palsy due to, 507–508

N-Acetyl galactose-aminidase defects, 469

N-Acetylaspartate excess, 461

N-Acetylglucosamine-1-phosphotransferase
defects, 471

Acid maltase defects, 463

Acidemias
encephalopathy in, 337
organic, 425, 438–442

Acidosis, in neurometabolic disorders, 416

Adenine phosphoribosyl transferase deficiency,
454–455

Adenosine deaminase deficiency, 449,
454–456

Adenylosuccinate lyase defects, 454–455

ADP-ribosyl protein lyase deficiency, 461

Adrenoleukodystrophy, 466

Aldolase deficiency, 459

Alexander disease, 461, 465

Alopecia, in neurometabolic disorders, 416

Alzheimer disease, in Down syndrome, 485

Ambulation, in cerebral palsy, life expectancy
and, 549–551

Aminoacidopathies, 442–447, 456

Aminolevulinic aciduria, 450–451

Amniotic fluid, meconium stained, cerebral
palsy and, 340

Amylo-1,6-glucosidase defects, 463

Amylo-1,4,6-transglucosidase defects, 463

Anderson disease, 463

Anemia, stroke in, cerebral palsy due to, 374

Angelman syndrome, cerebral palsy in,
493–494

Angiography, magnetic resonance, in arterial
ischemic stroke, 369–370

Anticoagulants, for stroke, 380

Apgar score, in asphyxia, 340

Apolipoprotein C-II defects, 452–453

Apoptosis, of neurons, bilirubin causing, 391

Appendicitis, maternal, cerebral palsy due
to, 319

Aqueductal stenosis, hydrocephalus in, 520

Arginase defects, 444–445

Argininemia, 444–445

Argininosuccinase defects, 444–445

Argininosuccinate synthetase defects,
444–445

Argininosuccinic aciduria, 444–445

Arrhinencephaly, in Patau syndrome, 486

Arrhythmias, stroke in, cerebral palsy due
to, 375

Artane, for kernicterus, 403

Arterial ischemic stroke, cerebral palsy in,
367–386
definition of, 367
diagnosis of, 369–372
differential diagnosis of, 371
epidemiology of, 367
in preterm infants, 367–368
in sinovenous thrombosis, 369
outcome of, 376–379
pathophysiology of, 371, 373–376
presumed, 367–369
treatment of, 379–381

Changing Your Address?

Make sure your subscription changes too! When you notify us of your new address, you can help make our job easier by including an exact copy of your Clinics label number with your old address (see illustration below.) This number identifies you to our computer system and will speed the processing of your address change. Please be sure this label number accompanies your old address and your corrected address—you can send an old Clinics label with your number on it or just copy it exactly and send it to the address listed below.

We appreciate your help in our attempt to give you continuous coverage. Thank you.

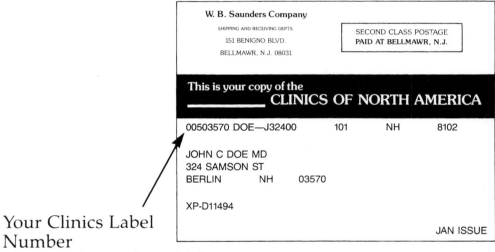

Your Clinics Label Number
Copy it exactly or send your label
along with your address to:
W.B. Saunders Company, Customer Service
Orlando, FL 32887-4800
Call Toll Free 1-800-654-2452

Please allow four to six weeks for delivery of new subscriptions and for processing address changes.